Ewles & Simnett's

Promoting
Health

A PRACTICAL GUIDE

EIGHTH EDITION

Ewles & Simnett's

Promoting Health

A PRACTICAL GUIDE

Angela Scriven BA, Cert Ed, MEd.

Retired academic, formally Reader in Health Promotion at Brunel University,
London, UK

James Woodall BSc, MSc, PhD

Reader in Health Promotion,
School of Health, Leeds Beckett University,
Leeds, UK

Gareth Morgan Bsc, MPhil, MPH, D.Prof,

Service Planning and Improvement Lead
Public Health, Hywel Dda University Health Board
Llanelli, Carmarthenshire, Wales

ELSEVIER

First edition 1985
Second edition 1992
Third edition 1995
Fourth edition 1999
Fifth edition 2003
Sixth edition 2010
Seventh edition 2017

Notices

Practitioners and researchers must always rely on their own experience and knowledge in evaluating and using any information, methods, compounds or experiments described herein. Because of rapid advances in the medical sciences, in particular, independent verification of diagnoses and drug dosages should be made. To the fullest extent of the law, no responsibility is assumed by Elsevier, authors, editors or contributors for any injury and/or damage to persons or property as a matter of products liability, negligence or otherwise, or from any use or operation of any methods, products, instructions, or ideas contained in the material herein.

ISBN: 978-0-323-88186-9

Content Strategist: Robert Edwards
Content Project Manager: Taranpreet Kaur/Suthichana Tharmapalan
Design: Amy Buxton
Marketing Manager: Deborah Watkins

Printed in India

Last digit is the print number: 9   8   7   6   5   4   3   2   1

Working together
to grow libraries in
developing countries

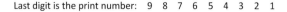

www.elsevier.com • www.bookaid.org

CONTENTS

Events in recent years have shone a light on public health and health promotion as never before. Placing our profession firmly in the public eye, the COVID-19 pandemic has demonstrated the importance of an expert workforce not only equipped to tackle the most serious threats to health but one able to deliver effective, equitable interventions to improve health.

Standing at the forefront of one of the most significant global events we have seen in modern history, the public health workforce has met the challenges of the COVID-19 pandemic with skill, determination, and a resolute commitment to safeguarding the health of populations across the globe.

Public health always shines in a crisis, and in tackling the global pandemic, we have seen rapid innovations in public health practice, as well as a deepening of cross-system working on a global scale. Underpinning these developments is the outstanding, collaborative leadership of the public health workforce.

This edition of *Promoting Health: A Practical Guide* could not have come at a more significant time for public health. As we emerge from our immediate response to the COVID-19 pandemic, we must now seek to deliver an equitable, health-focussed recovery which promotes better health for all.

Communities across the globe have been devastated by the pandemic, not only by the virus itself but by loss of earnings, stagnant economies, cuts to essential services, poor mental health, and a plethora of other long-term impacts.

These issues are compounded by events playing out on the global stage – climate change, international conflict, and global inequity – all of which demand our consideration as public health professionals.

The challenges facing us then remain many and varied. Whilst in public health we know it is a question of 'when' rather than 'if' we will face our next pandemic or other major incident, until – and indeed when – that time arrives, there are many other issues competing for our attention. Life expectancy is stalling in the UK, even declining in some areas, whilst health inequalities are widening, and early years' health is worsening. The cost-of-living crises in our country and across the world will have devastating effects, particularly on those living in the most deprived circumstances.

With domestic and global health needs becoming increasingly complex, we must continue to adapt our responses to these challenges to safeguard health for generations to come. This latest edition of *Promoting Health: A Practical Guide* represents this evolution of practice in health promotion, and I commend it to all readers.

Professor Maggie Rae, FFPH, FRSPH, FRCP (Hon), FRCP Edin, FRCPath (Hon), FFOM (Hon), FFSRH (Hon)
President of the Epidemiological and Public Health Section of the Royal Society of Medicine and immediate past President Faculty of Public Health

PREFACE

The aim of this book is to provide an accessible, practical guide for public health practitioners and health promoters. It was first published in 1985, and in response to demand, a new updated edition has been produced approximately every five years. This is the eighth edition. Earlier editions have also been published in German, Hungarian, Finnish, Greek, Indonesian, Italian and Swedish.

The book is addressed to all those who promote health, including health promotion specialists and public health practitioners and other members of public health teams; hospital, community and occupational health nurses; health visitors and midwives; hospital doctors and general practitioners; dentists and dental hygienists; pharmacists; health service managers and the professions allied to medicine; and health trainers and champions. It is also for the wide range of health promoters in statutory and non-statutory agencies, for example, local authority staff such as environmental health officers and social workers, voluntary organisations, youth and community workers, teachers with a health education remit in schools, colleges and universities, probation officers, prison officers and police officers.

Health promotion and public health encompass a wide variety of disciplines and activities with the common purpose of improving the health of individuals and communities. This book is concerned with the what, why, who and how of health promotion and public health practice. It aims to help you explore important questions such as the following:

How do we define and measure health and well-being?

What are the determinants of health and well-being?

What constitutes 21st-century health promotion and public health practice?

How does it fit with the wider public health movement?

Who are the agents and agencies with remits for public health and health promotion?

How are the population and individual needs identified when promoting health?

How are priorities set for evidence-informed practice?

How are health-promoting public health campaigns and projects planned, managed and evaluated?

How can health promoters and public health practitioners best carry out health promotion?

What are the competencies they require?

What are the key issues for public health and health promotion in the 21st century, and how has the COVID-19 pandemic impacted public health strategies and priorities?

There is a focus on the theories, principles and competencies for practice, whatever your background and wherever you work. The range of health issues and the settings for health promotion (such as communities, schools, workplaces, GP surgeries and hospitals) is wide-ranging, but it is beyond the scope of this book to cover all these in depth. Different professional groups will all have their own areas of expert knowledge and specialist skills to be employed alongside the specific competencies in promoting health addressed in this book.

The book is organised into three parts.

Part 1. Thinking About Health, Health Promotion, and Public Health deals with essential ideas of what health, health promotion, public health and health education are about and the different approaches and ethical issues that need to be considered. The agencies and people who have a part to play in health promotion and public health are identified.

Part 2. Planning and Managing Health Promotion and Public Health Practice focuses on planning and evaluation at the level of a health promoter's daily work, beginning with a basic planning and evaluation framework. This is followed by a discussion of how to identify and assess needs and priorities and develop skills to manage yourself and your work effectively.

Part 3. Competencies in Health Promotion and Public Health Practice examines how you can develop your competence in carrying out a range of activities, including enabling people to learn in one-to-one and group settings, enabling people towards healthier living, working with communities and changing policies and practices. The fundamentals of communication and of using communication tools are also addressed.

This eighth edition is fully revised and updated to account for the new challenges and the changing context in which health is promoted as we move through the 21st century. The text will examine the national strategies for health and new policies that have a bearing on the promotion of health. It is important to note, however, that priorities, policies and strategies for health frequently change, particularly when governments change, and there will be a general election in the United Kingdom (UK) during the life of this eighth edition. The UK is no longer a member of the European Union, and this has had an impact on public health, the extent of which will emerge during the coming years. Furthermore, there has been a global pandemic since the last edition, with COVID-19 challenging public health capacity and capabilities, with legislative action dominating global strategies to protect communities. Because of its significance, the COVID-19 pandemic is a permeating theme throughout the book. At the time of writing, the cost-of-living crisis in the UK is also creating a public health emergency and will impact significantly the work and priorities of those engaged in promoting population health.

New issues that are highlighted in the eighth edition are:

Changes to the structure and organisation of public health in the UK.

COVID-19 and its public health impact and legacy.

Economic and cost of living influences on population health.

New health data plus recent research on the comparative effectiveness of different approaches to health promotion and public health practice.

The internet's role and impact on public health, including social media misinformation. Websites, webinars, blogs and other relevant social media will be referenced at the end of each chapter. Social media such as Facebook, Twitter, Instagram and YouTube will be considered in terms of their use as both health-promoting assets and for their negative influences on wellbeing and health.

As in previous editions, several terms have been used to describe the people that health promotion targets. These terms include 'patients' (referring mainly to those who receive their health promotion in a healthcare environment), 'clients' (for patients and nonpatients) or simply users, individuals or community and population groups. The term 'health promoters' is used to cover the multidisciplinary workforces that have remits for promoting health that were listed at the beginning of this Preface. It also covers those with a specialist remit to promote health. Since the sixth edition of the book, the term most commonly used in England to describe the specialist workforce is '**public health practitioners**'. Throughout this edition, the term 'health promoter' is used alongside the term 'public health practitioner' to reflect the multidisciplinary workforce that the book is targeting (see Chapters 2 and 3 for a detailed discussion on who promotes health and what the differences are between health promotion and public health).

The user-friendly style adopted in the previous editions has been retained. The overall aim of the book is the same, to keep you involved so that studying this book will be an active educational experience. Exercises are included that can be undertaken as an individual or in a group, and examples and case studies are provided to help you to apply ideas to your own situation. Often, the exercises and the practice points at the end of each chapter are designed to stimulate thought and discussion, and there may be no right answers. You will need to think it through, talk it over and reflect. In this way, the answers will have personal meaning and application.

ACKNOWLEDGEMENTS

Linda Ewles and Ina Simnett, the authors of the first five editions of this book, produced a seminal text that has been used in the training and education of health promoters over the last 35 years. The book has shaped health promotion and public health practice in the United Kingdom over this time. I have been the author of the sixth and seventh editions of the book, and for this eighth edition, I would like to thank Dr James Woodall and Dr Gareth Morgan for joining me in updating the chapters and bringing to it their understanding and knowledge in the field of public health and health promotion. I would also like to thank Professor Maggie Rae for her Foreword. Professor Rae has had a distinguished career in health promotion and public health and has been instrumental in leading developments in the field. Her opening contribution to the book is compelling and clearly lays out the challenges ahead. Finally, I would like to thank the health promoters who have provided case studies of their work and Elsevier for their support and encouragement throughout the process of producing this new edition.

Angela Scriven

Thinking About Health, Health Promotion, and Public Health

PART CONTENTS

PART SUMMARY

Part 1 has three purposes:
- It sets the context for the whole book by introducing key concepts, principles and ideas, and providing you with a common language in which to communicate about health promotion and public health.
- It offers an introduction to the dimensions of health and the domains and scope of public health and health promotion, which enables you to focus on the wide range of activities and approaches being utilised by health promoters.
- It highlights important philosophical and ethical issues, which are explored in a practical context later in the book.

Health is an extremely difficult word to define, but it is clearly important that you know the competing explanations and definitions. This is discussed in Chapter 1, along with a description of the major influences on health and inequalities in health. There is also a historical overview of some of the international and national movements that have worked towards better health.

In Chapter 2, health promotion and public health are defined and shown to encompass a wide range of activities. Frameworks are given for classifying the major areas of health promotion action. Public health competencies are outlined, and an exercise is provided to help you explore the scope of your health promotion and public health practice work.

In Chapter 3, the agents and agencies of health promotion and public health practice are identified, and there is an opportunity to clarify your own health-promoting role.

In Chapter 4, the aims and values associated with different approaches to promoting health are analysed, a number of ethical dilemmas are examined, and guidance is provided on how to make ethical decisions.

What Is Health?

Angela Scriven

SUMMARY

This chapter starts with an exercise which enables you to examine what being healthy means to you and reviews the wide variation in perceptions and concepts of health. The interaction of the dimensions of health is considered (physical, mental, emotional, social, spiritual, cultural, environmental and societal), and health is explored as a holistic concept. Factors that influence health are identified, with a particular focus on medicine and inequalities in health. Case studies illustrate the factors that shape the health of people in differing circumstances, including a pandemic, such as COVID-19. In the final section, there is an overview of the contribution of international and national movements towards better health.

WHAT DOES BEING HEALTHY MEAN TO YOU?

Being healthy means different things to different people. There is extensive literature about lay concepts based on research about people's varying perceptions, beliefs and concepts of health (for example, Cross, 2020). It is important that public health practitioners and health promoters explore and define what being healthy means and what it might mean to the individuals and groups that you work with.

Exercise 1.1 generally indicates that people can hold very different perceptions of health. What you choose is often a reflection of your particular circumstances, your experiences and/or your professional background. For example, if you are a member of the LGBT community, a migrant or a refugee, you may consider living free of prejudice and within your own sociocultural milieu important to health and wellbeing, or if you work in a COVID-19 vaccine rollout capacity, you may prioritise being double vaccinated as a crucial aspect of being healthy. As your life stage, professional circumstances or global public health priorities change, your idea of what being healthy means to you might also change.

EXERCISE 1.1   What Does Being Healthy Mean to You?

In **Column 1**, tick any of the statements that describe important aspects of your health.

In **Column 2**, tick the six statements you consider to be the most important aspects of being healthy.

In **Column 3**, rank these six in order of importance – put one by the most important, two by the next most important and so on down to six.

If you are working in a group, compare your responses with others. Discuss the similarities and differences and the reasons for your choices. Analyse what your choices tell you about your perception of health.

(Continued)

EXERCISE 1.1   What Does Being Healthy Mean to You?—Cont'd

For me, being healthy involves:	Column 1	Column 2	Column 3
1. Being able to connect with family, friends, social networks and/or community	☐	☐	☐
2. Living to old age	☐	☐	☐
3. Feeling generally happy, in control and able to manage stress	☐	☐	☐
4. Having an adequate income	☐	☐	☐
5. Not being reliant on tablets or medicines	☐	☐	☐
6. Being the ideal weight for my height	☐	☐	☐
7. Taking regular exercise and feeling fit	☐	☐	☐
8. Living in my own sociocultural milieu	☐	☐	☐
9. Avoiding health risks, e.g. wearing a mask and being vaccinated against COVID-19; not smoking	☐	☐	☐
10. Not experiencing ill health or disease	☐	☐	☐
11. Having good levels of health literacy	☐	☐	☐
12. Being resilient and able to adapt to life's challenges	☐	☐	☐
13. Drinking only recommended safe levels of alcohol	☐	☐	☐
14. Having a home and a secure community to live in	☐	☐	☐
15. Having my body in good functional order	☐	☐	☐
16. Getting on well with other people most of the time	☐	☐	☐
17. Eating a nutritious diet and having access to clean water	☐	☐	☐
18. Enjoying some form of relaxation or recreation	☐	☐	☐
19. Having a job or meaningful occupation	☐	☐	☐
20. Having a good work-life balance	☐	☐	☐

CONCEPTS OF HEALTH AND WELLBEING

Health is a difficult concept to define in absolute terms. The meaning can be culturally and professionally determined, with definitions and explanations changing over time and being influenced by a number of factors, including our digital society (Larsen, 2021; Svalastog et al., 2017).

Lay Perceptions

1. It is important to understand the way lay people think about health and wellness, as this may impact their health and wellness-related behaviours. Researchers have found a wealth of complex lay notions about health. Some lay perceptions are based on pragmatism, where health is regarded as a relative phenomenon, experienced and evaluated according to what an individual finds reasonable to expect, given their age, medical condition, and social situation. For them, being healthy may just mean not having a health problem which interferes with their everyday lives. The development and validation of a measure of lay definitions of health, the wellness beliefs scale, confirmed three distinct wellness beliefs: belief in the importance of biomedical (absence of illness), functional (ability to carry out daily tasks) and wellbeing (vitality) indicators of wellness. Whatever the lay understandings of health and wellbeing are based on, however, they illustrate that lay accounts are unique and influenced by multiple factors, including social media (see Wang et al., 2021), for a discussion of how lay health beliefs linked to COVID-19 are being influenced by social media). Further examples of differences in lay health explanations include the health and illness beliefs of the oldest, which demonstrate that wellbeing and physical and mental health are closely connected and linked to life satisfaction, feelings of happiness, having a sense of purpose and meaning in life (Halaweh et al., 2018).

2. Although generally willing to discuss health inequalities, many of the lay study participants tended to

explain health inequalities in terms of individual behaviours and attitudes rather than social/structural conditions (Smith and Anderson, 2018).

Concepts and understanding of health, illness and disease have generally been linked with people's social and cultural situations. Knowledge of illness, prevention and treatment can also be powerful in shaping people's concept of health. Standards of what may be considered healthy also vary. An elderly woman may say she is in good health on a day when her chronic arthritis has eased up enough to enable her to get to the shops. A man who smokes may not regard his early morning cough as a symptom of ill health because, to him, it is normal. People assess their own health subjectively, according to their own norms and expectations, and may also trade off different aspects of health. A common example is that individuals may accept the physical health damage from smoking as the price they pay for the emotional and/or social benefits.

Because of the variety and complexity of how health and wellbeing are perceived, it is difficult to objectively measure health when based on lay accounts.

For more about measuring health, see Chapter 7, which focuses on finding and using evidence.

Concepts of Health

Concepts of health have changed over time. In the late 19th and 20th centuries, as medical discoveries were made and medical practice developed, there was a pre-occupation with a mechanistic view of the body and, consequently, physical health. Earlier still, there have been centuries of many philosophies of health in different civilisations, such as Greek, where a more holistic view of health has been held. See Ashton and Levin (2021) for a fascinating overview of public health concepts, issues and reflections presented in the form of aphorisms. Since the 1970s, the concept of health has been thoroughly discussed within the philosophy of medicine, with several categories of definitions developed ranging from merely physiological interpretations to more holistic, including a number of dimensions, such as mental and/or social, with the inclusion of the term wellbeing. Three levels of health have been explored by Lerner and Berg (2017): One Health, Planetary and EcoHealth. But they argue that only One Health at the individual level might be seen as a true concept of health and that health at the other levels is more a tool for the surveillance and measurement of processes or states. One way of examining the various meanings and understandings that have been given to the term health is to use broad categories or models. Five models are identified in the following text and include the *medical model*, the *holistic model*,

the *biopsychosocial model*, the *ecological model*, and the *wellness model*.

The Medical Model

- The medical model (sometimes called a biomedical model) dominated thinking about health for most of the 20th century.
- Health is defined and measured as the absence of disease and the presence of high levels of function.
- This approach uses the sciences such as physiology, anatomy, pathophysiology, pharmacology, biology, histopathology and biochemistry.
- In its most extreme form, the medical model views the body as a machine to be fixed when broken.
- It emphasises treating specific physical diseases, does not accommodate mental or social problems well, and de-emphasises prevention or prevention is seen as disease prevention rather than tackling the wider determinants of health or promoting optimal wellbeing. It is often referred to as reductionist.

The Holistic Model

- The holistic model was exemplified by the World Health Organisation (WHO) constitution, which referred to health as a state of complete physical, mental and social wellbeing and not merely the absence of disease or infirmity (WHO, 1948).
- This broadened the medical model perspective and highlighted the idea of positive health, although the WHO did not originally use that term and linked health to wellbeing and a range of dimensions, not just physical.
- Holistic health is difficult to measure. This is less because of the complexity of measuring wellbeing (see the wellness model in the following text) but more because doing so requires some subjective assessments that contrast sharply with the objective indicators favoured by the medical model.

The Biopsychosocial Model

- The biopsychosocial model (see Fig. 1.1) advances the medical model by incorporating some aspects of the holistic model, specifically the social, psychological and emotional dimensions.
- It recognises that health and wellbeing cannot be understood in isolation from the social and cultural environment.
- It acknowledges and takes into account individual and group circumstances that might affect health. See Engel's (1978) seminal work for the origins of this model and Bolton and Gillett (2019) for a detailed assessment of its relevance in the 21st century.

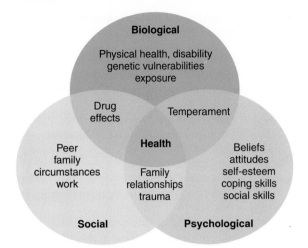

Fig. 1.1 The biopsychosocial model (Source: http://www.pierlu-
igimasini.it/2016/02/01/lapproccio-biopsicosociale-in-medicina/)

The Ecological Model

Social ecology provides a framework for understanding how individuals and their social environments mutually affect each other. The ecological health model (sometimes referred to as the socioecological health model) informs public health and health promotion as it emphasises the linkages between multiple factors (or determinants) affecting health across the lifespan. Typically, they are grouped into categories:

- **Individual**, sometimes called intrapersonal factors, such as genetics and individual behaviours.
- **Interpersonal**, which includes social support, family, friends and peer characteristics.
- **Institutional and community environments**, for example, work sites, schools, service systems and transportation. Risk factors to health here may include the level of unemployment, population density or the existence of a local drug trade.
- **Broader social, economic and political influences**, which could encompass a range of factors from social policies that maintain socioeconomic inequalities, laws and regulations and social and cultural norms to racism and discrimination (McCartney et al., 2019).

The Wellness Model

In 1984, a WHO seminal discussion document proposed moving away from viewing health as a state toward a dynamic model that presented it as a process or a force (WHO, 1984). This was amplified in the influential *Ottawa Charter for Health Promotion*, which proposed that health is the extent to which an individual or group is able to realise aspirations and satisfy needs and to change or cope with the environment, with health seen as a positive concept, emphasising social and personal resources (WHO, 1986).

Related to this is the notion of resiliency, such as the success with which individuals and communities adapt to changing circumstances (see Antonovsky's seminal work, 1979 and 1987, sense of coherence theory and Riopel, 2021 for a critical update). Overall, therefore, there has been a change from measuring health as the absence of disease or illness to equating health with wellbeing, which is influenced by a diverse range of conditions, such as quality of life, material circumstances and various types of capital. There is a growing interest in population wellbeing as an objective of governments. The Organisation for Economic Cooperation and Development (OECD) has been instrumental in producing a framework for measuring wellbeing in populations (see Fig. 1.2) and a range of wellbeing indicators (OECD 2020). The United Kingdom (UK) has measurements against national indicators of wellbeing (Office for National Statistics [ONS], 2019), and there have been moves to not just see the measure of wellbeing as the end goal but to use wellbeing indicators to inform government policy (see Chapter 16) and to even use population wellbeing as a measure of national performance (Hardoon et al., 2020; Newson, 2020).

There are advantages and disadvantages to each of the five models and explanations of the meaning of health. The medical model has credence because diseases represent a major global public health problem, and disease states need to be treated and can be readily diagnosed and counted. But this approach is narrow, negative and reductionist, and in an extreme form implies that people with disabilities are unhealthy and that health is only about the absence of morbidity. A further potential limitation of the medical model is its omission of a time dimension. Should we consider as equally healthy two people in equal functional status, one of whom is carrying a fatal gene that may lead to an early death?

The holistic, psychosocial, ecological and wellness models recognise a wider set of determinants of health. Bradley et al. (2018) explore these more contemporary definitions of health, which recognises that disease and disability often coexist with wellness. In the new conceptions, health is more than just a state which requires the absence of disease but is a dynamic quality which emphasises the fullness of life and quality of living. Fallon and Karlawish (2019) question whether the WHO definition of health is still appropriate, particularly in relation to older adults. They argue that our definitions of health should acknowledge that managing disease, and not solely its absence, is a means to a healthy life. One disadvantage of this move to a more holistic conception of health is the

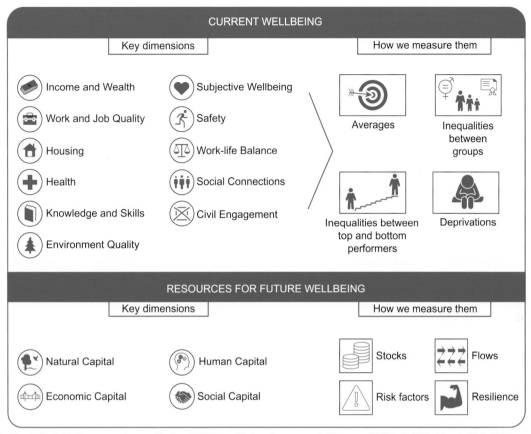

Fig. 1.2 How's life? 2020: measuring wellbeing **OECD wellbeing framework** (Source: OECD. (2020). *How's life? 2020: measuring well-being.* Paris, OECD Publishing. https://doi.org/10.1787/9870c393-en)

risk of excessive breadth, but the measurements of wellbeing are now more established (see for example, Rugeri et al. (2020) for a multidimensional analysis of wellbeing across 21 countries).

It is important to note that the WHO (1948) constitution definition of health mentioned under the holistic model has been heavily criticised, mainly on two grounds; it is unrealistic and idealistic and implies a static position. Some criticisms of the WHO definition focus on its lack of operational value and the problem created by the use of the word *complete*. An editorial in the *Lancet* (2009) is just one example of the range of criticisms levied against the WHO definition. Nonetheless, the WHO's focus on wellbeing encourages nations to expand the conceptual framework of their health systems beyond the traditional boundaries set by the physical condition of individuals and their diseases, and it challenges political, community and professional organisations devoted to improving or preserving health to pay more attention to wellbeing and

the social determinants of health (see for example, WHO (2021) for evidence of this).

In exploring the concept of health further, it is useful to consider the identification of the different dimensions of health which began with the WHO definition but have been subsequently expanded. The dimensions now include the following:

Physical health. This is perhaps the most obvious dimension of health and is concerned with the mechanistic functioning of the body.

Mental health. Mental health refers to the ability to think clearly and coherently. It can be distinguished from emotional and social health, although there is a close association between the three.

Emotional health. This means the ability to recognise emotions such as fear, joy, grief and anger and to express such emotions appropriately. Emotional (or affective) health also means coping with stress, tension, depression and anxiety.

Social health. Social health means the ability to make and maintain relationships with other people.

Spiritual health. For some people, spiritual health might be connected with religious beliefs and practices; for other people, it might be associated with personal creeds, principles of behaviour and ways of achieving peace of mind and being at peace with oneself.

Societal health. So far, health has been considered at the level of the individual, but a person's health is inextricably related to everything surrounding that person. It is impossible to be healthy in a sick society that does not provide the resources for basic physical and emotional needs. For example, people obviously cannot be healthy if they cannot afford necessities like food, clothing and shelter, but neither can they be healthy in countries of extreme political oppression where basic human rights are denied. Women cannot be healthy when their contribution to society is undervalued, and neither black nor white people can be healthy in a racist society where racism undermines human worth, self-esteem and social relationships. Unemployed people cannot be healthy in a society that values only people in paid employment, and it is very unlikely that health can be fully achieved in areas that lack basic resources such as clean water or services and facilities such as health care, transport, and recreation.

The identification of these wider social determinants of health (Public Health England, 2021a and b) is a useful exercise in raising awareness of the complexity and holistic nature of health. But in practice, it is obvious that dividing people's health into categories, such as physical and mental,

can impose artificial divisions and unhelpful distortions. Sexual health, for example, can cross all these boundaries, proving that the dimensions of health are interrelated.

When the WHO broadened its definition, as noted in the wellness model outlined earlier in the chapter, they also identified key aspects of health, encompassing ideas of:

- Personal growth and development (realise aspirations).
- Meeting personal basic needs (satisfy needs).
- The ability to adapt to environmental changes (resilience to change and ability to cope with the environment).
- A means to an end, not an end in itself (a resource for everyday life, not the objective of living).
- Not just the absence of disease (a positive concept).
- A holistic concept (social and personal resources, including physical capacities).

These aspects of health have much to offer the public health practitioner and health promoter. They recognise that health is a dynamic state, that each person's potential is different and that each person's health needs vary. Working for health is both an individual and a societal responsibility and involves empowering people to improve their quality of life. Table 1.1 sums up this section by offering a broad comparison of the medical and social models of health.

Exploring the concepts and competing explanations of health is a preliminary stage in understanding the determinants of health. Before moving on to a consideration of what affects health, it might be useful to undertake Exercises 1.2 and 1.3 and answer the associated questions.

TABLE 1.1   Comparison of the Medical and Social Models of Health

Medical Model	Social Model
Negative (health is the absence of disease, illness, infirmity or disability)	Positive (health is more than the absence of disease, illness, infirmity or disability and is associated with wellbeing)
Narrow or simplistic understanding of health (reductionist)	Broad, multidimensional and complex understanding of health (holistic)
Medically orientated definitions focusing on the absence of disease, illness, infirmity or disability-health as equilibrium	More holistic definitions of health taking a wider range of factors into account, such as mental, social, spiritual and environmental dimensions of health
Does not take into account the broader determinants of health	Takes into account wider influences on health, such as the environment and the impact of inequalities
Strongly influenced by scientific knowledge and is expert-led, top-down in approach	Takes into account lay knowledge and understanding and can be bottom-up in approach
Emphasises personal, individual responsibility for health	Emphasises collective, social responsibility for health

Source: Adjusted from Warwick-Booth et al. (2012).

EXERCISE 1.2   Dimensions of Health and Wellbeing

1. Go back to your answers in Exercise 1.1, 'What does being healthy mean to you?' Tick if any of the following dimensions of health are reflected in the statements you ticked in column 1:

   Physical ☐   Emotional ☐

   Mental ☐   Spiritual ☐

   Social ☐   Societal ☐

   Cultural ☐   Environmental ☐

2. Are any of these dimensions more important to you than the others? How do these dimensions relate to each other?
3. Consider Table 1.1. Do you think you have more of an affinity with a social or a medical model of health?
4. Which of the five models of health outlined earlier in the chapter would fit under the social model of health and why?
5. If you have had professional training in health or a related area of work, what difference has this made to your conceptions of health?
6. What do you think being healthy may mean to someone who:
   - Has a permanent physical disability such as deafness or paralysis?
   - Has an illness or infection for which there is currently no known cure, such as diabetes, arthritis, long COVID or schizophrenia?
   - Lives in poverty?
7. Identify three or four key ideas about being healthy that you have learned from this exercise.
8. Finally, how might the COVID-19 pandemic have changed your and others' perception of health?

EXERCISE 1.3   What Shapes People's Health and Wellbeing?

Read the case studies and answer the following questions:
- What factors might be affecting the health and wellbeing of each of the people in these case studies?
- Which statement in Exercise 1.1 do you think each would choose as important to them?
- What might be done to promote and improve their health and wellbeing?
- Construct a list of the health and wellbeing determinants emerging from each of the case studies.

Jane is 75, single and has always lived in the same small town. She has no immediate family but is active in the local community. The COVID-19 pandemic lockdowns have made her feel isolated and extremely lonely. Moreover, having worked all her adult life, she had thought that her state pension and her small occupational pension would be sufficient in her retirement, but she is finding paying the bills difficult. She is worried about her fuel bills, which increase each year, and has recently sold her car, as she can't afford the running costs.

Linda, 46, and **Andy**, 48, live together in a small bungalow which they rent. Due to their disabilities, they have both been unable to work and rely heavily on care and support services. They have mounted up considerable debts. The couple is extremely anxious because of a current cost of living crisis and about facing a review of their benefits that could cut their income.

Mary is 40 and exhausted from working long hours for the minimum wage to try to provide for her two children, aged eight to 16, and her 80-year-old mother, who is in the early stages of Alzheimer's. The three generations of the family share a damp and overcrowded three-bedroom social housing flat in the centre of a large city. Mary finds it difficult to pay for school uniforms and school trips. Her 16-year-old son is a member of the LGBT community and has been bullied at school to the point where he has become withdrawn and depressed.

John is 19 and lives in a town where there are 12 times as many people claiming job seeker's allowance as there are job vacancies. Despite having passed a number of GCSEs and A-levels and having applied for hundreds of jobs over the last two years, John is still unemployed, and because of the COVID-19 restrictions, he lost hope of finding a job. He has to live with his parents and has found this increasingly difficult, particularly through COVID-19 lockdowns. He wants his independence. He smokes cigarettes and front loads and binge drinks when he goes out with his mates on the weekend.

Fiona is a high-earning and successful criminal lawyer and a partner in a large law firm. She is 39 and works very long hours, often sleeping in the office overnight. To cope with stress, she exercises every day for at least an hour. She is often too busy to eat and just grabs coffee and snacks when she can. Her weight has dropped to the point where her body mass index (height-to-weight ratio) is dangerously low. She has no time to socialise, and although she would like to have a partner and start a family, her work-life balance doesn't allow for this.

(Continued)

EXERCISE 1.3   What Shapes People's Health and Wellbeing?—Cont'd

Ahmed is 39 and is a refugee. He is a single parent and unemployed. He lives with his two sons, both of whom have learning difficulties. The family has lived in temporary accommodation since arriving in the UK just before the COVID-19 pandemic. Ahmed has no family or friends in the area and feels isolated and anxious. He is in recovery from COVID-19 and still feels exhausted and is worried he may have long COVID. He has refused to be vaccinated against COVID-19 as he has read negative reports about the vaccine on social media. He also does not want his two sons vaccinated.

Some of the case studies are adjusted from the Poverty and Social Exclusion Website referenced under the websites at the end of the chapter.

DETERMINANTS OF HEALTH AND WELLBEING

A state of health or wellbeing or ill health, however defined, is the result of a combination of factors having a particular effect on individuals or population groups at any one time. To work towards better health, we need to identify these influential factors.

Exercise 1.4 will have identified a range of factors which affect health and wellbeing. These might include genetics, gender, family, religion, culture, friends and social networks, income, advertising, public health campaigns, social media, health literacy, social cohesion and inclusion, socioeconomic grouping, race, age, employment, working and living conditions, health and social services, self-esteem, access to leisure facilities and other resources, education, national public health and social policies, geographical location, environmental pollution, war, migration, global pandemics such as COVID-19 and many more. For further details, Public Health England (2021a) provides an extensive overview of the wider determinants of health and wellbeing and their implications for the promotion of health, whilst the United States Office for Disease Prevention and Health Promotion (2021) offers a set of pointers as to what they consider to be the social determinants of health and how they will address them in their Healthy People 2030 policy.

Health and Medicine

There is much debate about the relative importance of the many and varied social determinants of health and wellbeing (see the extensive work of Marmot, for example, Marmot et al., 2020a). There have also been concerns that medicine and healthcare might have less effect on the population's overall health improvement than promoting lifestyle changes or socioeconomic reforms, although the arguments are complex. Whilst governments argue that prevention is better than cure (see, for example, Department of Health and Social Care, 2018), the National Health Service (NHS) in the UK has often been seen as a

EXERCISE 1.4   A Framework for the Determinants of Health?

Many models and frameworks have been developed over time, which categorises and explain the interaction between the various factors that influence health and wellbeing. See for example, Fig. 1.3, which has been taken from the Australian Institute of Health and Welfare, 2014 and forms part of their report on Understanding Health and Illness:

- Critically assess the framework in Fig. 1.3. Do you feel all the determinants have been included? Are there determinants which are missing, or are there some that you would remove or modify?
- Undertake an internet search to consider other frameworks and models of determinants. Construct a model/framework that categorises the determinants in your particular geographical region or community.

---

treatment and care service for people who are ill, not as the major means of improving public health. There are moves, however, to associate the NHS with prevention policies (see NHS Long Term Plan Chapter 2, 2019, and Snell, 2019).

Some people have claimed that the practice of scientific medicine has, in fact, done considerable harm. Examples are the side effects of treatment, complications that set in after surgery, and patient dependence on prescribed drugs. But more important, perhaps, is that control over health and illness has been taken away from people themselves, who become dependent on doctors and medical drugs. Aspects of life that are natural, such as pregnancy and childbirth, menopause and ageing, have become medicalised, and the responsibility for health has shifted from the lay public to the medical profession. These arguments that medicine is, at best, a treatment and care service for the ill and, at worst, a means of undermining people's competence and confidence to improve their health reached a peak around 1980, led in part by

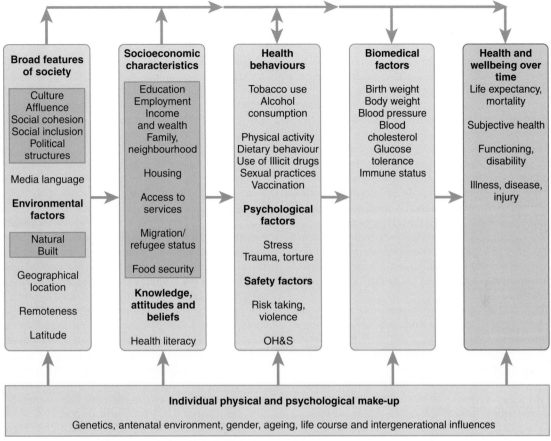

Fig. 1.3 An example of a framework for the determinants of health *Note:* Shading highlights selected social determinants of health. (Source: Australian Institute of Health and Welfare, 2014)

the seminal work of Illich (1977), but they are still relevant today (Russell, 2019).

The Wider Determinants of Health

In the UK, the landmark publication, The Black Report (Townsend and Davidson, 1982), showed that, for almost every kind of illness and disability in the UK, people in the upper socioeconomic groups had a greater chance of avoiding illness and staying healthy than those in the lower socioeconomic groups. It also established the differences in the risks to men and women and variations in the apparent health consequences of living in different parts of the country.

All this pointed to the fact that the major determinants of health were socioeconomic conditions, geographical location and gender. Evidence from the late 1990s (Acheson, 1998) demonstrated that the health

gap was widening so that whilst overall population health may be improving, the rate of improvement is not equal across all sections of society. The gap in the health status between the lower socioeconomic groups and the higher socioeconomic groups continues to increase.

Work comparing data across different countries has shown another slant on the issue of inequalities. It is not the richest societies with the best health, but those with the smallest income differences between the rich and poor. It is the *relative* difference in income levels which is crucial. The reason seems to be that small income differences across society mean an egalitarian society that has a strong community life and better quality of life in terms of strong social networks, less social stress, higher self-esteem, less depression and anxiety and more sense of control (see Bambra, 2021, who discusses five global examples of levelling up in terms of health inequalities and Marmot, 2021 who sets out a framework to reduce health inequities).

Marmot's work (Marmot et al., 2020a) on UK inequalities has resulted in a range of calls for action (for example, Kings Fund, 2021). There are also practice resources aimed at local action by directors of public health, public health teams and all those working to improve health (NHS England and Public Health England, 2021).

One way of addressing health inequalities and inequities is by building *social capital*. Social capital is the term used to describe investment in the social fabric of society so that communities develop high levels of trust and many networks for the exchange of information, ideas and practical help. Social capital is produced when, for example, there are neighbourhood schemes of child care and crime prevention, community groups and social activities that engage a wide range of interests and people. Low social and other capital levels have been linked to socioeconomic inequalities in health (Veenstra and Abel, 2019).

Differences in health experience may not be due entirely to socioeconomic determinants. There are important differences in rates of illness and death between ethnic groups, including deaths associated with COVID-19, which may be related to differences in income, education and living conditions, cultural factors or genetic makeup. There are also differences associated with age, sex, occupation and where people live (ONS, 2021). Addressing the distribution of wealth in society, reducing the gap between rich and poor and tackling socioeconomic disadvantage are clearly political issues, with Public Health England (2021a) reflecting the UK government's commitment to reducing health inequalities.

IMPROVING HEALTH – HISTORICAL OVERVIEW

A number of conclusions can be drawn from the previous discussion. First, health is a complex concept, meaning different things to different people. Second, health status is linked with people's ability to reach their full potential. Finally, health is affected by a wide range of factors, which may be broadly classified as:

- Lifestyle factors to do with individual health and risk-taking behaviour (which may be strongly influenced by socioeconomic and cultural experiences).
- Broader social, economic, cultural, political and environmental factors such as whether people live in an egalitarian society, what social support networks are available, and how they live in terms of employment, income and housing.

Early public health work in the first half of the 20th century in the UK concentrated on structural reforms such as slum clearance, improved sanitation and clean air. Then in the 1950s and 1960s, the focus shifted towards the need for changes in individual health behaviour, for example, family planning, venereal disease (the original term to describe sexually transmitted infections), accident prevention, immunisation, cervical smear checks, weight control, alcohol consumption and smoking. This emphasis on the lifestyle approach meant a concentration of effort on health education, which was reflected in government statements at the time (see for example, Department of Health and Social Security, 1976). Over time, this emphasis has been heavily criticised because it distracts attention from the social and economic determinants of health and tended to blame individuals for their own ill health. For example, people with heart disease could be blamed for it because they were overweight and smoked, but the complex social reasons for being overweight and smoking, what Marmot (2018) refers to as the causes of the causes, were ignored. Reasons may have included lack of education, no help available to stop smoking, eating and smoking used as a way of coping with stresses such as poor housing or unemployment, lack of availability of cheap, nutritious foods, and so on. This blaming people for their health behaviour became known as ***victim-blaming*** (see Caraher, 1995 and Dougherty, 1993 for early discussions of victim-blaming and Pennington, 2021 for a more recent critique of the term). In the 1980s, a broader approach was used in conjunction with what was called the new public health movement (WHO, 1986). It encompassed health education but also political and social action to address issues such as poverty, employment, discrimination and the environment in which people live. It also, importantly, focused on the grass-roots involvement of people in shaping their own health destiny.

See Chapter 3 for information on people and organisations working to improve public health.

INTERNATIONAL INITIATIVES FOR IMPROVING HEALTH

More is said about the role of the WHO and other international organisations in Chapter 3.

The WHO took a leading role in the evolution of health promotion in the 1980s and 1990s. It stated in 1978 that the main target of governments in the coming decades should be the attainment for all citizens of the world by the year 2000 of a level of health that will permit them to lead a socially and economically productive life (WHO, 1978).

This was the beginning of what came to be known as the *Health for All* (HFA) movement. It led to the development of a strategy for the WHO European Region in 1980 (WHO, 1985).

This regional strategy called for fundamental changes in the health policy of member countries, including a much higher priority for health promotion and disease prevention. It called for not only health services but all public sectors with a potential impact on health to take positive steps to maintain and improve health. Specific regional targets were published; these have been subsequently updated, and the movement is now called *Health 21* (see Rifkin, 2018 for an assessment of HFA in a contemporary context). The targets emphasise the following HFA principles:

- Reducing inequalities in health.
- Positive health through health promotion and disease prevention.
  Community participation.
- Cooperation between health authorities, local authorities and others with an impact on health.
- A focus on primary healthcare as the main basis of the healthcare system.

A major milestone for health promotion was the publication in 1986 of the Ottawa Charter, launched at the first WHO international conference on health promotion held in Ottawa, Canada (WHO, 1986). This identified five key themes for health promotion:

1. Building healthy public policies.
2. Creating supportive environments.
3. Developing personal skills through information and education in health and life skills.
4. Strengthening community action.
5. Reorienting health services toward prevention and health promotion.

(See Thompson et al., 2018, and Wilberg et al., 2021, for an overview of the continuing influence of the Ottawa Charter on health promotion.)

The Jakarta declaration in 1997 (WHO, 1997) reiterated the importance of the *Ottawa Charter* principles and added priorities for health promotion in the 21st century: to promote social responsibility for health.

- Increase investment in health development.
- Expand partnerships for health promotion.
- Increase community capacity and empower the individual.
- Secure infrastructure for health promotion.

The Bangkok Charter for Health in a Globalised World is the most recent WHO declaration (WHO, 2005). The Charter builds on Ottawa by asserting that progress towards a healthier world requires strong political action, broad participation and sustained advocacy.

- The call is to ensure that health promotion's established repertoire of proven effective strategies will need to be fully utilised, with all sectors and settings acting to **advocate** for health based on human rights and solidarity.
- **Invest** in sustainable policies, actions and infrastructure to address the determinants of health.
- **Build capacity** for policy development, leadership, health promotion practice, knowledge transfer and research, and health literacy.
- **Regulate and legislate** to ensure a high level of protection from harm and enable equal opportunity for health and wellbeing for all people.
- **Partner and build alliances** with public, private, non-governmental and international organisations and civil society to create sustainable actions.

It is clear that the Charters briefly outlined previously are targeting the wider determinants of health and are not focused on a narrow understanding of health and how it can be achieved.

NATIONAL INITIATIVES

See Chapter 3, a section on national health strategies, for more about national strategies for health and how they are implemented.

Influenced by the WHO Charters, an important development for the UK in the early 1990s was the advent of national strategies for health improvement. The first was *The Health of the Nation* in England (Department of Health, 1992) and comparable strategies for Wales, Scotland and Northern Ireland. These were the first national strategies to focus on health and health gain rather than illness and health services and to take a broader view of health. The most recent of these strategies are:

- 2019 Public Health England Strategy 2020–2025 In England (Public Health England, 2019).
- 2021 Welsh Government A Healthier Wales: Our Plan for Health and Social Care (Welsh Government, 2021).
- 2014: Department of Health Northern Ireland. Making Life Better 2013–2023 is the 10-year public health strategic framework providing direction for policies and actions to improve the health and wellbeing of people in Northern Ireland (Department of Health Northern Ireland, 2014).
- 2020: Public Health Scotland. A Scotland where everyone thrives: Public Health Scotland's three year strategy to improve and protect the health and wellbeing of people in Scotland (Public Health Scotland, 2020).

WHERE ARE WE NOW?

As this book is being written, we are two years into the COVID-19 pandemic, which has challenged public health systems globally, draining resources and impacting on public health priorities. Notwithstanding, it is clear from the discussions in this chapter that there is a broad understanding of the wider determinants of individual and population health, and there are international and national health strategies which recognise socioeconomic determinants. There remains a strong international, national and local emphasis on prevention, health improvement and reducing inequalities, with health promotion and public health playing a bigger part in the remits of many health and social welfare professions. In the UK, health and wellbeing issues feature in public policy debates at central and local government and across the health services. But as yet, these positive developments have failed to narrow the health gap between socioeconomic groups both between and within nations. Health promoters and public health practitioners in the UK still encounter entrenched inequalities in health and huge problems of poverty, unemployment and homelessness (Marmot et al., 2020b; Williams et al., 2020). In conclusion, public health is a significant issue for governments with inequalities in health and the impact of COVID-19 through the lens of health inequalities being the focus of much political debate (see Balogun et al., 2020; Bibby et al., 2020; Marmot et al., 2020b).

PRACTICE POINTS

- Health and being healthy mean different things to different people, and you need to explore and understand what they mean to you and to the individuals and population groups with which you work.
- A wide range of factors at many levels influence and determine people's health, including pandemics, climate change, conflict and other environmental and social issues.
- There are wide inequalities in the health status of people from different socioeconomic and ethnic groups, age groups, sexes and people who live in different geographical locations.
- Improving people's health means addressing the social, environmental, political and economic factors that affect their health, as well as individual health behaviour and lifestyle.
- International and national strategies and movements have emerged to tackle the complex lifestyle, socioeconomic and environmental interrelating determinants of health and to target the reduction of inequalities in health.

References

Acheson, D. (1998). *Independent inquiry into inequalities in health*. London: The Stationery Office.

Antonovsky, A. (1979). *Health, stress and coping*. San Francisco: Jossey-Bass.

Antonovsky, A. (1987). *Unravelling the mystery of health – how people manage stress and stay well*. San Francisco: Jossey-Bass.

Ashton, J., & Levin, L. (2021). *Public health explored: 50 stories to change the world*. London: Critical Publishing Ltd.

Australian Institute of Health and Wellbeing. (2014). *Understanding health and illness*. http://www.aihw.gov.au/australias-health/2014/understanding-health-illness/

Balogun, B., Rough, E., Loft, P., Harker, R., & Powell, T. (2020). *Opposition day debate: health inequalities*. London: UK Parliament House of Commons Library.

Bambra, C. (2021). Levelling up: global examples of reducing health inequalities. *Scandinavian Journal of Public Health, 50*(7), 908–913 https://doi.org/10.1177/14034948211022428.

Bibby, J., Everest, G., & Abbs, I. (2020). *Will COVID-19 be a watershed moment for health inequalities?*. London: The Health Foundation.

Bolton, D., & Gillett, G. (2019). *The biosocial model of health and disease*. London: Palgrave Pivot.

Bradley, K. L., Goetz, T., & Viswanathan, S. (2018). Towards a contemporary definition of health. *Military Medicine, 183*(Suppl 3), 207. https://doi.org/10.1093/milmed/usy213.

Caraher, M. (1995). Nursing and health education: victim blaming. *British Journal of Nursing, 4*(20), 1190–1192. 1209–1213. https://doi.org/10.12968/bjon.1995.4.20.1190.

Cross, R. (2020). Understanding the importance of concepts of health. *Nursing Standard*. https://doi.org/10.7748/ns.2020.e11539.

Department of Health, (1992). *The health of the nation: a strategy for health in England*. London: The Stationery Office.

Department of Health Northern Ireland, (2014). *Making life better 2013–2023*. Belfast: DoH.

Department of Health and Social Care, (2018). *Prevention is better than cure: our vision to help you live well for longer*. London: The Stationery Office.

Department of Health and Social Security, (1976). *Prevention and Health: Everybody's Business*. London: The Stationery Office.

Dougherty, C. J. (1993). Bad faith and victim-blaming: the limits of health promotion. *Health Care Analysis, 1*(2), 111–119. https://doi.org/10.1007/BF02197104.

Engels, G. L. (1978). The biopsychosocial model and the education of health professionals. *Annals of the New York Academy of Sciences, 310*, 169–181. https://doi.org/10.1111/j.1749-6632.1978.tb22070.x.

Fallon, C. K., & Karlawish, J. (2019). Is the WHO definition of health aging well: frameworks for "health" after three score years and 10. *American Journal of Public Health, 109*(8), 1104–1106. https://doi.org/10.2105/AJPH.2019.305177.

Halaweh, H., Dahlin-Ivanoff, S., Svantesson, U., & Willen, C. (2018). Perspectives of older adults on aging well: a focus group study. *Journal of Aging Research 2018*, Article ID 9858252, 9 pages. https://doi.org/10.1155/2018/9858252.

Hardoon, D., Hey, N., Brenetti, S. (2020). *Wellbeing evidence at the heart of policy*. https://whatworkswellbeing.org/wp-content/uploads/2020/02/WEHP-full-report-Feb2020_.pdf

Illich, I. (1977). *Limits to medicine – medical nemesis: the expropriation of health*. Harmondsworth: Pelican.

Kings Fund, (2021). *Health inequalities: our position*. London: Kings Fund.

The Lancet Editorial. What is health? The ability to adapt. Mar 07, 2009 Volume 373 Number 9666 p781-866. https://doi.org/10.1016/S0140-6736(09)60456-6

Larsen, L. T. (2021). Not merely the absence of disease: a genealogy of the WHO's positive health definition. *History of Human Sciences, 35*(1). https://doi.org/10.1177/095269512199535.

Lerner, H., & Berg, C. (2017). A comparison of three holistic approaches to health: One health, ecohealth and planetary. *Frontiers in Veterinary Science, 4*, 163. https://doi.org/10.3389/fvets.2017.00163.

McCartney, G., Hearty, W., Arnot, J., Popham, F., Cumbers, A., & McMasters, R. (2019). *Impact of Political Economy, 109*(6), 1–12. https://doi.org/10.1016/S0140-6736(17)32848-9.

Marmot, M. (2018). Inclusion health: addressing the causes of the causes. *Lancet, 391*(10117), 186–188. https://doi.org/10.3389/fvets.2017.00163.

Marmot, M., Allen, J., Boyce, T., Goldblatt, P., & Morrison, J. (2020a). *Health equity in England: the Marmot review 10 years on*. Institute of Health Equity www.instituteofhealthequity.org/the-marmot-review-10-years-on.

Marmot, M., Allen, J., Goldblatt, P., Herd, E., & Morrison, J. (2020b). *Build back fairer: the COVID-19 Marmot review*. London: The Health Foundation and Institute of Health Equity.

Marmot, M. (2021). *Framework to reduce inequalities for future generations launched by Professor Sir Michael Marmot*. http://www.ucl.ac.uk/news/2021/jun/framework-reduce-inequalities-future-generations-launched-proffesor-sir-michael-marmot

Newson, N. (2020). *Wellbeing as an indicator of national performance debate on 12 March 2020*. London: House of Lords Library Briefing.

NHS. (2019). *Long term plan chapter 2*. https://www.longtermplan.nhs.uk/wp-content/uploads/2019/08/nhs-long-term-plan-version-1.2.pdf

NHS England and Public Health England. (2021). *Reducing health inequalities resources*. https://wwwengland.nhs.uk/about/equity/equity-hub/resources/

Office for National Statistics. (2019). *Measures of national wellbeing dashboard*. https://www.ons.gov.uk/peoplepopulationandcommunity/wellbeing/articles/measuresofnationalwellbeingdashboard/2018-04-05

Office for National Statistics. (2021). *All data related to health and wellbeing*. https://www.ons.gov.uk/peoplepopulationandcommunity/healthandsocialcare/healthandwellbeing/datalist?=datasets&page=2

Organisation for Economic Cooperation and Development, (2020). *How's life? 2020 measuring well-being*. Paris: OECD Publishing.

Pennington, C. (2021). Micro-psychology in public health promotion. *Online Journal of Complementary and Alternative Medicine, 6*(3). https://doi.org/10.33552/OJCAM.2021.06.000638.

Public Health England, (2019). *PHE strategy 2020-2025*. London: Public Health England.

Public Health England, (2021a). *Place based approaches for reducing health inequalities: main report*. London: Public Health England.

Public Health England. (2021b). *Wider determinants of health*. https://www.gov.uk/government/statistics/wider-determinants-of-health-may-2021-update/wider-determinants-of-health-data-to-be-included-5-may-2021

Public Health Scotland, (2020). *A Scotland where everyone thrives: Public Health Scotlands three year strategy to improve and protect the health and wellbeing of people in Scotland*. Edinburgh: Public Health Scotland.

Rifkin, S. B. (2018). Health for all and primary health care 1978-2018: a historical perspective on policies and programs over 40 years: *The Oxford Research Encyclopedia, Global Public Health*. Oxford: Oxford University Press.

Riopel, L. (2021). *What does it mean to have a sense of coherence. Positive psychology*. https://positivepsychology./com/sense-of-coherence-scale/

Ruggeri, K., Garcia-Garzon, E., Macquire, A., Matz, S., & Huppert, F. A. (2020). Well-being is more than happiness and life satisfaction: a multidimensional analysis of 21 countries. *Health Quality of Life Outcomes, 18*, 192. https://doi.org/10.1186/s12955-020-01423-y.

Russell, C. (2019). Does more medicine make us sicker. *Gaceta Sanitaria, 33*(6), 579–583. https://doi.org/10.1016/j.gaceta.2018.11.006.

Smith, K. E., & Anderson, R. (2018). Understanding lay perspectives on socioeconomic health inequalities in Britain: a meta analysis. *Sociology of Health and Illness, 40*(1), 146–170. https://doi.org/10.1111/1467-9566.12629.

Snell, A. (2019). *Prevention is better than cure, so lets do more of it*. https://england.nhs.uk/prevention-is-better-than-cure-so-lets-do-more-of-it/

Svalastog, A. L., Donev, D., & Gajovic, S. (2017). Concepts and definitions of health and health related values in the knowledge landscapes of the digital society. *Croatian Medical Journal, 58*(6), 431–435. https://doi.org/10.3325/cmj.2017.58.431.

Thompson, S. R., Watson, M. C., & Tilford, S. (2018). The Ottawa charter 30 years on: still an important standard for health promotion. *International Journal of Health Promotion and Education, 56*(2), 73–84. https://doi.org/10.1080/14635240.2017.1415765.

Townsend, P., & Davidson, N. (1982). *Inequalities in health: Black report*. Harmondsworth: Penguin.

United States Office for Disease Prevention and Health Promotion. (2021). *Social determinants of health*. https://health.gov/healthypeople/priority-areas/social-determinants-health

Veenstra, G., & Abel, T. (2019). Capital interplays and social inequalities in health. *Scandinavian Journal of Public Health*, *47*(6), 631–634. https://doi.org/10.1177/1403494818824.

Wang, H., Yikuan, L., Hutch, M., Naibech, A., & Luo, Y. (2021). Using tweets to understand how Covid-19-related health beliefs are affected in the age of social media: Twitter data analysis study. *Journal of Medical Internet Research*, *23*(2). https://doi.org/10.2196/26302.

Warwick-Booth, L., Cross, R., & Lowcock, D. (2012). *Contemporary health studies: an introduction*. Cambridge: Polity Press.

Welsh Government, (2021). *A healthier Wales: our plan for health and social care*. Cardiff: Welsh Government.

Wilberg, A., Saboga-Nunes, L., & Stock, C. (2021). Are we there yet? Use of the Ottawa Charter action areas in perspective of European health promotion professionals. *Journal of Public Health*, *29*, 1–7. https://doi.org/10.1007/s10389-019-01108-x.

Williams, E., Buck, D., & Babalola, G. (2020). *What are health inequalities*. London: Kings Fund.

World Health Organisation. (1948). *Constitution of the World Health Organisation*. www.who.int/governance/eb/who_constitution_en.pdf

World Health Organisation, (1978). *Alma Ata Declaration*. Geneva: World Health Organisation.

World Health Organisation, (1984). *Health promotion: a discussion document on the concepts and principles*. Copenhagen: World Health Organisation.

World Health Organisation, (1985). *Regional targets for health for all*. Geneva: World Health Organisation.

World Health Organisation, (1986). *The Ottawa charter for health promotion*. Geneva: World Health Organisation. http://www.who.int/hpr/hpr/documents/ottawa.html.

World Health Organisation, (1997). *The Jakarta declaration on leading health promotion into the 21st century*. Geneva: World Health Organisation. http://www.who.int/hpr/hpr/documents/jakarta/english.html.

World Health Organisation, (1999). *Health 21: health for all in the 21st century*. Copenhagen: World Health Organisation.

World Health Organisation, (2005). *The Bangkok charter for health promotion in a globalized world*. Geneva: World Health Organisation. http://www.who.int/health-promotion/conferences/6gchp/bangkok_charter/en/index.html.

World Health Organisation, (2021). *Its time to build a fairer, healthier world for everyone, everywhere by taking action on the social determinants of health to advance equity*. Geneva: World Health Organisation.

Websites

NHS. *Equality and health inequalities hub*. http://www.englan.nhs.uk/about/equality/equality-hub/

The Health Foundation. *Social determinants of health*. https://www.health.org.uk/topics/social-determinants-of-health

Poverty and Social Exclusion. https://www.poverty.ac.uk

OECD. *How's life? Reveals improvements in well-being, but persistent inequalities*. www.oecd.org

Blogs

Merrifield, K., & Nightingale, G. (2021). *Five tests for levelling up health*. The Health Foundation. https://ww.health.org.uk/new-and-comment/blogs/five-tests-for-levelling-up-health.

Facebook

World Health Organisation. For up to date global health information, media briefings and coverage of issues such as COVID-19 and the way social media might impact on wellbeing and our understanding of health.

Twitter and Instagram

World Health Organisation

What Is Health Promotion?

Angela Scriven

SUMMARY

This chapter starts with a discussion of the definitions of health promotion, public health and the related terms of health improvement, health development, health education and social marketing. This is followed by an examination of the position of health promotion within the multidisciplinary public health movement. An outline of the scope of health promotion work is offered, with frameworks for activities for promoting health. Broad areas of practice covered by professional health promoters and the core competencies needed are set out with an outline of the framework for national occupational standards and skills for health. Exercises are included to help you explore the range of public health and health promotion activities and the extent of your own health promotion and public health practice work.

DEFINING HEALTH PROMOTION

Health promotion as a term was used for the first time in the mid-1970s (Lalonde, 1974) and quickly became an umbrella term for a wide range of strategies designed to tackle the wider determinants of health. There is no clear, universally adopted consensus of what is meant by health promotion. Some definitions focus on activities, others on values and principles and are often imprecisely defined. Health promotion involves promoting the health and wellbeing of individuals, communities and whole population groups. Promotion in this context means improving, advancing, supporting, advocating for, empowering and placing health higher on personal, public and political agendas.

Given that major socioeconomic determinants of health are often outside individual or even collective control, a fundamental aspect of health promotion is that it aims to empower people to have more control over aspects of their lives that affect their health. These twin elements of improving health and having more control over it are fundamental to the aims and activities of health promotion. The World Health Organisation (WHO) definition of health promotion, as it appears in the Ottawa Charter, has been widely adopted and encompasses this: Health promotion is the process of enabling people to increase control over and to improve their health (WHO, 1986). The WHO Health Promotion glossary of terms (WHO, 2021) reiterates this definition but expands by stating that health promotion represents a comprehensive social and political process directed at strengthening the skills and capabilities of individuals and actions directed at changing the social, environmental and economic determinants of health. It could be argued that this definition is too elusive and, as such, is unfit for purpose. The WHO, however, accompanied their definition with a logo and an explanation which indicated more clearly what the process of enabling people to increase control over and improve their health would entail (Fig. 2.1).

The logo and the Ottawa Charter present five key action areas and three strategies for health promotion, which further explain the nature and purpose of health promotion (see Box 2.1 for further details):

Action Areas
- Build healthy public policy.
- Create supportive environments for health.

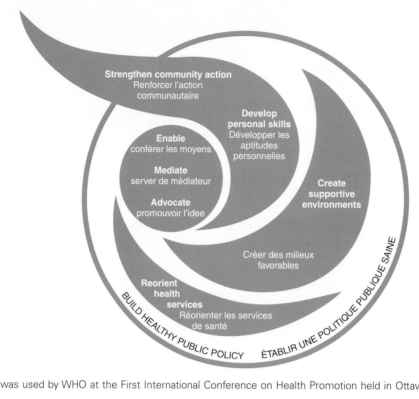

Fig. 2.1 The logo was used by WHO at the First International Conference on Health Promotion held in Ottawa, Canada, in 1986. (WHO, 1986).

- Strengthen community action for health.
- Develop personal skills.
- Reorient health services.

Strategies

- Enable.
- Mediate.
- Advocate.

It has been argued that the Ottawa Charter has established an international agenda for public health and has not lost any of its significance (Nutbeam et al., 2021). However, the social model of health (see Chapter 1) that health promotion embraces can be in sharp contrast to a more medically dominated public health approach. To counteract this, the new Office for Health Promotion in England is designed to help ministers operationalise a step change in public health policy which recognises and tackles the wider determinants of health (Department of Health and Social Care, 2021)

EXERCISE 2.1

Consider the definition, logo, action areas and strategies previously outlined and expanded on in Box 2.1, and answer the following questions:

1. How relevant do you feel the Ottawa Charter is to public health action in the 21st century?
2. Consider the local, national and international public health policies that you are familiar with, including those relating to the COVID-19 pandemic, and assess whether both the ideas and values contained within the Ottawa Charter are influencing public health policy development.
3. Are there any of the action areas and strategies outlined in the Ottawa Charter which are embedded in your professional remit and/or practice, and if so, what are they?
4. Do you consider yourself to be a health promoter? Please explain your answer.

BOX 2.1 The Ottawa Charter

Build Healthy Public Policy – Health promotion goes beyond healthcare. It puts health on the agenda of policymakers in all sectors and at all levels, directing them to be aware of the health consequences of their decisions and to accept their responsibilities for health. Health promotion policy combines diverse but complementary approaches, including legislation, fiscal measures, taxation and organisational change. It is coordinated action that leads to health, income and social policies that foster greater equity. Joint action contributes to ensuring safer and healthier goods and services, healthier public services and cleaner, more enjoyable environments. Health promotion policy requires the identification of obstacles to the adoption of healthy public policies in non-health sectors and ways of removing them. The aim must be to make the healthier choice, the easier choice for policymakers as well.

Create Supportive Environments – Our societies are complex and interrelated. Health cannot be separated from other goals. The inextricable links between people and their environment constitute the basis for a socioecological approach to health. The overall guiding principle for the world, nations, regions and communities alike is the need to encourage reciprocal maintenance – to take care of each other, our communities and our natural environment. The conservation of natural resources throughout the world should be emphasised as a global responsibility. Changing patterns of life, work and leisure have a significant impact on health. Work and leisure should be a source of health for people. The way society organises work should help create a healthy society. Health promotion generates living and working conditions that are safe, stimulating, satisfying and enjoyable. Systematic assessment of the health impact of a rapidly changing environment – particularly in areas of technology, work, energy production and urbanisation – is essential and must be followed by action to ensure positive benefits to the health of the public. The protection of the natural and built environments and the conservation of natural resources must be addressed in any health promotion strategy.

Strengthen Community Actions – Health promotion works through concrete and effective community action in setting priorities, making decisions, planning strategies and implementing them to achieve better health. At the heart of this process is the empowerment of communities – their ownership and control of their own endeavours and destinies. Community development draws on existing human and material resources in the community to enhance self-help and social support and to develop flexible systems for strengthening public participation in and direction of health matters. This requires full and continuous access to information, learning opportunities for health, as well as funding support.

Develop Personal Skills – Health promotion supports personal and social development by providing information and education for health and enhancing life skills. By so doing, it increases the options available to people to exercise more control over their own health and over their environments and to make choices conducive to health. Enabling people to learn throughout life to prepare themselves for all its stages and to cope with chronic illness and injuries is essential. This must be facilitated in school, home, work and community settings. Action is required through educational, professional, commercial and voluntary bodies and within the institutions themselves.

Reorient Health Services – The responsibility for health promotion in health services is shared among individuals, community groups, health professionals, health service institutions and governments. They must work together towards a healthcare system which contributes to the pursuit of health. The role of the health sector must move increasingly in a health promotion direction beyond its responsibility for providing clinical and curative services. Health services need to embrace an expanded mandate which is sensitive and respects cultural needs. This mandate should support the needs of individuals and communities for a healthier life and open channels between the health sector and broader social, political, economic and physical environmental components. Reorienting health services also requires stronger attention to health research and changes in professional education and training. This must lead to a change of attitude and organisation of health services which refocuses on the total needs of the individual as a whole person.

Moving Into the Future – Health is created and lived by people within the settings of their everyday life, where they learn, work, play and love. Health is created by caring for oneself and others, by being able to take decisions and has control over one's life circumstances, and by ensuring that the society one lives in creates conditions that allow the attainment of health by all its members. Caring, holism and ecology are essential issues in developing strategies for health promotion. Therefore, those involved should take as a guiding principle that, in each phase of planning, implementation and evaluation of health promotion activities, women and men should become equal partners.

(WHO, 1986).

Connection Between Health Promotion and Public Health

There has been considerable debate about the relationship between health promotion as a set of professional activities – internationally guided by WHO charters and declarations such as the Ottawa Charter previously discussed – and public health, which in England is regulated by the Faculty of Public Health.

What Is Public Health?

In the United Kingdom (UK), the Faculty of Public Health (FPH) defines public health as the science and art of promoting and protecting health and wellbeing, preventing ill health and prolonging life through the organised efforts of society (FPH, 2021).

The faculty's approach is that public health:
- Is population based
- Emphasises collective responsibility for health, its protection and disease prevention
- Recognises the key role of the state, linked to a concern for the underlying socioeconomic and wider determinants of health, as well as disease
- Emphasises partnerships with all those who contribute to the health of the population

The faculty proposes three domains of public health outlined in Table 2.1 and nine areas of public health practice.

The nine key areas are:
- Surveillance and assessment of the population's health and wellbeing
- Assessing the evidence of the effectiveness of health and healthcare interventions, programmes and services
- Policy and strategy development and implementation
- Strategic leadership and collaborative working for health
- Health improvement
- Health protection
- Health services
- Public health intelligence
- Academic public health

Functions of the Local Public Health System can be found on the FPH website (see the reference at the end of the chapter), in addition to current manifestos and details on public health standards.

Internationally, public health is seen as multi-faceted and targeting numerous social, environmental and behavioural determinants, including the impacts of globalisation, economic constraints, living conditions, demographic changes and unhealthy lifestyles (European Commission (EC), 2020). The World Federation of Public Health Associations (WFPHA), in collaboration with the WHO, has developed a Global Charter for the Public's Health, and in doing so they point to the major influence of the Ottawa Charter for Health Promotion (WHO, 1986) in improving health throughout the world. The purpose of the public health charter is to provide a succinct and practical implementation guideline to public health associations to work with other non-government organisations, universities, civil societies and governments to plan and implement strategies for better health outcomes. The WFPHA conceptualises global public health as a new

TABLE 2.1   Faculty of Public Health—Domains of Public Health

THREE DOMAINS OF PUBLIC HEALTH PRACTICE		
Health Improvement	**Improving Services**	**Health Protection**
• Inequalities	• Clinical effectiveness	• Infectious diseases
• Education	• Efficiency	• Chemicals and poisons
• Housing	• Service Planning	• Radiation
• Employment	• Audit and Evaluation	• Emergency response
• Family/community	• Clinical Governance	• Environmental health hazards
• Lifestyles	• Equity	
• Surveillance and monitoring of specific diseases and risk factors		
• Clinical effectiveness		
• Efficiency		
• Service planning		
• Audit and evaluation		
• Clinical governance		
• Equity		

Source: Adjusted from FPH (2016).

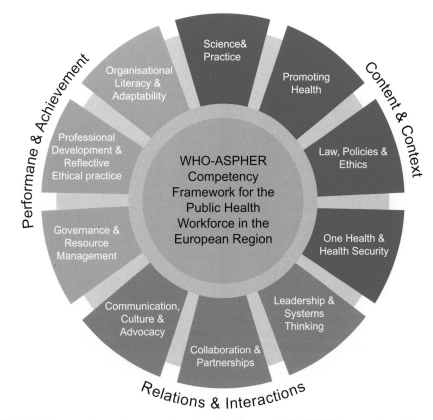

Fig. 2.2 The WHO-ASPHER competency framework categories. Source WHO-ASPHER competency framework for the public health workforce in the European Region (2020) .

health era, more dedicated to preventive solutions rather than a disease-specific focus. The Global Charter for the Public's Health provides new insights into the direction of public health and provides guidance for a group of core services: protection, prevention and promotion, and a group of enabler functions: governance, advocacy, capacity and information (ASPHER, 2022; WFPHA, 2016; 2022; see Fig. 2.2).

See Chapter 3 for an overview of the health promotion and public health workforce.

It is important to note that, in addition to health promotion and public health, a range of other terms have been used to describe the process of enabling individuals and communities to improve their health. These include health development, health improvement, health education and social marketing. Health development is used in several ways. There are public health teams and units that refer to themselves as health development departments and there is a Health Development Consultancy (HDC), which supports health promoters

EXERCISE 2.2

Examine the UK FPH public health domains plus their nine key areas of public health and the WHO-ASPHER competency framework for the public health workforce in the European Region 2020 in Fig. 2.2 and answer the following:

- Which FPH domains and key areas of practice do you not consider to be health promotion, and why?
- Where does health promotion fit in the WFPHA global public health charter?
- What conclusions can you draw from Exercises 2.1 and 2.2 in terms of the difference between public health and health promotion?
- Do you consider yourself working in health promotion, public health, or both? Explain your answers.

and public health practitioners by producing a range of courses (HDC, 2022). Health improvement is frequently used by health departments (see NHS Greater Glasgow and Clyde, 2020). The term covers a wide range of activities, principally focused on improving the health and wellbeing of individuals and communities (much like health promotion). Health education comprises the consciously constructed opportunities for learning involving some form of communication designed to improve health literacy, including improving knowledge and developing life skills which are conducive to individual and community health. It can be considered a core public health discipline and has strong links to health literacy and digital health communication (Stock, 2022). In the 1970s, the range of activities undertaken to pursue better health began to diverge from health education. There was also criticism that the health education approach was too narrow, focused too much on behavioural change and could become victim-blaming (see Chapter 1, Historical overview) and increasingly, work was being undertaken on wider issues such as political action to change public policies. Such activities went beyond the scope of traditional health education, and the term 'health promotion' came into use to describe the wider range of health interventions used to tackle the broader determinants of health.

Like health education, social marketing is a health-promoting strategy to achieve and sustain behaviour goals on a range of social issues. There are several definitions of social marketing, but the National Social Marketing Centre (NSMC) in the UK describes social marketing as a proven tool to develop activities aimed at changing or maintaining people's behaviour for the benefit of individuals and society (NSMC, 2022).

THE SCOPE OF HEALTH PROMOTION

The questions in Exercise 2.3 give examples of the wide range of activities that may be classified as health promotion. Answering 'yes' to each one indicates a broad view of what may be included: mass media advertising, campaigning on health issues, patient education, self-help, environmental safety measures, public policy issues, health education, preventive and curative medical procedures, codes of practice on health issues, health-enhancing

---

EXERCISE 2.3   Exploring The Scope of Health Promotion

Consider each of the following activities and decide whether you think each is or is not health promotion:

	Yes	No
1. Using TV, radio, cinema and social media for advertisements to encourage people to drink safely.	☐	☐
2. Campaigning for a tax on sugar.	☐	☐
3. Explaining to patients how to carry out their doctor's advice.	☐	☐
4. Setting up a self-help group for people who have been sexually abused as children.	☐	☐
5. Providing advice on environmental threats, including pollution and noise.	☐	☐
6. Leading on the development, implementation and evaluation of health improvement programmes across organisations, partnerships and communities to improve population health and wellbeing and reduce health inequalities.	☐	☐
7. Identifying the causes and distribution of ill health, interpreting the results and reporting on their implications.	☐	☐
8. Immunising population groups against infectious diseases such as COVID-19.	☐	☐
9. Protesting to local and national politicians about a breach in the voluntary code of practice for alcohol advertising.	☐	☐
10. Running low-cost gentle exercise classes for older people at local leisure centres.	☐	☐
11. A celebrity chef advocating for healthier menu choices at school canteens.	☐	☐
12. Teaching a school-based programme of personal, social, economic and health education.	☐	☐
13. Providing support to people with learning disabilities living in the community.	☐	☐
14. Tackling community issues based on local needs assessment, such as childhood obesity and smoking.	☐	☐
15. Legislating for a whole population lockdown during a pandemic.	☐	☐

Explain your reasons for deciding whether an activity is or is not 'health promotion'?

facilities in local communities, workplace health policies and personal and social education for young people. Answering 'no' indicates that you identify criteria that you believe exclude these activities from the realms of health promotion. For example, you may have said 'no' to item 2 because a sugar tax might impact negatively on families living in poor financial circumstances, thus putting their health more at risk.

Frameworks and models for classifying health-promoting activities have helped to determine the scope of health promotion. See for example the seminal model in Tannahill (2009). Drawing on these, Fig. 2.3 identifies the activities that contribute to health gain and maps out all those activities which aim to improve people's health and wellbeing. There are two sets of activities: those about providing services for people who are ill or who have disabilities, and positive health activities, which

are about personal, social and environmental changes aiming to prevent ill health, to improve wellbeing and develop healthier living conditions and lifestyles. These two sets of activities overlap because they both contribute to health gain, and they are often closely related in practice. Ten categories of activities are identified, comprising two illness and disability services and eight types of positive health activities.

Illness and Disability Services

Personal social services. This includes all those social services aimed at addressing the needs of sick people and people with disabilities or disadvantages whose health, wellbeing and quality of life is improved by those services.

This includes, for example, community care of mentally ill people.

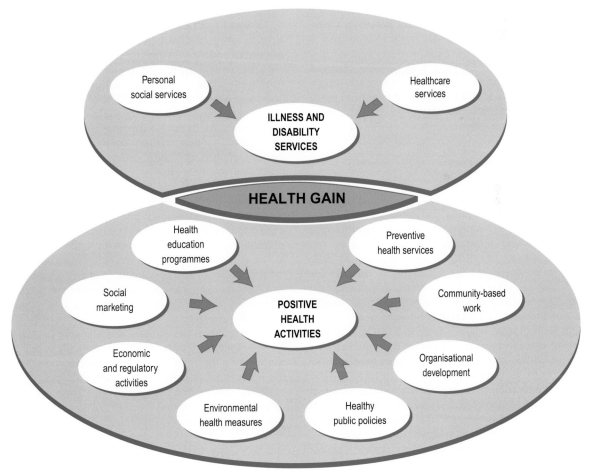

Fig. 2.3 Health-promoting actions.

Healthcare services. This includes the major work of health services: treatment, cure and care in primary care and hospital settings.

An important question when considering the boundaries of service provision by health promoters is, 'If all illness and disability services improve health and produce varying amounts of health gain, are they all called health promotion?' For example, is giving someone with osteoarthritis a full hip replacement considered health promotion?

It is helpful to go back to the WHO (1986) definition of health promotion, which is about enabling people to increase control over and improve their health. Are things that need to be done to people (like a full hip replacement) excluded from this definition, so it is not health promotion? They are health gain activities. What about those aspects of care and treatment that are about enabling people to take control over their health and improve it (such as educating patients in the skills of diabetes self-care)? Creating a health-promoting environment by, for example, modifying a home to make it suitable for a person with disabilities or providing affordable housing for homeless people might also be seen as health promotion.

During the COVID-19 pandemic, a wide range of approaches was used, but the most dominant was legislative action, such as forced lockdowns, compulsory mask-wearing and social distancing. Would you describe these as health-promoting actions?

Positive Health Activities

Health Education Programmes

These are planned opportunities for people to learn about health and wellbeing and to undertake voluntary changes in their behaviour. Such programmes may include providing information, exploring values and attitudes, making health decisions and acquiring skills to enable behaviour change to take place. They involve developing self-esteem and self-empowerment so that people are enabled to take action about their health. This can happen on a personal one-to-one level, such as health visitor/client, teacher/pupil; in a group such as a smoking cessation group or exercise class; or reaching large population groups through the mass media, social media, health fairs or exhibitions.

Health education programmes may also be a part of healthcare and personal social services, and because of this, it is useful to understand the concepts of primary, secondary, tertiary and quaternary health education.

Primary health education. This would reflect McKinley's (1979) seminal vision of upstream, preventive activity. It is directed at healthy people and aims to prevent ill health from arising. Most health education for children and young people falls into this category, dealing with such topics as sexual health, nutrition and social skills and personal relationships, aiming to build up a positive sense of self-worth in children. Primary health education is concerned not merely with helping to prevent illness but with positive wellbeing.

Secondary health education. There is also often a major role for health education when people are ill. It may be possible to prevent ill health from moving to a chronic or irreversible stage and to restore people to their former state of health. This is known as secondary health education, educating patients about their condition and what to do about it. Restoring good health may involve the patient changing behaviour (such as stopping smoking) or complying with a therapeutic regime and, possibly, learning about self-care and self-help. Clearly, health education of the patient is of great importance if treatment and therapy are to be effective and illness is not to recur.

Tertiary health education. There are, of course, many patients whose ill health has not been, or could not be, prevented and who cannot be completely cured. There are also people with permanent disabilities. Tertiary health education is concerned with educating patients and their carers about how to make the most of the remaining potential for healthy living and how to avoid unnecessary hardships, restrictions and complications. Rehabilitation programmes contain a considerable amount of tertiary health education with a focus on improving quality of life.

Quaternary (meaning final stage) health education. This focuses on facilitating optimal states of empowerment and emotional, social and physical wellbeing during a terminal stage of disease. It differs from quaternary prevention, which is the action taken to identify patients at risk of overmedicalisation, to protect them from new medical invasion and to suggest to them interventions which are more ethically acceptable (Martins et al., 2018). Quaternary health education would be a strong tool in quaternary prevention.

It is not always easy to see where people fit into this primary, secondary or tertiary framework because a person's state of health is open to interpretation. For example, is educating an overweight person who appears to be perfectly well, despite being overweight, primary or secondary health education?

Social Marketing

The NSMC identifies the primary aim of health-related social marketing as the achievement of a social good (rather than commercial benefit) in terms of specific, achievable and manageable behaviour goals relevant to improving health and reducing health inequalities. Social marketing is a systematic process using a range of marketing techniques and approaches (a marketing mix) phased to address short-, medium- and long-term issues. The following six features and concepts are pertinent to understanding social marketing:

Customer or consumer orientation. A strong customer orientation with importance attached to understanding where the customer is starting from, their knowledge and attitudes and beliefs, along with the social context in which they live and work.

Behaviour and behavioural goals. A clear focus on understanding existing behaviour and key influences upon it, alongside developing clear behavioural goals. These can be divided into actionable and measurable steps, or stages phased over time.

Intervention mix and marketing mix. Using a mix of different interventions or methods to achieve a particular behavioural goal. When used at the strategic level, this is commonly referred to as the intervention mix, and when used operationally, it is described as the marketing mix.

Audience segmentation. Clarity of audience focus using audience segmentation to target effectively.

Exchange. Use of the exchange concept, understanding what is being expected of people, and the real cost to them.

Competition. This means understanding factors that impact on people and that compete for their attention and time (adjusted from NSMC 2022 planning guide and toolkit).

Social marketing uses the total process planning model summarised in Fig. 2.3. The front-end scoping stage drives the whole process. The primary concern is establishing clear, actionable and measurable behaviour goals to ensure focused development across the rest of the process. The ultimate effectiveness and success of social marketing rests on whether it is possible to demonstrate a direct impact on behaviour. It is this feature that sets it apart from other communication or awareness-raising approaches, such as health education, where the main focus is on imparting information and enabling people to understand and use it. For more details on how to engage in health-related social marketing, refer to the NSMC website referenced at the end of this chapter and an example of the evaluation of a social marketing campaign in Nosi and Barbarossa (2021).

Preventive Health Services

These include medical services that aim to prevent ill health, such as vaccinations for COVID- 19 and other communicable diseases, family planning and personal health checks, as well as wider preventive health services, such as child protection services for children at risk of abuse.

Community-Based Work

This is a bottom-up approach to health promotion, working with and for people, involving communities in health work such as local campaigns for better facilities. It includes community development, which is essentially about communities identifying their own health needs and taking action to address them. The sort of activities that may result could include forming self-help and pressure groups and developing local health-enhancing facilities and services.

See Chapter 15, Working with communities.

Organisational Development

This is about developing and implementing policies within organisations to promote the health of staff and customers. Examples include implementing policies on equal opportunities, providing healthy food choices at places of work and working with commercial organisations to develop and promote healthier products.

See Chapter 16, Influencing and implementing policy.

Healthy Public Policies

Developing and implementing healthy public policies involves statutory and voluntary agencies, professionals and the public working together to develop changes in the conditions of living. It is about seeing the implications for health in policies about, for example, equal opportunities, housing, employment, transport and leisure. Good public transport, for example, would improve health by reducing the number of cars on the road, decreasing pollution, using less fuel and reducing the stress of the daily grind of travelling for commuters. It could also reduce isolation for those who do not own cars and enable people to have access to shopping and leisure facilities, all measures that improve wellbeing (see Greszczuk (2019) for detailed examples and lessons of healthy public policies around the world).

See Chapter 16, Influencing and implementing policy.

Environmental Health Measures

Environmental health is about making the physical environment conducive to health, whether at home, at work or in public places. It includes public health measures such as ensuring clean food and water and controlling traffic and other pollution.

Economic and Regulatory Activities

These are political and educational activities directed at politicians, policymakers and planners involving lobbying for and implementing legislative changes such as food labelling regulations, pressing for voluntary codes of practice such as those relating to alcohol advertising or advocating financial measures such as increases in tobacco taxation.

A FRAMEWORK FOR HEALTH PROMOTION ACTIVITIES

Building on Fig. 2.3, there are two points to make about the use of the framework of health promotion activities in Fig. 2.4. The first is that it illustrates that health promotion

has an established relationship to both public health and health and social care practice, but it also includes a specialist field of activities that are vital to the public health agenda and population health and wellbeing. The second point to consider when using the framework is that health promotion does not always fall neatly into categories. For example, would a public health practitioner who was supporting a local women's health group be engaged in a health education programme because they provided health information to the group and set up stress management sessions, or in community-based work because some members of the group had got together to lobby

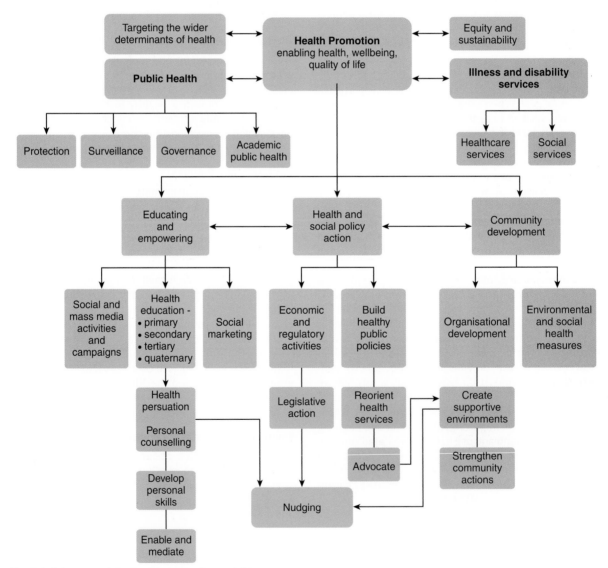

Fig. 2.4 A framework for health promotion activities.

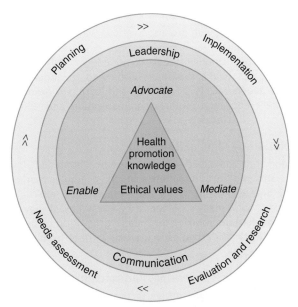

Fig. 2.5 CompHP core competencies framework for health promotion. (Source: IUHPE, 2016).

their local health services for better sexual health advice clinics for young people?

Obviously, areas of activity overlap, but this is not important. What is important is to appreciate the range of activities encompassed by health promotion, the link between health promotion, public health, healthcare and social services and the many ways in which you can contribute to health improvements.

This framework reflects planned, deliberate activities, but it is important to recognise that a great deal of health promotion happens informally and incidentally. For example, health-related depictions in TV soaps and dramas are becoming more authentic and prompt people to seek support (Bhebhe, 2022), and product advertising campaigns can have strong health messages, such as promoting positive associations around moderate drinking choices and the establishment of alcohol-free beer as "cool" (McCarthy, 2020). There are, therefore, health promotion activities which are not likely to be planned with specific health promotion aims in mind. There may, however, be significant influences for behavioural and lifestyle changes.

See Chapter 11, a section on mass media, for more detail.

AREAS OF COMPETENCIES IMPORTANT TO PROMOTING HEALTH

To engage in the activities outlined in the framework in Fig. 2.4, health promoters and public health practitioners require a range of competencies. Competencies can be defined as a combination of the essential knowledge, abilities, skills and values necessary for the practice of health promotion. Core competencies are the minimum set of competencies that constitute a common baseline for all health promotion roles. There are two aspects of health promotion work to consider. One is the specialist aspect, such as immunising a child, taking a cervical smear test, recording blood pressure, or undertaking microbiological tests for food hygiene purposes. All of these are the subject of specialist training and are outside the scope of this book.

The other aspect of promoting health is about working with people to promote health and wellbeing in many different situations with a variety of different aims. To do this, health promoters need to have knowledge of methods and acquire specialist competencies through training. The IUHPE competencies framework (IUHPE, 2016) covers a range of areas (for a review of their effectiveness, see Battel-Kirk and Barry, 2019) as indicated in Fig. 2.5, with all of these competencies covered in this book, including the following:

Managing, Planning and Evaluating

All these are addressed in Part 2: Planning and managing for effective practice, Chapters 5, 6, 7, 8 and 9.

Managing resources for health promotion and public health practice, including budgets, materials, time and people/teams, is crucial. Systematic planning is needed for effective and efficient health promotion. All health promotion work also requires evaluation, and different evaluative methods are appropriate for different approaches.

Communicating and Educating

Communication and educating are addressed in Chapters 8, 9, 10, 11, 12, 13 and 14.

Health promotion is about people, so competence in communication is essential and fundamental. A high level of competence is needed in one-to-one communication and in working with groups in various ways, both formal and informal.

Effective communication is an educational competence, but health promoters also need to understand how people receive information and learn. For example, patient education requires communication and educational competencies.

Marketing and Publicising

Marketing and publicising are covered in Chapter 11.

This requires competence in, for example, marketing and advertising, using social media, local radio and getting local press coverage of health issues. It may be used when undertaking any health promotion or public health practice activities that would benefit from wider publicity.

Facilitating, Networking, Partnership Working

This means enabling others to promote their own and other people's health, using various means such as sharing skills and information and building up confidence and trust. These competencies are particularly important when working with communities. They are also vital for working with other agencies and forming partnerships for health that cross barriers of organisations and disciplines.

Facilitating, networking and partnership working are addressed in Chapters 9, 13 and 15.

Influencing Policy and Practice

Influencing policies and practices that affect health can be at any level, from national (such as policies set by the government or political parties about, for example, COVID-19, housing, transport and future directions for the NHS) to the level of day-to-day work (such as what sort of health promotion programmes will be run in a GP practice, or what resources will be devoted to specific health promotion activities in an environmental health department).

Influencing policy and practice is addressed in Chapter 16.

COMPETENCIES IN PUBLIC HEALTH AND HEALTH PROMOTION

Several initiatives in the UK and Europe have resulted in a clear set of competencies for public health and health promotion. At an international level, the Galway Consensus Statement based on building global capacity in health promotion sets out eight domains of core competency in health promotion, and these have been consolidated in the CompHP discussed earlier and now incorporated

into the IUHPE (2016) (for further mention of the Galway Consensus Statement and a wider discussion of the value of competency-based approaches in health promotion see Battel-Kirk and Barry, 2019).

The UK Public Health Skills and Knowledge Framework (PHSKF) (PHE, 2016), with an overview in Table 2.2, is applicable to all those in the multidisciplinary public health workforce. PHSKF is reflective of the prevailing public health landscape and is an important tool in developing public health capabilities needed in the future. Bornioli et al. (2020) provide an evaluation of the framework and an analysis of its value for developing international competency frameworks. The UK Framework (which may soon be revised following consultation with the public health force (FPH, 2022) consists of three areas (A. Technical, B. Context, C. Delivery), each with a set of four or five functions, with each function having approximately six subfunctions. Function A2 is about the enterprise behind health promotion, including community development, advocacy, behaviour change and sustainable efforts to address the wider determinants of health. Within these functions are references to elements of WHO's Ottawa Charter for Health Promotion (WHO, 1986) and to proportionate universalism (PU) and efforts to reduce health inequalities (for a discussion of the theoretical and practical challenges of PU, see Francis-Oliviero et al., 2020). All public health workers will be contributing to some of these functions. It is noted, however, that there is a specialist workforce who are particularly knowledgeable and skilled in this area.

EXERCISE 2.5   Mapping Your Health Promotion and Public Health Work Against the UK PHSKF

Study Table 2.2 and note with the appropriate numbers from the PHSKF your level of activity in the public health areas and functions using the following Likert scale. If you currently do not have a health promotion or public health role, identify those areas where you would like further training.

Very high level	High level	Fair level	Some level	No activity

What were the results of this mapping in terms of your understanding of the differences between health promotion and public health?

Explain the difference between public health and health promotion.

TABLE 2.2 UK PHSKF

Function	Area A Technical					
A1 Measure, monitor and report population health and wellbeing; health needs; risks; inequalities; and use of services	A1.1 Identify data needs and obtain, verify and organise that data and information	A1.2 Interpret and present data and information	A1.3 Manage data and information in compliance with policy and protocol	A1.4 Assess and manage risks associated with using and sharing data and information, data security and intellectual property	A1.5 Collate and analyse data to produce intelligence that informs decision-making, planning, implementation, performance monitoring and evaluation	A1.6 Predict future data needs and develop data capture methods to obtain it
A2 Promote population and community health and wellbeing, addressing the wider determinants of health and health inequalities	A2.1 Influence and strengthen community action by empowering communities through evidence-based approaches	A2.2 Advocate public health principles and action to protect and improve health and wellbeing	A2.3 Initiate and/or support action to create environments that facilitate and enable health and wellbeing for individuals, groups and communities	A2.4 Design and/or implement universal programmes and interventions while responding proportionately to levels of need within the community	A2.5 Design and/or implement sustainable and multi-faceted programmes, interventions or services to address complex problems	A2.6 Facilitate change (behavioural and/or cultural) in organisations, communities and/or individuals
A3 Protect the public from environmental hazards, communicable diseases and other health risks while addressing inequalities in risk exposure and outcomes	A3.1 Analyse and manage immediate and longer-term hazards and risks to health at an international, national and/or local level	A3.2 Assess and manage outbreaks, incidents and single cases of contamination and communicable disease, locally and across boundaries	A3.3 Target and implement nationwide interventions designed to offset ill health (e.g. screening, immunisation)	A3.4 Plan for emergencies and develop national or local resilience to a range of potential threats	A3.5 Mitigate risks to the public's health using different approaches such as legislation, licensing, policy, education, fiscal measures	

(Continued)

TABLE 2.2   UK PHSKF—Cont'd

Function	Area A Technical					
A4 Work to and for the evidence base, conduct research and provide informed advice	A4.1 Access and appraise evidence gained through systematic methods and through engagement with the wider research community	A4.2 Critique published and unpublished research, synthesise the evidence and draw appropriate conclusions	A4.3 Design and conduct public health research based on current best practice and involving practitioners and the public	A4.4 Report and advise on the implications of the evidence base for the most effective practice and the delivery of value for money	A4.5 Identify gaps in the current evidence base that may be addressed through research	A4.6 Apply research techniques and principles to the evaluation of local services and interventions to establish local evidence of effectiveness
A5 Audit, evaluate and re-design services and interventions to improve health outcomes and reduce health inequalities	A5.1 Conduct economic analysis of services and interventions against health impacts, inequalities in health and return on investment	A5.2 Appraise new technologies, therapies, procedures and interventions and the implications for developing cost-effective, equitable services	A5.3 Engage stakeholders (including service users) in service design and development to deliver accessible and equitable person-centred services	A5.4 Develop and implement standards, protocols and procedures, incorporating national 'best practice' guidance into local delivery systems	A5.5 Quality assurance and audit services and interventions to control risks and improve their quality and effectiveness	

Function	Area B Context				
B1 Work with and through policies and strategies to improve health outcomes and reduce health inequalities	B1.1 Appraise and advise on global, national or local strategies in relation to the public's health and health inequalities	B1.2 Assess the impact and benefits of health and other policies and strategies on the public's health and health inequalities	B1.3 Develop and implement action plans with and for specific groups and communities, to deliver outcomes identified in strategies and policies	B1.4 Influence or lead on policy development and strategic planning, creating opportunities to address health needs and risks, promote health and build approaches to prevention	B1.5 Monitor and report on the progress and outcomes of strategy and policy implementation, making recommendations for improvement

B2 Work collaboratively across agencies and boundaries to improve health outcomes and reduce health inequalities	B2.1 Influence and coordinate other organisations and agencies to increase their engagement with health and wellbeing, ill health prevention and health inequalities	B2.2 Build alliances and partnerships to plan and implement programmes and services that share goals and priorities	B2.3 Evaluate partnerships and address barriers to successful collaboration	B2.4 Collaborate to create new solutions to complex problems by promoting innovation and the sharing of ideas, practices, resources, leadership and learning	B2.5 Connect communities, groups and individuals to local resources and services that support their health and wellbeing	
B3 Work in a competitive contract culture to improve health outcomes and reduce health inequalities	B3.1 Set commissioning priorities balancing particular needs with the evidence base and the economic case for investment	B3.2 Specify and agree on service requirements and measurable performance indicators to ensure the quality provision and delivery of desired outcomes	B3.3 Commission and/or provide services and interventions in ways that involve end users and support community interests to achieve equitable person-centred delivery	B3.4 Facilitate positive contractual relationships managing disagreements and changes within legislative and operational frameworks	B3.5 Manage and monitor progress and deliverables against outcomes and processes agreed upon through a contract	B3.6 Identify and de-commission provision that is no longer effective or value for money
B4 Work within political and democratic systems and with a range of organisational cultures to improve health outcomes and reduce health inequalities	B4.1 Work to understand, and help others to understand, political and democratic processes that can be used to support health and wellbeing and reduce inequalities	B4.2 Operate within the decision-making, administrative and reporting processes that support political and democratic systems	B4.3 Respond constructively to political and other tensions while encouraging a focus on the interests of the public's health	B4.4 Help individuals and communities to have more control over decisions that affect them and promote health equity, equality and justice	B4.5 Work within the legislative framework that underpins public service provision to maximise opportunities to protect and promote health and wellbeing	

(Continued)

TABLE 2.2   UK PHSKF—Cont'd

Area C Delivery

Function					
C1 Provide leadership to drive improvement in health outcomes and the reduction of health inequalities	C1.1 Act with integrity, consistency and purpose, and continue my own personal development	C1.2 Engage others, build relationships, manage conflict, encourage contribution and sustain a commitment to deliver shared objectives	C1.3 Adapt to change, manage uncertainty, solve problems and align clear goals with lines of accountability in complex and unpredictable environments	C1.4 Establish and coordinate a system of leaders and followers engaged in improving health outcomes, the wider health determinants and reducing inequalities	C1.5 Provide vision, shape thinking, inspire shared purpose and influence the contributions of others throughout the system to improve health and address health inequalities
C2 Communicate with others to improve health outcomes and reduce health inequalities	C2.1 Manage public perception and convey key messages using a range of media processes	C2.2 Communicate sometimes complex information and concepts (including health outcomes, inequalities and life expectancy) to a diversity of audiences using different methods	C2.3 Facilitate dialogue with groups and communities to improve health literacy and reduce inequalities using a range of tools and technologies	C2.4 Apply the principles of social marketing and/or behavioural science to reach specific groups and communities by enabling information and ideas	C2.5 Consult and listen to individuals, groups and communities likely to be affected by planned intervention or change

C3 Design and manage programmes and projects to improve health and reduce health inequalities	C3.1 Scope programmes/projects stating the case for investment, the aims, objectives and milestones	C3.2 Identify stakeholders, agree requirements and programme/project schedule(s) and identify how outputs and outcomes will be measured and communicated	C3.3 Manage programme/project schedule(s), resources, budget and scope, accommodating changes within a robust change control process	C3.4 Track and evaluate programme/project progress against schedule(s) and regularly review quality assurance, risks and opportunities to realise benefits and outcomes	C3.5 Seek independent assurance throughout programme/project planning and processes within organisational governance frameworks
C4 Prioritise and manage resources at a population/systems level to achieve equitable health outcomes and return on investment	C4.1 Identify, negotiate and secure sources of funding and/or other resources	C4.2 Prioritise, align and deploy resources towards clear strategic goals and objectives	C4.3 Develop workforce capacity and mobilise the system-wide paid and volunteer workforce to deliver public health priorities at scale	C4.4 Design, implement, deliver and/or quality assure education and training programmes to build a skilled and competent workforce	C4.5 Adapt capability by maintaining flexible service learning and development systems for the workforce

Source: Adjusted from Public Health England (2016, 2019).

Exercise 2.5 is designed to encourage you to think about your health promotion and public health practice work and how it contributes to the wider public health function. It will also help you consider the differences between health promotion and public health.

PRACTICE POINTS

- Health promotion and public health practice encompass a wide range of approaches that are united by the same goal, to enable people to increase control over and improve their health.
- It is important for you to identify the full scope of your health promotion and public health practice work and to see how this fits with the work of your organisation or employer and the wider remits of public health.
- IUHPE provides a competencies and standards map, and UKFPH provides PHSKF, which can be used by organisations, managers, education and training providers, and individuals to improve the quality of public health and health promotion work.

References

ASPHER. (2022). *Video gallery: a message for ASPHER: the global charter for the public's health*. https://www.aspher.org/video,a-message-for-aspher-the-global-charter-for-the-publics-health,24.html

Battel-Kirk, B., & Barry, M. (2019). Has the development of health promotion competencies made a difference? A scoping review of the literature. *Health Education and Behavior*, 1–19.

Bhebhe, A. (2022). *Soap operas can deliver effective health education to young people- new research*. The Conversation. https://theconversation.com/soap-operas-can-deliver-effective-health-education-to-young-people-new-research-175087

Bornioli, A., Evans, D., & Cotter, C. (2020). Evaluation of the UK public health skills and knowledge framework (PHSKF): implications for international competency frameworks. *BMC Public Health*, 20, 956. https://doi.org/10.1186/s12889-020-09024-6.

Department of Health and Social Care. (2021). *Press release 29 March 2021: new office for health promotion to drive improvement of nation's health*. https://www.gov.uk/government/news/new-office-for-health-promotion-to-drive-improvement-of-nations-health

EC. (2020). *EU public health policy*. https://health.ec.europa.eu/eu-health-policy/overview_en

Faculty of Public Health. (2021). *Functions and standards of a public health system*. Faculty of Public Health. http://www.fph.org.uk

Faculty of Public Health. (2022). *Public health skills and knowledge framework*. https://www.fph.org.uk/professional-development/workforce/public-health-skills-and-knowledge-framework/

Frances-Oliviero, F., Cambon, L., Wittwer, J., Marmot, M., & Alla, F. (2020). Theoretical and Practical challenges of proportionate universalism: a review. *Rev Panam Salud Publica*, 15(44), E110. https://doi:10.26633/RPSP.2020.110.

Greszczuk, C. (2019). Implementing health in all policies: lessons from around the world. London: The Health Foundation.

Health Development Consultancy. (2022). *Courses*. http://www.healthdc.co.uk/courses/

Heineken. (2016). *Moderate drinkers wanted TV, cinema, and internet commercial*. https://www.tvadsongs.uk/heineken-advert-song-i-need-a-hero-commercial/.

IUHPE, (2016). *Core competencies and professional standards for health promotion: full version*. Geneva: IUHPE.

Lalonde, M. (1974). *A new perspective on the health of Canadians*. Ottawa: Information Canada. http://www.phac-aspc.gc.ca/ph-sp/pdf/perspect-eng.pdf.

Martins, C., Godycki-Cwirko, M., & Brodersen, J. (2018). Quaternary prevention: reviewing the concept. *European Journal of General Practice*, 24(1), 106–111. https://doi:10.1080/13814788.2017.1422177.

McKinlay, J. B. (1979). A case for refocusing upstream: the political economy of health. In E. G. Jaco (Ed.), *Patients, physicians and illness*. Basingstoke: Macmillan.

McCarthy, J. (2020). *How Heineken's using the biggest ever non-alcoholic beer sponsorship to grow the category*. The Drum. https://www.thedrum.com/news/2020/08/11/how-heineken-s-using-the-biggest-ever-non-alcoholic-beer-sponsorship-grow-the

NHS Greater Glasgow and Clyde (2020). *Health improvement*. Nhsggc.org.uk

Nosi, C., & Barbarossa, C. (2021). Evaluating a social marketing campaign on health nutrition and lifestyle among primary-school children: a mixed-method research design. *Evaluation and Program Planning*, 89. https://doi:10.1016/j.evalprogplan.2021.101965.

NSMC. (2022). *Planning guide and toolkit*. https://thensmc.com/toolkit

Nutbeam, D., Corbin, J. H., & Lin, V. (2021). *Health Promotion International*, 36(Suppl 1), 1–13. https://doi.org/10.1093/heapro/daab150

Public Health England. (2016). *Public health skills and knowledge framework*. https://www.gov.uk/government/uploads/system/uploads/attachment_data/file/545012/Public_Health_Skills_and_Knowledge_Framework_2016.pdf

Public Health England. (2019). *Public health skills and knowledge framework: August 2019 update*. https://www.gov.uk/government/publications/public-health-skills-and-knowledge-framework-phskf/public-health-skills-and-knowledge-framework-august-2019-update

Tannahill, A. (2009) Health promotion: the Tannahill model revisited. *Public Health*. May;123(5):396–9. http://doi:10.1016/j.puhe.2008.05.021.

Stock, C. (2022). Grand challenges for public health Education and Promotion. *Frontiers in Public Health*, 10, 917685. https://doi.org/10.3389/fpubh.2022.917685.

World Federation of Public Health Associations. (2016 and 2022). *A global charter for the public's health*. http://www.wfpha.org/wfpha-projects/14-projects/171-a-global-charter-for-the-public-s-health-3

World Health Organisation. (1986). *The Ottawa Charter for health promotion*. Geneva: World Health Organisation. https://www.who.int/teams/health-promotion/enhanced-well-being/first-global-conference.

World Health Organisation, (2021). *Health promotion glossary of terms 2021*. Geneva: World Health Organisation.

WHO-ASPHER (2020) *Competency framework for the public health workforce in the European Region 2020*. https://www.euro.who.int/__data/assets/pdf_file/0003/444576/WHO-ASPHER-Public-Health-Workforce-Europe-eng.pdf

Websites

ASPHER. https://www.aspher.org/video,a-message-for-aspher-the-global-charter-for-the-publics-health,24.html

Functions of the Local Public Health System. https://www.fph.org.uk/media/3031/fph_systems_and_function-final-v2.pdf

Blogs

Faculty of Public Health Blog. *Better health for all*. https://betterhealthforall.org/

The National Social Marketing Centre Blog. https://www.thensmc.com/blog/understanding-covid-19-vaccine-hesitancy (interesting blog by John Landels on understanding COVID-19 vaccine hesitancy)

Facebook

Royal Society for Public Health. https://www.facebook.com/royalsocietyforpublichealth/

World Health Organisation (WHO). https://www.facebook.com/WHO/videos/924934254833664. For a range of live videos and up to briefings

Twitter

Faculty of Public Health FPH@FPH.

Association of Directors of Public Health ADPH@ADPHUK.

YouTube

American Public Health Foundation. Webinar on changes to core competencies in public health. Useful as a comparison to the core competencies used in this chapter. https://www.youtube.com/watch?v=d3bMGqGgoME. Accessed September 2022.

UK Faculty of Public Health. https://www.youtube.com/watch?v=d3bMGqGgoME. President of the FPH

Who Promotes Health?

Angela Scriven

SUMMARY

In this chapter, some of the key agents and agencies of public health and health promotion are identified, and their roles discussed. Included are international and national organisations, the government, local authorities, the National Health Service (NHS) and voluntary and non-government organisations (NGOs). The chapter ends with an exercise on identifying and mapping key local health promoters and public health professionals in your geographical area.

This chapter provides an overview of the people and organisations that support and enable better individual and population health. The aim here is to identify the agents and agencies through which planned, deliberate public health and health promotion programmes and policies are delivered. It must be recognised that these agents and agencies change over time and that there are frequent government reorganisations of health and public health systems. Moreover, COVID-19 will have impacted the resources and functions of all the public health organisations discussed below. Those working to promote health need to be very familiar with local and national systems. At the time of writing, the four countries that make up the United Kingdom (UK) – England, Wales, Scotland, and Northern Ireland – have slightly different health and public health systems. Box 3.1 sums up the current organisational structures in the four countries. Many of the health promoters and public health practitioners discussed later in the chapter either work in these health and public health systems or establish collaborative partnerships with the people who do.

NATIONAL PUBLIC HEALTH AGENCIES

The Government

The national public health strategies for health in England, Wales, Scotland, and Northern Ireland demonstrate a commitment towards the pursuit of improved health and a reduction in health inequalities for the populations they serve. To this end, in England, key public health agencies have been established, such as the National Institute for Health and Care Excellence (NICE) and the Office for Health Improvement and Disparities, which is part of the Department of Health and Social Care. The government tackles health issues such as drug and substance

EXERCISE 3.1

1. Critically compare the different health structures outlined in Box 3.1 and identify the key differences in the organisation of public health between England, Wales, Scotland, and Northern Ireland.
2. If you were a government minister for health, how would you structure the statutory health promotion and public health services? For example, would you have a lead agency for public health and if so, what would you call it? Would you locate responsibility for public health within the NHS or the local authority? What areas of public health would you prioritise? Offer a rational for each of your decisions.

(Continued)

BOX.3.1   An Overview of the Uk Health and Public Health Systems

England

The NHS provides healthcare services through NHS trusts, foundation trusts (including mental health and ambulance trusts), and some charities and social enterprises. All GPs in England are part of a clinical commissioning group which is responsible for planning and commissioning (buying) the services their patients need.

NHS England

A national body - NHS England - oversees the NHS commissioning budget of approximately £80 billion, and its area teams are responsible for commissioning the following:

- GP
- Dental
- Pharmacy
- Some optical services

NHS England's area teams also have overall responsibility for screening and immunisation programmes.

Public Health in England

Public health services in England are primarily delivered through:

- The OHID
- Local authorities that have public health responsibilities.

The OHID's mission is to protect and improve the nation's health and wellbeing and reduce health inequalities.

The Health and Social Care Act (2012) gave some local authorities mandatory requirements for commissioning public health services such as sexual health, NHS health checks and the National Child Measurement Programme, and for providing public health advice through clinical commissioning groups. Each such local authority has a health and wellbeing board which sets the local strategic direction for public health and a strategy based on the needs of the local population. The Health and Social Care Act (2022) is resulting in structural and funding changes.

Local authorities also have statutory responsibilities to ensure systems are in place to protect the health of the population and to provide information and advice in the event of a health protection incident or outbreak.

The Health and Social Care Act (2022) is resulting in structural and funding changes to the NHS in England (see Fig. 3.1 and the Kings Fund website referenced at the end of the chapter for further details).

Wales

As a devolved administration, Wales receives a grant from the UK central government, which is then distributed between the different departments, including NHS Wales. The main difference for patients in Wales is that prescriptions for medicines are free for everyone.

NHS Wales

Health services in Wales are delivered through seven health boards and three NHS trusts, each one responsible for delivering all healthcare services within a particular geographical area. The three NHS trusts in Wales with an all-Wales focus are:

- The Welsh Ambulance Services Trust for emergency services.
- Velindre University NHS Trust offers specialist services in cancer care.
- Public Health Wales.

The seven health boards work together with community health councils which represent patients and user groups.

Scotland

As a devolved administration, Scotland receives a block grant from the UK central government, which is then distributed between the different departments, including NHS Scotland.

NHS Scotland

NHS Scotland is made up of 14 health boards which are responsible for delivering the acute and primary healthcare services their populations need. There are also eight special health boards that cover services such as ambulance services, Scotland's health improvement agency (called NHS Health Scotland) and NHS Education for Scotland. They also have their own careers website.

Public Health in Scotland

Each health board has a public health department where responsibility lies for monitoring and improving the health of their populations.

NHS Health Scotland is one of the special health boards, and its overall aim is to improve Scotland's health by focusing on the inequalities that prevent health from being improved by all. NHS Health Scotland is the main health improvement agency in Scotland and covers every aspect of health improvement across all health topics, settings, and life stages.

BOX.3.1   An Overview of the Uk Health and Public Health Systems—Cont'd

More than 50 organisations are involved in health protection in Scotland over two 'tiers':

- Local authorities and NHS boards
- Government, NHS special boards, Scottish Environment Protection Agency, Scottish Water, the Food Standards Agency and the Health and Safety Executive.

Health Protection in Scotland

Health Protection Scotland provides advice and services to the rest of NHS Scotland. It:

- Provides the national blood transfusion service.
- Provides advice on healthcare environments and equipment.
- Monitors hazards and exposures affecting people's health.
- Provides guidance on tackling healthcare-associated infections.
- Coordinates screening programmes.

Northern Ireland

The health system differs in Northern Ireland in that both health and social care are provided through an integrated service, and prescriptions for medical care are free for everyone.

Northern Ireland receives a block grant from the UK Treasury, which funds the Department of Health, Social Services and Public Safety for Northern Ireland (DHSSPS).

The DHSSPS has overall responsibility for providing health and social care services in Northern Ireland, including public health and public safety.

Health and Social Care Board

Working under the DHSSPS, a Health and Social Care Board is responsible for commissioning services, resource management, performance management, and service improvement. The Health and Social Care Board works to identify and meet the needs of the Northern Ireland population through its five local commissioning groups. The local commissioning groups cover the same geographical areas as five health and social care trusts that deliver health and social care services. A separate trust – Northern Ireland Ambulance Trust – provides ambulance services across Northern Ireland.

Public Health in Northern Ireland

The Public Health Agency is responsible for the following:

- Health protection
- Screening
- Health and social care research and development
- Safety and quality
- Improving health and social wellbeing

It also provides public health, nursing, and allied health professional advice to support the Health and Social Care Board and its local commissioning groups.

Source Health Careers. (2022a). https://www.healthcareers.nhs.uk/working-health/uk-health-systems/uk-health-systems.

misuse (Department of Health [DoH], 2018) and obesity and healthy eating (Department of Health and Social Care [DHSC], 2020a, 2020b) and strategies linked to the COVID-19 pandemic (HM Government, 2022). In relation to obesity, the government action in England involves giving people advice on a healthy diet and physical activity through the better health programme; improving the labelling of food and drink to help people make healthy choices with a consistent front-of-pack labelling system that makes it clear what is in food and drink; and encouraging restaurant businesses to include calorie information on their menus so that people can make healthy choices. For full details on the obesity strategy for adults and children, see DHSC (2020a, 2020b).

The National Institute for Health and Care Excellence (NICE)

The National Institute for Health and Care Excellence (NICE) is a non-departmental public body providing national guidance and advice to improve health and social care in England. The way NICE was established in legislation means that the guidance is officially England-only. However, there are agreements to provide certain NICE products and services to Wales, Scotland, and Northern Ireland. Decisions on how the guidance applies in these countries are made by the devolved administrations, who are often involved and consulted during the development of NICE guidance. NICE also provides resources to help maximise the use of evidence and guidance for key groups, including general practitioners (GPs), local government, and public health professionals (NICE, 2021). Their evidence sections, lifestyle and wellbeing and population groups and COVID-19, are of particular importance to those promoting health with guides on topics and approaches such as behaviour change (see Chapter 8 for more about evidence-informed practice and Chapter 14 for behaviour change approaches).

The Office for Health Improvement and Disparities (OHID)

The Office for Health Improvement and Disparities (OHID) is part of the Department of Health and Social Care. The

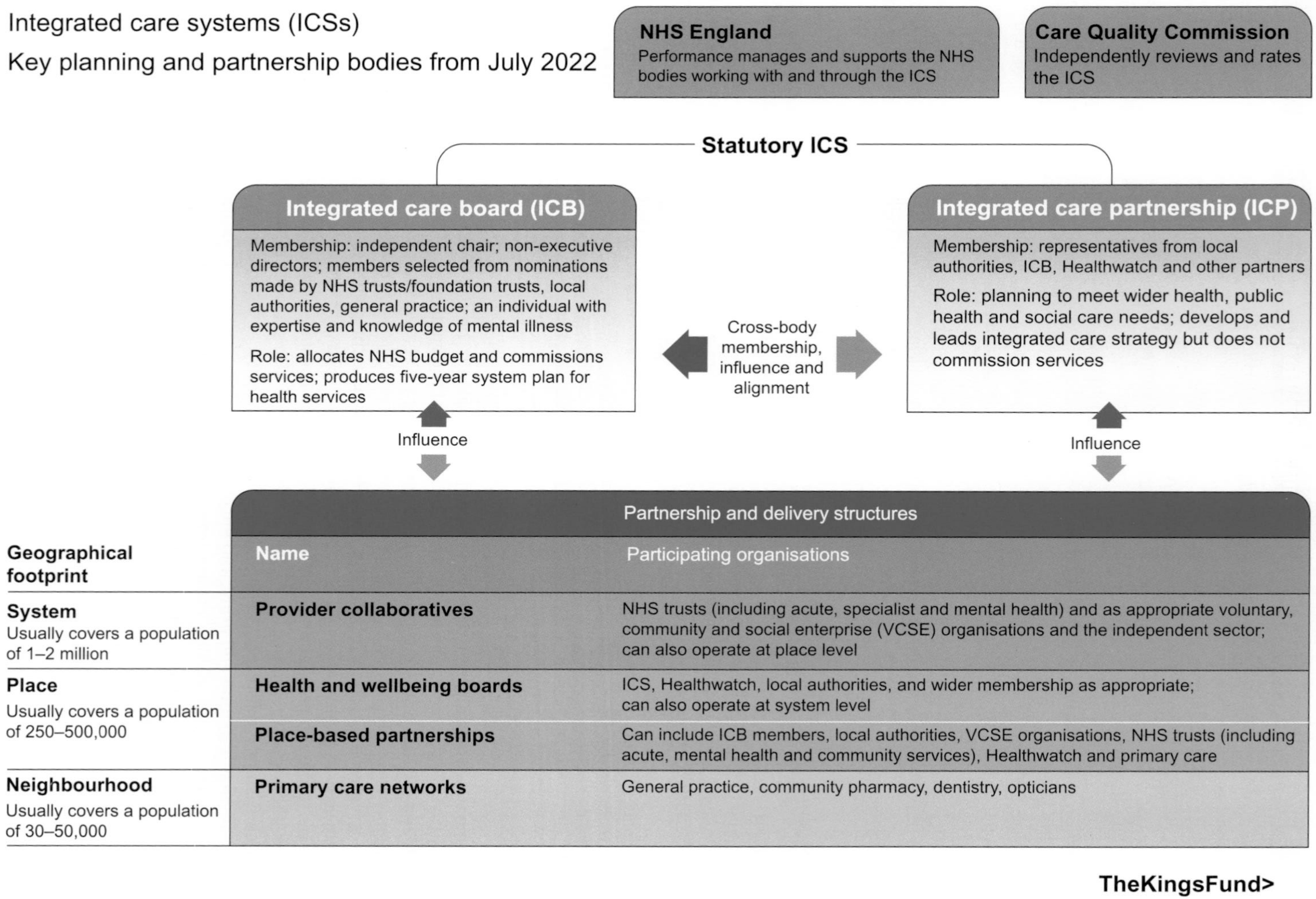

Integrated care systems (ICSs)
Key planning and partnership bodies from July 2022

NHS England
Performance manages and supports the NHS bodies working with and through the ICS

Care Quality Commission
Independently reviews and rates the ICS

———— Statutory ICS ————

Integrated care board (ICB)

Membership: independent chair; non-executive directors; members selected from nominations made by NHS trusts/foundation trusts, local authorities, general practice; an individual with expertise and knowledge of mental illness

Role: allocates NHS budget and commissions services; produces five-year system plan for health services

Integrated care partnership (ICP)

Membership: representatives from local authorities, ICB, Healthwatch and other partners and as appropriate voluntary, public health and social care needs; develops and leads integrated care strategy but does not commission services

Role: planning to meet wider health, public health and social care needs; develops and leads integrated care strategy but does not commission services

Cross-body membership, influence and alignment

Influence

Influence

Partnership and delivery structures

Geographical footprint	Name	Participating organisations
System Usually covers a population of 1–2 million	**Provider collaboratives**	NHS trusts (including acute, specialist and mental health) and as appropriate voluntary, community and social enterprise (VCSE) organisations and the independent sector; can also operate at place level
Place Usually covers a population of 250–500,000	**Health and wellbeing boards**	ICS, Healthwatch, local authorities, and wider membership as appropriate; can also operate at system level
	Place-based partnerships	Can include ICB members, local authorities, VCSE organisations, NHS trusts (including acute, mental health and community services), Healthwatch and primary care
Neighbourhood Usually covers a population of 30–50,000	**Primary care networks**	General practice, community pharmacy, dentistry, opticians

TheKingsFund>

Fig. 3.1 The structure of the NHS in England from July 2022. (Source: Kings Fund, 2022).

TABLE 3.1   The Public Health and Health Promotion Priorities, Responsibilities and Functions of the OHID

Priorities
- To identify and address health disparities, focusing on those groups and areas where health inequalities have the greatest effect.
- To act on the biggest preventable risk factors for ill health and premature death, including tobacco, obesity, and harmful use of alcohol and drugs.
- To work with the NHS and local government to improve access to the services which detect and act on health risks and conditions as early as possible.
- To develop strong partnerships across government, communities, industry, and employers to act on the wider factors that contribute to people's health, such as work, housing and education.
- To drive innovation in health improvement, harnessing the best of technology, analytics, and innovations in policy and delivery, to help deliver change where it is needed most.

RESPONSIBILITIES

National Health Improvement, Prevention of Poor Health, and Tackling Health Disparities	Public Health Analysis	Regional Public Health	Public Health Advice
Functions 1. Build the scientific evidence, lead and develop the policy, and deliver core services around: healthy weight, healthy diet, and physical activity, the health of children and families, smoking, addiction and the health of vulnerable groups. 2. Lead the policy development and support the effective delivery of prevention services, helping individuals to better understand and manage their health 3. Build the scientific evidence on public mental health	1. Lead public health data management and analysis, publishing official statistics, statistical reports, and analytical products 2. Deliver system-wide leadership, skills, and knowledge transfer in public health analysis, epidemiology, and data science 3. Lead surveillance of non-communicable disease	Support the delivery of national and regional priorities for prevention and health inequalities and ensure a joined-up approach to public health, building strong interfaces with different teams, and areas of public health across the regional system	Under the leadership of the Chief Public Health Nurse, lead international and national public health advice on nursing, midwifery and allied health professionals

Source: Adjusted from The Office of Health Improvement and Disparities. (2022). https://www.gov.uk/government/organisations/office-for-health-improvement-and-disparities/about#responsibilities.

OHID focuses on a) improving the nation's health so population groups can expect to live more of life in good health and b) on levelling up health disparities to break the link between socioeconomic circumstances and prospects for a healthier life (see Table 3.1 for more detail on the priorities, responsibilities and functions of OHID). OHID are charged with working across government, local government, the healthcare system, and industry with an emphasis on preventing ill health, particularly in those communities where there are the most health disparities (OHID, 2022)

The Office for Health Promotion

The Office for Health Promotion (OHP) was established in 2021 with a brief to lead national efforts to improve and level up the population health. It will help ministers design and operationalise a step change in public health policy with action across government to improve the nation's health by tackling obesity, improving mental health, and promoting physical activity.

The OHP reports jointly to the Health Secretary and the Chief Medical Officer. The office's remit is to systematically tackle the top preventable risk factors causing death and ill health in the UK by designing and implementing health-promoting strategies and tracking the delivery. It brings together a range of skills to lead a new era of public health polices, leveraging modern digital tools, data, and actuarial science and delivery experts that will enable more joined-up, sustained action between national and local government, the NHS, and cross-government, where much of the wider determinants of health sit. The OHP informs cross-government agenda, which will look to track the wider determinants of health and implement policies in other departments where appropriate. The office combines health improvement expertise with existing DHSC health policy capabilities to promote and deliver better health to communities nationwide (DHSC, 2021).

Health Services

Statutory health services are very important agents for public health and the promotion of health globally, nationally, and locally. The UK has a government-sponsored universal healthcare system called the NHS. The NHS consists of a series of publicly funded healthcare systems in the UK. It includes the NHS (England), NHS Scotland, NHS Wales, and Health and Social Care in Northern Ireland. The pandemic radically reshaped the delivery of health services, and there will likely be long term impacts. What the implications will be for how the NHS is organised in the long term remain to be seen, but beyond lessons for the future pandemic response, the NHS will need to carefully prioritise resources as it returns to normal activity. There are likely to be significant implications for recently introduced strategies to improve clinical outcomes and tackle workforce issues, as well as greater urgency to calls for social care reform. Other existing trends, such as closer working between local health and care providers, and the move to online working, have been accelerated by system-wide responses to COVID-19. Some changes to ways of working that have been introduced in the NHS during the pandemic response may become a 'new normal' (Powel et al., 2020). Fig. 3.1 shows the structure of the health services in England following the Health and Care Act 2022; a greater emphasis has been placed on integrated working (Kings Fund, 2022). Community services include health centres, clinics, and services in people's homes. Mental health services provide health and social care for people with mental health problems. These services are provided through primary care, such as GP services, or through more specialist care. This might include counselling and other psychological therapies, community and family support, or general health screening. For example, people experiencing bereavement, depression, stress or anxiety can get help from their GP and be referred to a specialist mental health service (NHS, 2019)

Hospital services employ medical teams and a range of other health-promoting professions, such as physiotherapists, radiographers, podiatrists, speech and language therapists, counsellors, occupational therapists, and psychologists.

Primary care is the first point of health services contact for most people and includes GPs, dentists, pharmacists, and optometrists, as well as NHS walk-in centres and the NHS 111 telephone service. Secondary care is a range of specialist services, usually based in a hospital as opposed to being in the community, and patients are usually referred to secondary care by a primary care provider such as a GP. Both primary and secondary care services have health promotion functions. To see more on priorities and operational planning guidelines, see the publication (NHS, 2022a). In the NHS Long Term Plan (Charles et al., 2019; NHS, 2019), areas of work include prevention, ageing well, and starting well, with an emphasis on the prevention of avoidable illness. NHS primary and secondary care services deliver health-promoting and other preventative strategies.

The structures in Scotland, Wales, and Northern Ireland differ (see Box 3.1 for the overview). In addition to Box 3.1, Understanding the NHS Long Term Plan (NHS, 2019) and Nicholson and Shuttleworth (2020) offer a succinct outline of the provision in these three countries. At the time of writing, there is a major review and transition of health services (see Anderson et al., 2022 for further details) and a crisis in workforce capacity, so systems are adapting and changing. In the interests of keeping the text in this book short, the examples used are drawn from England, but readers in all countries will need to familiarise themselves with the structure in the country where they work by undertaking Exercise 3.2

Online Public Health Resources

There are many online public health resources that are easily accessible to the public. For example, the NHS webpage offers multiple categories of public health advice and guidance, including information on a range of health issues, a directory of local services and a live well section which offers a wide range of health promotion information and advice to help users improve their lifestyle. There is information on alcohol, smoking, physical activity, healthy eating, sexual health, and much more. The live well section also offers advice on healthy weight, exercise and offers tools to support lifestyle changes, such as alcohol units and body mass index calculators. There are online

TABLE 3.2   Mapping the Core Public Health Roles in England

Health Visitors

Public Health Practitioners

Environmental Health Professionals

School Nurses

Public Health Scientists

Public Health Consultants, Specialists and Registrars, Including Directors of Public Health

Intelligence and Knowledge Professionals

Public Health Managers

Other Public Health Nurses

Public Health Academics

Source: Adjusted from Centre for Workforce Intelligence (2014).

exercise videos relating to improving strength and flexibility and very useful advice (see for example NHS, 2021).

Non-Government Organisations

There are several NGOs concerned specifically with public health and health promotion in the UK, such as The Royal Society for Public Health, the UK Public Health Association and The Institute of Health Education and Health Promotion.

The Royal Society for Public Health (RSPH). The RSPH is an independent organisation dedicated to the promotion and protection of population health and wellbeing. It advises on policy development; provides education and training services; encourages scientific research; disseminates information through publications, reports, blogs, Facebook, Twitter, and webpages; and runs public health campaigns. The RSPH is the largest multidisciplinary public health organisation in the UK and advocates for the importance of specialised health promotion and public health practitioners within public health. Their campaigns demonstrate their commitment to the principles of health promotion, for example, their 'Dream it. Try it. Live it.' The RSPH (2017) campaign aimed to empower young people to adopt healthy behaviours and raise awareness of the benefits of living healthier, more active lives. The campaign covered a range of topics, including mental wellbeing, physical activity, healthy eating, body image, and the importance of sleep, and it is led by a team of young volunteers linked to the youth health champion qualification with support from RSPH staff. These volunteers directed the campaign, conducted interviews and research, made and edited promotional videos, wrote blogs, and worked

EXERCISE 3.2   Finding Out About Your Local NHS, Local Authority, and the Wider Range of Public Health Agents and Agencies

Exercise 3.2 is designed to help you determine how your local public health system is organised and identify the health promotion agents and agencies that are important for your work. There is much to gain by having good local knowledge of health promoters you can refer clients to or work in partnerships.

1. Find out about the structure of the public health teams in the area where you work:

- What is the name and function of the local statutory organisation with responsibility for public health?
- What regional and/or national organisations are responsible for public health where you work? Find out about the agencies and agents on your patch:
- Think of the geographical patch where you work and identify its boundaries as clearly as you can. It might be the area served by a GP practice, the catchment area of a hospital or the population of a Local Authority or Health Trust.
- Identify as many health promotion agents and agencies on your patch as you can using Fig. 3.2 and the information about agents and agencies in health promotion in this chapter as checklists.

It is likely that you will know some very well and others not at all. Identify those you would find it helpful to know more about and plan to find out about them. If there are some you know nothing about, such as the voluntary and community groups on your patch, identify people who are likely to know about them (such as health promotion or public health practitioners/specialists) and contact them to find out more.

Finally, assess how the COVID-19 pandemic has had an impact on the agents and agencies who promote health.

with a wide range of public health and corporate organisations. It was a multimedia campaign using Twitter, Instagram, YouTube, and Snapchat. Updates were also posted on the youth health movement website. See website references at the end of this chapter.

The Institute of Health Promotion and Education (IHPE). The IHPE is a professional association with charitable status which brings together people with a professional interest in health education and health promotion. The Institute offers comprehensive information resources (such as the International Journal of Health Promotion and Education) and professional development support. You can subscribe to their newsletter (IHPE, 2022).

Voluntary and Charitable Organisations and Pressure Groups

There are many international and national voluntary and charitable organisations concerned with public health and health promotion. National examples of these are The Advisory Council on Alcohol and Drug Education (TACADE) and the National Association for Mental Health (MIND). Most of these organisations produce educational material, and some run training courses for professionals and/or the public. Some organisations act mainly as pressure groups, such as Friends of the Earth. See the editorial in the *Lancet Editorial*, 2020 for a critical review of the role of charities in supporting health services and how the COVID-19 pandemic has impacted on this vital role, and Corry (2018) for a discussion of the role of the charity sector in supporting individual and population health in the UK.

Professional Associations

Professional associations such as the British Medical Association, the Royal College of Nursing (RCN), the Chartered Institute for Environmental Health (CIEH) and the Faculty of Public Health (FPH) have been highly influential in policy and legislative changes and in practice support and training of their members in public health and health promotion.

Trade Unions

Trade unions are active in promoting health, wellbeing, and safety at work, both through negotiating workplace conditions and through their health and safety representatives. For example, for a discussion of how unions can support mental health in the UK, see Frith (2022). The Health and Safety Executive also oversees the implementation of health and safety at work legislation and provides a range of resources and information on workplace health.

Commercial and Industrial Organisations

These have a role in safeguarding public health. Examples include companies providing water and refuse removal. In recent years in the UK, some facilities with a public health protection function have been privatised. This has raised public health dilemmas, for example, 'Should water companies have the right to cut off supplies to consumers who are unable to pay their bills when a possible consequence of this is the occurrence and spread of infectious diseases such as dysentery?'

Manufacturers and Retailer

Manufacturers and retailers are a powerful influence on public health. For example, millions of families in the UK use a major supermarket every week. Food manufacturers have both the technical expertise to make healthier products and the marketing expertise to influence purchasing habits. If the full strength of these skills is directed towards activities to encourage and enable people to make healthier food choices, the public health benefits could be great. The government established the public health responsibility deal to maximise these benefits. By working in partnership, public health, commercial, and voluntary organisations agreed on practical actions to secure more progress, more quickly, with less cost than legislation across a range of public health issues, including food, alcohol, physical activity, and health at work (see Knai et al. (2018), Laverty et al. (2017) and Mwatsama et al. (2019) for qualification of the impact of the Public health responsibility deal on a number of health outcomes).

The Mass Media

The mass media refers to all major outlets distributing public health information across a variety of formats, including television, print, radio, and online. Mass media can facilitate targeted health campaigning or can contribute indirectly. The trend towards developing an online presence and the traditional newspapers or TV channels demonstrates a move towards the immediacy of web-based communications. The mass media are intensively employed in public health, including the production and distribution of booklets, pamphlets, exhibits, newspaper, and magazine articles, and radio and television programmes, plus the various online and social media outlets (such as YouTube, Facebook, Twitter, websites, and Instagram). These media are employed to promote the uptake of health information and knowledge, to change health attitudes and values, and to encourage the establishment of new health behaviour (Stead et al., 2019). Schillenger et al. (2020) argue that during the COVID-19 pandemic, social media was a source of toxic 'infodemics' as well as providing a valuable tool for the promotion of public health. They then proceed to present a novel framework to guide any investigation and assessment of the role of social media on public health. See Chapter 11 for more about the mass media and social media in public health and health promotion, including a consideration of some of the negative influences.

Churches and Religious Organisations

Churches and religious organisations can play an important part in influencing the communities they serve with the values, attitudes, and beliefs that affect health.

Moreover, Roberts (2019) argues that religious involvement is associated with better health outcomes, including greater longevity, coping skills, health-related quality of life, and less depression and suicide. In addition, faith-based delivery of health promotion and public health activities and programmes can reach community groups who may be underserved by public health services. For an example of a faith-based physical activity programme, see Haughton et al. (2020).

INTERNATIONAL PUBLIC HEALTH AGENCIES

The European Community

Ranging from influence over world trade laws affecting health to population health issues such as obesity to the use of comparative data to affect health policy, the European Union's (EU) public health policies are an important influence on national and local policies across the European Member Countries (European Parliament, 2021a).

On 31 January 2020, the UK officially left the EU and, at the same time, was battling the largest public health crisis in a century, the COVID-19 pandemic. For a full mapping out of the health areas that have been affected by exiting the EU and the identification of the policy issues and dilemmas, and possible impacts, plus how these may be tracked over time, see Dayan et al. (2020).

The EU4Health programme 2021–2027 (European Parliament, 2021b; EC Public Health EU4 Health Programme, 2021–2027) is a vision for a healthier EU and was adopted as a response to the COVID-19 pandemic. Its goal is to reinforce crisis preparedness in the EU because of the pandemic, highlighting the fragility of national health systems. EU4Health brings an EU-added value and complements the policies of the Member States to pursue four general objectives representing the ambitions of the programme and ten specific objectives representing the areas of intervention:

- Improve and foster health
  - Health promotion and disease prevention, in particular, cancer
  - International health initiatives and cooperation
- Protect people
  - Prevention, preparedness, and response to cross-border health threats
  - Complementing national stockpiling of essential crisis-relevant products
  - Establishing a reserve of medical, healthcare, and support staff
- Access to medicinal products, medical devices, and crisis-relevant products
  - Ensuring that these products are accessible, available, and affordable

- Strengthen health systems
  - Reinforcing health data, digital tools, and services, digital transformation of healthcare
  - Enhancing access to healthcare
  - Developing and implementing EU health legislation and evidence-based decision-making
  - Integrated work among national health systems (EC, 2022)

The World Health Organization (WHO)

The WHO has a significant role in guiding European and global health policy. It has issued many statements in the form of declarations and charters addressing important and broad areas of health promotion and public health-related policy. It is responsible for Health 2020, the European policy for health and wellbeing (See Zuidberg et al. (2020) for an assessment of the progress of Health 2020) and coordinates European networks such as school and youth health/health-promoting schools and healthy cities.

The WHO's role in guiding the promotion of health is discussed in Chapter 1.

Other International Agencies

The International Union for Health Promotion and Education (IUHPE)

The IUHPE is a unique worldwide, independent, and professional association of individuals and organisations committed to improving the health and wellbeing of the people through education, community action and the development of healthy public policy. It is a leading global network working to promote health and contribute to the achievement of equity in health between and within countries. It advances the knowledge base and improves the quality and effectiveness of health promotion and health education practice. The IUHPE works across all continents and decentralises its activity through regional offices. It works in close cooperation with the major inter-governmental and NGOs, such as the WHO, to influence and facilitate the development of health promotion strategies and projects.

As an international health promotion agency, it works towards:

- Greater equity in the health of populations between and within countries of the world.
- Effective alliances and partnerships to produce optimal health promotion outcomes.
- Accessible, evidence-based knowledge to inform practice.
- Excellence in policy and practice for effective quality health promotion.

- High levels of capacity in individuals, organisations, and countries to undertake health promotion activities.

To achieve these goals, the IUHPE pursues the following objectives:

- Increased investment in health promotion by governments, intergovernmental and NGOs, academic institutions, and the private sector.
- An increase in organisational, governmental and intergovernmental policies, and practices that result in greater equity in health between and within countries.
- Improvements in policy and practice of governments at all levels, organisations, and sectors that influence the determinants of the health of populations.
- Strong alliances and partnerships among all sectors based on agreed ethical principles, mutual understanding and respect.
- Activities that contribute to the development, translation, and exchange of knowledge and practice that advance the field of health promotion (including world conferences).
- The wide dissemination of knowledge to health promotion practitioners, as well as to policymakers, government officials, and other key individuals and organisations.
- A strong and universally accessible knowledge base for effective, quality health promotion.
- Improved mechanisms for the exchange of ideas, experience, and knowledge that promote health and wellbeing.
- A global forum for mutual support and professional advancement of members.
- Capacity-building opportunities for individuals and institutions to better carry out health promotion initiatives and advocacy efforts (see IUHPE, 2023 for further details on the IUHPE mission statement, activities and governance structure).

In the dissemination of knowledge, the IUHPE is very active. It has an international journal, *Global Health Promotion*, and has associated journals which rank amongst the most important peer-reviewed journals in the field of health promotion (IUHPE, 2023).

European Public Health Alliance (EPHA)

EPHA is Europe's leading NGO advocating for better population health. It is a member-led organisation comprised of public health NGOs, patient groups, health professionals, and disease groups working together to improve health and strengthen the voice of public health in Europe. EPHA is a member of, among others, the Social Platform, the Health and Environment Alliance and the EU Civil Society Contact Group. Their mission is to bring together the public health community to provide thought leadership and facilitate change, to build public health

capacity, to deliver equitable solutions to European public health challenges and to improve health and reduce health inequalities.

Their vision is of a Europe with universal good health and wellbeing where all have access to a sustainable and high quality health system; a Europe whose policies and practices contribute to health, both within and beyond its borders.

What they do:

- Monitor the policy-making process within the EU institutions and support the flow of information on health promotion and public health policy developments amongst all interested players, including politicians, civil servants, NGOs, stakeholders, and the public.
- Promote greater awareness amongst European citizens and NGOs about policy developments and programme initiatives that effect the health of those living in the EU, allowing them to contribute to the policy-making process.
- Train, mentor and support NGOs, local health organisations, and those working with disadvantaged communities, and enable engagement with the EU.
- Participate in policy debates and stakeholder dialogues to raise the profile of health in all policy areas, supporting collaboration and partnerships between NGOs and other organisations active at European, national and local levels on health promotion, and public health (EPHA, 2022).

World Federation of Public Health Associations (WFPHA)

The WFPHA is an international NGO composed of multidisciplinary national public health associations. It is the only worldwide professional society representing and serving the broad field of public health. WFPHA's mission is to promote and protect global public health. It does this throughout the world by supporting the establishment and organisational development of public health associations and societies of public health through facilitating and supporting the exchange of information, knowledge and the transfer of skills and resources, and through promoting and undertaking advocacy for public policies, programmes, and practices that will result in a healthy and productive world. WFPHA brings together public health professionals interested and active in safeguarding and promoting the public's health through professional exchange, collaboration, and action. WFPHA is accredited as an NGO in official relation with the WHO. It collaborates with the WHO to advance the field of public health through the promotion of pro-health policies, strategies, and best practices around the world. It is the only worldwide professional society representing and serving the broad area of public health as distinct from single disciplines or occupations. In relation to COVID-19, WFPHA hosted a historic meeting in February 2021 to initiate a coalition amongst leaders from international NGOs who share a common interest in equitable access for vaccines and treatment during COVID-19.

The organisations agreed to work together to build and sustain equity in global public health through increased advocacy for social protection and social development in vulnerable communities. Moreover, leaders expressed the need for an environmentally conscious and safe way to develop, distribute, and deliver vaccines, as this will also help reduce inequity following the pandemic by ensuring we do not exacerbate adverse climate effects. The coalition is committed to engaging with other organisations, governments, and key stakeholders to achieve a coordinated response to the pandemic. The organisations dedicate themselves to continue compiling resources, sharing evidence-based best practices, and using their collective voice to advocate for those who are disproportionately harmed by the pandemic, including chronically ill patients, individuals lacking access to healthcare services and medication, and marginalised communities (WFPHA, 2022). They have also developed the Global Charter for Public Health, which is discussed in Chapter 2.

Agents of Health Promotion

International, national, and local policy in the UK has focused on the development of a multidisciplinary public health workforce (see for example, Manyara et al. (2018) for an overview of organising the public health multidisciplinary teams across 12 countries). The extent and nature of the multidisciplinary public health workforce will vary within countries and be influenced by political changes. In England, the public health system is going through a transitional period following changes brought about by the Health and Social Care Act (2022) and the Health Education England Mandate: 2022 to 2023 (DHSC, 2022). These changes will take some time to become embedded.

In addition to the core public health workforce, many groups will contribute to health promotion and public health but will not necessarily have either public health or health promotion, or even health, in their professional titles. Fig. 3.2 identifies a broader range of agents and agencies with a remit for promoting statutory, non-statutory, national, and international public health. Most will have a variety of health-promoting functions or engage in a range of health-promoting activities.

The agents and agencies identified in Fig. 3.2 may work together in collaborative partnerships to make their work more effective. Partnership working has been a dominant theme in national and international health promotion

and public health policies, with government strategies and guidelines continuing to focus on the importance of partnerships for health between agencies and across government departments (see Chapter 9 for more on public health partnerships).

Directors of Public Health

The director of public health is the lead officer for public health functions within local authorities. They have specialist public health expertise and access to specialist resources spanning the three domains of public health: health improvement, health protection, and healthcare (such as the population health aspects of NHS-funded clinical services). The director has a critical role in public health needs assessment which drives commissioning and clinical commissioning. They will also lead on health protection and champion health across the whole of the authority's business (see DHSC (2020a, 2020b) for a full outline of the roles, responsibilities and context of the work of Directors of Public Health in England).

Health Promotion Specialists

Health promotion specialists (sometimes known by other professional titles such as public health practitioners; see the following section) are usually located within the public health teams. Health promotion specialists would normally hold graduate or postgraduate qualifications in health promotion or public health and would be responsible for the provision of expert advice, leadership, partnership development, training, programme development (including strategy and policy) and resources to support local health promotion initiatives. They liaise with other health promotion agents and agencies to ensure that public health activities, wherever initiated, are coordinated and supported. Health promotion specialists may be employed, for example, in the following roles:

- Health improvement practitioner.
- Health protection practitioner.
- Public health nutritionist.
- Smoking cessation adviser.
- Substance misuse worker.
- Teenage pregnancy coordinator.

For an overview of the work of health promotion specialists, see Target (2022).

Public Health Practitioners

The term 'public health practitioner' is used to describe members of the core public health workforce who work in various areas of public health, including health improvement, health protection, and healthcare public health. They may work in the public, private, and voluntary and community sectors. Although they work in a range of

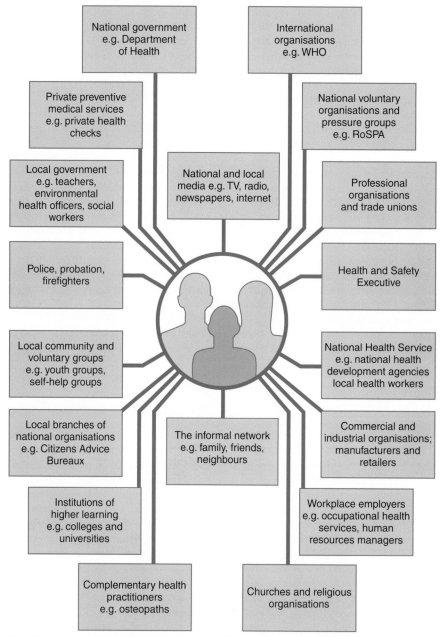

Fig. 3.2 Agents and agencies of health promotion and public health RoSPA: Royal Society for the Prevention of Accidents.

different areas of public health, public health practitioners all contribute to public health outcomes and improving the health and wellbeing of individuals, groups, communities, and populations. They work across the full breadth of public health, from health improvement and health protection to health information, community development and healthcare public health. They work in all settings: public service, voluntary and private sectors. Across the UK, thousands of practitioners work to protect and improve the health and reduce inequities. They are responsible for some of the most important health and social gains in the UK. Their roles are multidisciplinary, and they are responsible for individual and population-level interventions. Examples of the types of roles public health practitioners perform are similar to health promotion specialists and include:

Teenage pregnancy coordinator; Smoking cessation adviser; Substance misuse worker; Public health nutritionist; Health improvement practitioner; Advanced health improvement practitioner; Health improvement practitioner (specialist); Health improvement practitioner (advanced); and Health protection practitioner (FPH, 2022)

Public Health Specialists

Public health specialists work as system leaders at strategic or senior management levels in public health teams or at a senior level of expertise such as epidemiology. They come from a variety of professional backgrounds before entering a five-year training programme, which covers all aspects of public health, and are registered with the Faculty of Public Health and required to maintain registration through appraisal and revalidation. They have both leadership skills and technical skills and work across all of the three public health domains:

1. Health improvement: focusing on inequalities, wider determinants of health (education, housing, employment, and communities) and factors such as alcohol, tobacco, and obesity, as well as surveillance and monitoring of specific diseases, risk factors, needs assessments, equity audit, and impact assessments.
2. Health protection: focusing on infectious diseases (e.g. COVID-19, flu, meningitis), chemicals, radiation, environmental health hazards, emergency response (e.g. flooding, major accident), screening and immunisation, vaccinations, and sustainability.
3. Healthcare public health (also known as health and social care quality): focusing on ensuring services meet the population's needs (prioritisation), are planned appropriately, are of high quality, and are equitable and efficient (return on investment) (see Chapter 2 and FPH (2022) for more details on public health specialists and Table 3.2 for a list of core public health roles in England).

Health Trainers and Community Health Champions

The health trainer service in England was introduced in 2004 and is now an integral part of the wider public health workforce. Since their introduction, health trainers have supported people to make positive lifestyle changes in areas such as smoking, physical activity, alcohol, diet, and emotional issues (RSPH, 2022). To undertake their role, HTs assist clients in assessing their lifestyles and wellbeing, set goals for improving their health, agree on action-plans, and provide practical support and information that will help people change their behaviour. This could include promoting the benefits of taking regular exercise and eating healthily, reducing alcohol intake, breastfeeding, practising safe sex, and stopping smoking and substances. Their role generally includes:

- Helping people identify how their behaviours may be affecting their health.
- Supporting individuals to create a health plan to help make changes to improve their health.
- Helping individuals to become more knowledgeable about things that can affect their health and wellbeing.
- Signposting to other agencies and professionals.

Health trainers are trained and knowledgeable about the health issues that affect the community they are working in. Their clients may be identified from the existing community and support groups, through referral (such as from a health professional at a children's centre) or via self-referral. Clients often come from hard to reach disadvantaged groups such as the homeless, travellers, and those with drug, alcohol, and addiction problems. Whilst much of a health trainer's work will be on a one-to-one basis, they sometimes work with groups of people, for example, delivering group sessions on behaviour change and health improvement. Health trainers may also be assisted in their work by members of the community who have been trained to be health trainer champions (HTCs). HTCs are usually volunteers who have undertaken health improvement training at level 2 with the Royal Society of Public Health and who can help health trainer services extend their reach within communities.

Health trainers often work for private companies that provide a health trainer service for the NHS or for a local authority. They may also work directly for the NHS, a local authority or a charity, in the prison service or the armed services (Health Careers, 2022b). See also Health Trainers England (2022a) for detailed descriptions of health trainers work across the regions of England and Case study 3.1 for an example of the work that they undertake in offender settings. A useful adjunct to Case study 3.1 is an evaluation of health trainer activity within community rehabilitation, which suggests that the services are an important strategic and tactical asset in reducing health inequality and that this workforce has an almost unique ability to leave a legacy with their clients in terms of improved health awareness and understanding (Webster, 2021).

Developing a health trainer service in prisons in Yorkshire and Humber. So far, HTCs are only operational in Everthorpe and Moorlands Open prisons, but Doncaster has trained staff who have just completed training prisoners, and HTCs will soon be operational. Staff have also been trained as trainers of HTCs at Full Sutton, where a

CASE STUDY 3.1   Offender Health–Jamal's Story

Jamal is a health trainer champion currently resident at Moorlands Open Prison near Doncaster. Jamal moved to Moorlands a few weeks ago to complete the last phase of his sentence. Before that, he was at Everthorpe prison near Hull. His story is told by Geof Dart, who works at Everthorpe as a Physical Education (PE) instructor but who is currently on secondment to the Yorkshire and Humber Improvement Partnership, where he is working to develop health trainers and HTCs in all 13 penal institutions in the region.

Geof trained the first HTCs in offender settings in the region when he was at Everthorpe. Jamal was picked out as someone who was already a prisoner mentor and who would be conscientious and reliable. Jamal jumped at the chance of undertaking the training, which was a 10 h course accredited with the Royal Society of Public Health.

What prisoners can do to improve their diet whilst in prison is somewhat limited, but they do have opportunities to improve their fitness as all prisons have gyms, and many have developed other physical activity options. Jamal was one of four HTCs at Everthorpe. Their role is to chat with other inmates about the options available, 'signpost' them, encourage them, and accompany them if appropriate. The prison has started 'walk to fitness' classes and a gym session specifically for health trainer champion clients who do not have the confidence to go to the gym when other inmates are there.

Jamal talked to Geof about one particular client who he was proud to have helped. George (not his real name) was doing nothing to keep fit, but Jamal got him interested and told him about the walking to fitness class. George was not confident enough to go along on his own, so Jamal went with him three times. George then felt confident enough to continue and is now going twice a week. Jamal kept a check on him and is really proud that he was able to help George make this behaviour change, particularly as in the prison setting, it involves an extra commitment to arrange to have exercise time together, and it is unusual for inmates to do something for nothing.

When Jamal was transferred to Moorlands, he asked if he could continue to work as a health trainer champion. The challenges are different as it is an open prison, and most inmates work outside the prison, so they are around less and have less time available for other activities. But the gym manager is supportive, and together he and Jamal are setting up a service. The gym manager and three other staff have trained as HTCs, and given most inmates are only at the prison for a short term before release, they will provide most of the service rather than offenders. They have set up sports and fitness classes and a stop smoking service, and there is a healthcare worker on site.

Jamal wants to continue as a health trainer champion on his release and is interested in training as a health trainer. He is already in touch with the health trainer service in his hometown, Bradford, where a pilot is just getting underway, working with the Probation Service to employ ex-offenders as health trainers to work with offenders, ex-offenders, and their families. Jamal will have to keep out of trouble for several months before he could apply to be a health trainer but could continue to work voluntarily as a health trainer champion upon his release.

Source Health Trainers England (2022b).

course for prisoners is full and will be complete in March and Hull, where again, a course is about to start. Leeds prisons (Armley, Wetherby, and Wealston) are taking a slightly different approach and have set up a 'health reps project'. Lindholme, Moorlands (closed), New Hall, and Wolds have trained staff, but training prisoners and setting up a service has been delayed due to staff shortages. There are no plans to set up a service at Wakefield, which is a category A prison where most inmates are sex offenders, but there are health trainers who go into the prison from the Wakefield District PCT health trainer service. Hull PCT also have a health trainer who works within Hull Prison. These health trainers are all trained to level 3 City and Guilds.

Collecting the evidence. Where health trainer champion/ health trainer services are operating, data is collected on the clients and what outcomes they achieve. This will be entered into the national health trainer data collection recording system. It will then be possible to draw off reports and map progress in relation to behavioural change outcomes.

Why offenders are a priority group. Offenders have an excessive burden of chronic illness, especially mental health problems, infections with blood-borne viruses, sexually transmitted diseases, and dependence on drugs and alcohol, compared to their peers in the community:

* 90% of all prisoners have a recognisable mental health problem, substance misuse problem or both.

- 66% of all prisoners admit to using drugs (other than alcohol) in imprisonment.
- 24% of prisoners reported having injected drugs- of these 20% were infected with hepatitis B and 30% with hepatitis C.
- 8% of a representative sample of prisoners tested positive for hepatitis B.
- 7% for hepatitis C, 0.3% of male prisoners are HIV positive, and 1.2% of females are HIV positive.
- Over 80% of prisoners smoke.
- The rate of suicide and self-harm in prison is higher than in the community.
- 20% of women prisoners ask to see a doctor each day.
- 38% will be homeless on release.
- 47% were in debt at the time of sentencing.
- 50% have poor reading levels.
- 80% have poor writing skills.

Meeting policy priorities. Working with offenders meets policy priorities within the NHS to reduce health inequalities and target 'hard to reach' groups and within the National Offender Management Service, which prioritised offender health.*

General Practitioners (GPs)

With its roots in the community, general practice has a unique role in identifying the individual and local determinants of illness. However, Beaney and Allen (2019) argue that GPs often miss opportunities to address the underlying causes of ill health in patients but that general practice still has a crucial role to play in improving the health of local communities beyond the consultation room. GPs have a responsibility for prevention set by their professional bodies, with a directive to help people to improve and maintain their health. Community orientation and the management of the health and social care of the practice population and local community are a priority. GPs provide a comprehensive range of diagnosis and treatment medical services for patients registered with their practice and for those outside the practice in an emergency. They refer patients to other healthcare workers as necessary, for example, to counsellors, practice nurses, health visitors, physiotherapists or consultants specialising in a particular disease area. Every consultation is an opportunity to detect early warning signs that could prevent illness and disease. Thomas et al. (2020) set out a critical assessment of how GPs could move from just supporting sick individuals to creating healthy communities. At the time of writing, however, there is a crisis in the GP workforce (Jefferson and Holmes, 2022), with particular focus

being placed on poor recruitment and retention, which has been exacerbated by the COVID-19 pandemic. GPs full potential in promoting population health will not be realised until a solution is found to serious workforce capacity issues.

Nurses and Midwives

Every nurse, health visitor, and midwife, not just those working in specialist public health roles, can become a health-promoting practitioner. They can use their knowledge and skills to make a personal and professional impact and to improve the health and wellbeing of the public. Every contact counts, from a healthy start right through to the end of life. Specialist public health nurses have specific health-promoting roles, but all nurses are key to ensuring information, understanding, and potential tools are available for individuals to make choices about their lifestyles (West, 2019). Midwives have key areas of health promotion, including infant feeding, smoking, screening, perinatal mental health, obesity, contraception, sexual health, Sudden Infant Death Syndrome (SIDs), immunisations, infection prevention, and a healthy lifestyle (Cutter, 2021). Fig. 3.3 demonstrates the range of roles of nurses in promoting health and wellbeing.

Other Health Professions

There are many other health professionals with health-promoting health functions, such as dentists (see for example, Allen et al., 2022), for an interesting discussion about educating students of dentistry to take on an active role in promoting health and health equity). Hospital and retail pharmacists are at the frontline of the health system, and thus in contact with the population, they have an undeniable role in population health. Their efforts in health promotion activities can lead to increased health levels of the population (Shirdel et al., 2021). Moreover, the full range of professions allied to medicine (Hindle, 2019) have a significant part to play in health promotion and disease prevention.

HEALTH PROMOTION AGENTS AND AGENCIES OUTSIDE THE NHS

Local Authorities

Local leadership and responsibility for public health in England lies with local authorities. The report 'Public health in local government: Celebrating ten years of transformation' (Local Government Association [LGA], 2022) reflects on ten years of public health in local authorities

---

*Written by Judy White, Yorkshire and Humber Regional Health Trainer Lead, based on an interview with Geof Dart and with the permission of Jamal, a health trainer champion at Moorlands Open Prison.

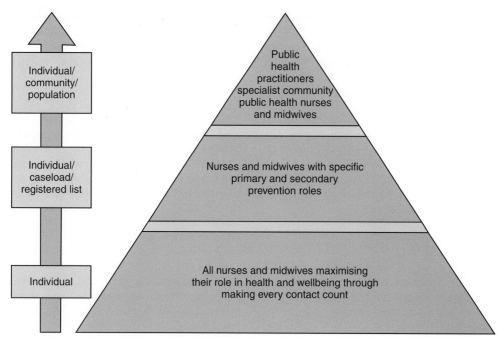

Fig. 3.3 Nurses' potential involvement in health promotion. (Source: Public Health England, 2013.)

covering the roles and responsibilities of the public health teams and looks forward to the opportunities and challenges of the coming years, including COVID-19 recovery. In addition to the public health teams, many local authority staff have health promotion functions such as recreation and leisure officers, housing officers, regeneration, youth and community workers, trading standards, and community safety officers.

Environmental Health Officers/Practitioners

Environmental health officers/practitioners are at the forefront of public health as every aspect of environmental health is designed to improve the public's health, wellbeing, and safety. Their work can make a real difference in people's health and wellbeing. For further details and case studies across the five disciplines of environmental health: environmental protection, food safety and integrity, health and safety, housing and community, and public health and protection, see CIEH (2022). The viewpoints in the case studies provide insights into the different ways in which Environmental Health Practitioners have responded to the pandemic by collaborating at local and national levels, working with organisations and companies in the public and private sectors on a mission to protect public health.

Personal, Social and Health, and Economic (PSHE) Teachers and Schools

Schools are an important setting to develop the knowledge, skills, and attributes young people need to keep themselves healthy and to thrive as individuals, family members, and members of society. Personal, social, health, and economic education is the curriculum area which develops these skills (Department of Education, 2021). The PSHE Association is a membership organisation and charity at the forefront of the development of PSHE (PSHE Association, 2021). The association provides a wide range of research, resources, training, advice, and guidance for teachers and schools. The health-promoting schools initiative (WHO, 2021) also strives to improve the health of school personnel, families, and community members, as well as pupils.

Social Services

The social services cover both social work and social care, providing an important range of health-promoting interventions to people who may fall outside the remit of health services. The client categories are the most vulnerable in society, including the mentally ill; the elderly; children who are abused, neglected or without support;

the physically sick and disabled; and people with learning disabilities. The services are provided within diverse settings, including people's homes, with social workers problem-solving (as an adviser, broker or advocate) and acting as key members of the workforce for health (Ross and de Saxe Zerden, 2020).

Complementary and Alternative Medicine Practitioners

Whilst there is no universally agreed definition of complementary and alternative medicine (CAM), NHS (2022b) suggests that when a non-mainstream practice is used together with conventional medicine, it is considered complementary, and when a non-mainstream practice is used instead of conventional medicine, it is considered complementary. Those practising CAM include homoeopaths, chiropractors, osteopaths, acupuncturists, reflexologists, and practitioners of herbal medicine, yoga, massage, and shiatsu, among others. These practitioners can play a part in promoting health, often using a more holistic approach. Therapies may be available from the NHS, either by a member of the primary care team or through referral to a complementary practitioner. There is potential for collaboration and closer integration between health promotion and complementary therapies, with Dalmolin and Heidemann (2020) highlighting how CAMS practitioners working in conjunction with primary care can improve the health of the public across a range of areas.

OTHER LOCAL ORGANISATIONS AND GROUPS

There are numerous individuals, groups, and organisations at the local level that promote aspects of health. Some notable ones are described below:

Universities and Colleges

Universities and colleges are not only responsible for the training of health promotion and public health professionals, but they are also key organisations for undertaking public health research. Moreover, The Healthy Universities Network, under its international charter, establishes that health-promoting universities and colleges are well placed to transform the health, wellbeing, and sustainability of our current and future societies (Doris et al., 2021).

Community, Voluntary, and Social Enterprise (CVSE) Sector

A huge range of CVSE groups exist and undertake health promotion activities on public health matters. In the UK, the government has clear aspirations for the voluntary and community sector as partners in public health, particularly in tackling health inequalities. The sector already operates extensively within health and social care, with the statutory sector spending significant sums of money per year on services provided by voluntary and community organisations (see Laverty et al., 2017 and the LGA website for case studies).

Employers

Employers can be active in developing and implementing health-promoting policies in the workplace. Human resource officers and occupational health staff are vital to implementing public health interventions in the workplace setting (Aldana, 2022).

Police, Probation, and Prison Officers

The police protect the public from crime and violence, take action to prevent the misuse of drugs and alcohol and help to ensure road safety. Prison officers and probation officers are involved in the health and wellbeing of prisoners and their families and may be involved in initiatives such as health-promoting prisons (Woodall et al., 2021).

Fire and Rescue Authorities (FRA)

The varied role of the FRAs in improving public health is clearly outlined in one FRAs service prevention programme (see Cheshire Fire and Rescue 2022 for more details). It is clear that FRAs have a key role to play in ensuring that their communities are safe through responding to emergencies and also through their extensive preventative work as diverse as falls prevention, in the home through their safe and well visits, to domestic violence and road safety.

It is clear from the wide range of health promotion and public health agencies and agents outlined in this chapter that some strategies, such as partnership working, are essential to improve capacity. The continued building of multi-professional understanding, partnerships and capabilities, and pulling together of the different professional groups under the banner of health promotion is vital to future success. To do this effectively, it is important to know who the health promotion and public health professionals are working within your area. Exercise 3.2 requires you to make a public health professional map of your locality.

PRACTICE POINTS

- It is important to understand the work of a whole range of agents and agencies with a health promotion and public health function, informal and formal, local, national and international.

- Think about and develop strategies for how you can best work collaboratively with other professionals and agencies.
- Ensure you are clear about your role and responsibilities in health promotion within the wider public health workforce.
- Consider how you could improve your health promotion and public health practice roles through education and training or through identifying what helps and hinders your health promotion and public health work and how your work could be improved.

References

Aldana, S. (2022). *7 reasons workplace health promotion programs work (Here is the proof)*. https://www.wellsteps.com/blog/2020/01/02/workplace-health-promotion-programs/

Allen, T. A., O'Loughlin, M., & Croker, F. (2022). Teaching health promotion competencies in undergraduate dentistry training: a unique pedagogical approach. *Health Promotion Journal of Australia*, *33*(1), 35–38. https://doi.org/10.1002/hpja.660.

Anderson, M., Pitchforth, E., Edwards, N., Alderwick, H., McGuire, A., & Mossialos, E. (2022). Health systems in transition vol. 24 no. 1: *United Kingdom Health System Review*. London: European Observatory on Health Systems and Policy.

Beaney, T., Allen, L. (2019). *What's the role of general practice in addressing population health*. https://www.kingsfund.org.uk/blog/2019/01/general-practice-population-health

Centre for Workforce Intelligence (2014). https://assets.publishing.service.gov.uk/government/uploads/system/uploads/attachment_data/file/507518/CfWI_Mapping_the_core_public_health_workforce.pdf

Charles, A., Ewbank, L., McKenna, H., & Wenzel, L. (2019). *The NHS long-term plan explained*. London: Kings Fund.

Chartered Institute of Environmental Health. (2022). *Visions of the future: the changing face of environmental health*. https://www.cieh.org/what-is-environmental-health/the-future-of-eh/

Cheshire Fire and Rescue Service. (2022). *Prevention*. https://www.cheshirefire.gov.uk/about-us/organisational-structure/prevention

Corry, D. (2018). *How charities help to keep the country well*. Blog/Public Health, The Health Foundation. https://health.org.uk/blogs/how-charities-help-to-keep-the-country-well.

Cutter, J. (2021). *Midwives play an essential role in promoting public health*. https://www.nursinginpractice.com/professional/the-key-role-midwives-play-in-promoting-public-health/

Dalmolin, I. S., & Heidemann, I. T. S. B. (2020). Integrative and complementary practices in primary care: unveiling health promotion. *Rev Lat Am Enfermagem*, *28*, e3277. https://doi.org/10.1590/1518-8345.3162.3277.

Dayan, M., Fahy, N., Hervey, T., McCarey, M., Jarman, H., & Greer, S. (2022). *Understanding the impact of Brexit on health in the UK*. London: Nuffield Trust.

Department for Education. (2021). *Guidance for personal, social, health and economic (PSHE) education*. https://www.gov.uk/government/publications/personal-social-health-and-economic-education-pshe/personal-social-health-and-economic-pshe-education

Department of Health, (2018). *New strategic direction for alcohol and drugs: phase 2*. London: The Stationery Office.

Department of Health and Social Care, (2020a). *Tackling obesity: empowering adults and children to live healthier lives*. London: Stationary Office.

Department of Health and Social Care, (2020b). *Directors of Public Health in local government: roles, responsibility and context*. London: The Stationary Office.

Department of Health and Social Care. (2021). *Press release: new office of health promotion to drive improvement of nations health*. https://www.gov.uk/government/news/new-office-for-health-promotion-to-drive-improvement-of-nations-health

Department of Health and Social Care, (2022). *Health education England mandate: 2022 to 2023*. London: The Stationery Office.

Doris, M., Powell, S., Parkin, D., & Ferrier, A. (2021). A health promoting universities: effective leadership for health, wellbeing and sustainability. *Health Education*, *121*(3), 295–310. https://doi.org/10.1108/HE-12-2020-0121.

EC Public Health EU4 Health Programme. (2021–2027) *A vision for a healthier European Union*. https://health.ec.europa.eu/funding/eu4health-programme-2021-2027-vision-healthier-european-union_en

European Parliament. (2021a). *Fact sheets on European Union public health*. https://www.europarl.europa.eu/factsheets/en/sheet/49/public-health

European Parliament. (2021b). Regulation (EU) 2021/522 establishing a programme for the union's action in the field of health ('EU4Health Programme') for the period 2021-2027. https://www.europeansources.info/record/proposal-for-a-regulation-on-the-establishment-of-a-programme-for-the-unions-action-in-the-field-of-health-for-the-period-2021-2027/

European Public Health Association. (2022). *About us*. http://epha.org/about-us/

Faculty of Public Health. (2022). *Public health practitioners*. https://www.fph.org.uk/media/3029/fph_ph_practitioner_09_20-v2.pdf

Faculty of Public Health. (2022). *The unique contribution of public health specialists*. https://www.fph.org.uk/media/3110/4-the-unique-contribution-of-public-health-specialists-sept16.pdf%20contribution%20of%20Public%20Health%20Specialists%20FINALSept16%20RA.pdf

Frith, N. (2022). *How unions can support your workplace mental health journey*. Mental Health at Work Blog. https://www.mentalhealthatwork.org.uk/blog/how-unions-can-support-your-workplace-mental-health-journey/

Haughton, J., Takemoto, M. L., & Arrrdondo, M. (2020). Identifying barriers, facilitators and implementation strategies for a faith based physical activity program. *Implementation Science Communication*, *1*, 51. https://doi.org/10.1186/s43058-020-00043-3.

Health Careers. (2022a). UK health systems: the four countries that make up the UK - England, Wales, Scotland and Northern Ireland - have slightly different health systems. https://www.healthcareers.nhs.uk/working-health/uk-health-systems/uk-health-systems

Health Careers. (2022b). *Health trainers*. https://www.healthcareers.nhs.uk/explore-roles/public-health/roles-public-health/health-trainer

Health and Social Care Act. (2022). https://www.legislation.gov.uk/ukpga/2022/31/contents/enacted

HM Government, (2022). *COVID-19 response: living with COVID-19*. London: Stationary Office.

Health Trainers England. (2022a). *Case studies*. https://sites.google.com/site/healthtrainersengland/case-studies

Health Trainers England. (2022b). *Case study: offender health - Jamal's story*. https://sites.google.com/site/healthtrainersengland/jamals-case-study

Hindle, L. (2019). *Allied health professionals have a major role to play in prevention*. https://ukhsa.blog.gov.uk/2019/05/09/allied-health-professionals-have-a-major-role-to-play-in-prevention/

International Union of Health Promotion and Education (IUHPE). (2023). *Mission statement*. https://www.iuhpe.org/index.php/en/iuhpe-at-a-glance/mission

Jefferson, L., & Holmes, M. (2022). GP workforce crisis: what can we do now? *British Journal of General Practice*, *72*(718), 206–207. https://doi.org/10.3399/bjgp22X719225.

Katibireddi, V., Hinds, K., Hilton, S., Lewis, S., Thomas, J., Campbell, M., Young, B., Bauld, L. (2019). Mass media to communicate public health messages in six health topic areas: a systematic review and other reviews of the evidence. *Public Health Research*, *7*(8). https://doi.org/10.3310/phr07080.

Kings Fund. (2022). What are the key organisations that make up the NHS? And how can they collaborate with partners in the health and care system to deliver joined-up care? https://www.kingsfund.org.uk/audio-video/how-does-nhs-in-england-work

Knai, C., Petticrew, M., Douglas, N., Durand, M. A., Eastmore, E., Nolte, E., & Mays, N. (2018). The public health responsibility deal: using a systems-level analysis to understand the lack of impact on alcohol, food, physical activity, and workplace health sub-systems. *International Journal of Environmental Research and Public Health*, *15*(12), 2895. https://doi.org/10.3390/ijerph15122895.

Lancet Editorial, (2020). Filling a gap in the UK health services: the role of charities. *Lancet*, *7*(10 October). https://doi.org/10.1016/S2352-3026(20)30295-7.

Laverty, A. A., Kypridemos, C., Seferidi, P., Vamos, E. P., Pearson-Stuttard, J., Collins, B., Capewell, S., & Local Government Association, (2017). *Public health working with the voluntary, community and social enterprise sector: 55 new opportunities and sustainable change*. London: Local Government Association.

Local Government Association, (2022). *Public health in local government: Celebrating 10 years of transformation*. London: Local Government Association.

Mwatsama, M., Cairney, P., Fleming, K., O'Flaherty, M., & Millett, C. (2019). Quantifying the impact of the public health responsibility deal on salt intake, cardiovascular disease and gastric cancer burdens: Interrupted time series and microsimulation study. *Journal of Epidemiology and Community Health*, *73*(9), 881–887. https://doi.org/10.1136/jech-2018-211749.

Manyara, A. M., Buunaaisie, C., Annett, H., Bird, E., Bray, I., Ige, J., Jones, M., Orme, J., Pilkington, P., & Evans, D. (2018). Exploring the multidisciplinary extent of public health career structures in 12 countries: an exploratory mapping. *Journal of Public Health*, *40*(4), e538–e544. https://doi.org/10.1093/pubmed/fdy057.

NHS. (2019). *Long term plan*. https://www.longtermplan.nhs.uk/areas-of-work/

NHS. (2021). *Physical activity guidelines for adults aged 19 to 64*. https://www.nhs.uk/live-well/exercise/exercise-guidelines/physical-activity-guidelines-for-adults-aged-19-to-64/

NHS. (2022a). *2022/23 Priorities and operational planning guidelines*. https://www.england.nhs.uk/wp-content/uploads/2022/02/20211223-B1160-2022-23-priorities-and-operational-planning-guidance-v3.2.pdf

NHS. (2022b). *Complementary and alternative medicine*. https://www.nhs.uk/conditions/complementary-and-alternative-medicine/

NICE, (2021). *NICE strategy 2021-2026: dynamic, collaborative, excellent*. London: NICE.

Nicholson, E., Shuttleworth, K. (2020). *Devolution and the NHS*. Institute for Government. https://www.instituteforgovernment.org.uk/explainers/devolution-nhs

Royal Society of Public Health. (2022). *Health trainers*. https://www.rsph.org.uk/our-work/policy/wider-public-health-workforce/health-trainers.html

Office of Health Improvements and Disparities. (2022). *About us*. https://www.gov.uk/government/organisations/office-for-health-improvement-and-disparities/about

Powel, T., Harker, R., Parkin, E. (2020). *The structure of the NHS in England*. https://commonslibrary.parliament.uk/research-briefings/cbp-7206/

PSHE Association. (2021). *We are the national body for PSHE education*. https://pshe-association.org.uk

Public Health England. (2013). Nursing and midwifery actions at the three levels of public health practice. Improving health and wellbeing at individual, community and population levels. London. Department of Health.

Roberts, N.F. (2019). Science says: Religion is good for your health. Forbes. Mar 29, Newsletter. https://www.forbes.com/sites/nicolefisher/2019/03/29/science-says-religion-is-good-for-your-health/?sh=108fd79d3a12

Ross, A. M., & de Saxe Zerden, L. (2020). Prevention, health promotion, and social work: aligning health and human service systems through a workforce for health. *American Journal of Public Health*, *110*(S2), S186–S190. https://doi.org/10.2105/AJPH.2020.305690.

Royal Society for Public Health. (2017). *Dream it, try it, live it*. https://www.youtube.com/watch?v=uH1 PytuN2CU

Schillenger, D., Chittamuru, D., & Ramirez, A. S. (2020). From "infodemics" to health promotion: a novel framework for the role of social media in public health. *American Journal of Public Health*, *110*(9). https://doi.org/10.2105/AJPH.2020.305746.

Shirdel, A., Poutteza, A., Daemi, A., & Ahmadi, B. (2021). Health-promoting services provided in pharmacies: a systematic review. *Journal of Education Health Promotion*, *10*, 234. https://doi.org/10.4103/jehp.jehp_1374_20.

Target. (2022). *Health promotion specialist: job description*. https://targetjobs.co.uk/careers-advice/job-descriptions/health-promotion-specialist-job-description

The Institute of Health Promotion and Education (IHPE). (2022). *Home page*. http://ihpe.org.uk/

Thomas, K., Barry, E., Watkins, S., Czauderna, J., & Allen, L. N. (2020). GP with an extended role in population health. *British Journal of General Practice*, *70*(697), 378–379. https://doi.org/10.3399/bjgp20X711821.

Webster, R. (2021). *Health trainers evaluation: community rehabilitation. Company evaluation series*. https://ingeus.co.uk/INGEUS/media/Documents/Justice/ingeus-justice-evaluation-series_health-trainers-evaluation.pdf

West, S. (2019). *Blog: A nurse's role in promoting health and preventing ill health (from the bedside to the bingo hall)*. https://www.nmc.org.uk/news/news-and-updates/blog-a-nurses-role-in-promoting-health-and-preventing-ill-health/

Woodall, J., Freeman, C., & Warwick-Booth, L. (2021). Health-promoting prisons in the female estate: an analysis of prison inspection data. *BMC Public Health*, *21*(1582), 2021. https://doi.org/10.1186/s12889-021-11621-y.

World Federation of Public Health Associations. (2022). *Coalition of international NGOs for equity*. https://www.wfpha.org/coalition-of-international-ngos-for-equity/

World Health Organisation, (2021). *Making every school a health promoting school- global standards and indicators*. Geneva: WHO.

Zuidberg, M. R. J., Shriwise, A., de Boer, L. M., & Johanson, A. S. (2020). Assessing progress under health 2020 in the European region of the World Health Organisation. *European Journal of Public Health*, *30*(6), 1072–1077. https://doi.org/10.1093/eurpub/ckaa091.

Websites

British Medical Association. http://www.bma.org.uk

CIEH. http://www.cieh.org

International Union of Health. *Promotion and health education for full details of the organisation's work*. http://www.iuhpe.org

Kings Fund. *What are the key organisations that make up the NHS? And how can they collaborate with partners in the health and care system to deliver joined-up care?* https://www.kingsfund.org.uk/audio-video/how-does-nhs-in-england-work

LGA website. https://www.local.gov.uk/

NHS. *111*. https://111.nhs.uk

NHS England. https://www.england.nhs.uk/

NHS Scotland. http://www.scot.nhs.uk/

NHS Wales. http://www.wales.nhs.uk/

NHS. https://www.nhs.uk.

NICE. *Evidence based public health and healthcare data and guidance*. https://www.nice.org.uk

Northern Ireland Health and Social Care. http://online.hscni.net/

Northern Ireland HSC Public Health Agency. https://www.publichealth.hscni.net/

Public Health Wales. http://www.publichealthwales.wales.nhs.uk/

Royal College of Nursing (RCN). http://www.rcn.org.uk

TACADE. http://www.tacade.com

The Health Foundation. *Wide range of up-to-date public health issues covered*. http://health.org.uk

UK Public Health Association. http://www.ukpha.org.uk/

Working Well Solutions. *Workplace health promotion*. https://workingwellsolutions.com/workplace-health-promotion/

Blogs

Health Foundation. Blog on health care improvement, quality, sustainability and population health. https://www.health.org.uk/news-and-comment/blogs

King's Fund Comment and analysis on the key issues in health and social care. https://www.kingsfund.org.uk/blog

NHS England Blog: World Health Day: can our stories change the world? https://www.england.nhs.uk/greenernhs/2022/04/blog-world-health-day-can-our-stories-change-the-world/

Values and Ethical Considerations in Health Promotion and Public Health

Angela Scriven

CHAPTER OUTLINE

SUMMARY

In this chapter, some key philosophical issues about aims and values in health promotion and public health practice will be identified and explored. Two fundamental dilemmas about the aims of health promotion will be addressed. First, whether health promoters and public health practitioners should aim to change the individual's lifestyle choices or to change society, and second, whether they should set out to ensure compliance with health promotion and public health programmes or enable clients to make an informed choice. A framework of five approaches to health promotion is provided as a tool for analysing key aims and values along with exercises and case studies. Ethical issues are discussed, four ethical principles are described, and there is a series of questions designed to help health promoters and public health practitioners make ethical choices. Exercises on making ethical decisions are included.

This chapter establishes some of the philosophical issues linked to the promotion of individual and population health. You are encouraged to think deeply about why you are engaging in specific activities, what values are reflected in your work and what ethical dilemmas are presented. Guidelines on how to approach ethical decision-making are considered, and some key principles of practice are explored.

If successful, health promotion and public health interventions will positively influence the lives of individuals and communities, and it would be irresponsible to develop and engage in health promotion and public health without understanding the values and ethics that should underpin interventions.

EXPLORING THE AIMS OF HEALTH PROMOTION AND PUBLIC HEALTH PRACTICE

Should health promoters and public health practitioners aim to change individual behaviour and lifestyles or instead aim to influence the socioeconomic determinants that directly influence people's lifestyles, behaviour and health, or both? Public health action often focuses on changing the attitudes and behaviour of individuals and communities towards healthier lifestyles, whilst neglecting the influence of the socioeconomic, political, and physical environments on people's lives, what Marmot (2020a) calls the causes of the causes. This focus on lifestyle influences on health and the need to change behaviour can result in victim blaming, which is a significant ethical dilemma that health promoters and public health practitioners need to address (see for example, Lewin, 2019).

It is important to note that individuals often can change their behaviour and may want to take responsibility to improve their health. Health promotion is an essential tool in enabling that process by promoting people's self-esteem and confidence, empowering them to take more control over their own health. Proponents of the lifestyle behavioural change approach also maintain that medical and health experts have knowledge that enables them to know what is in the best interests of their patients and the public at large and that it is their responsibility to persuade people to make healthier choices. Furthermore, society has vested that responsibility in health professionals, and the public often seeks advice and help in health matters; it is not necessarily a matter of persuading them against their will. Sometimes, too, individuals may not be able to take responsibility because they may, for example, be too young, too ill, or have severe learning difficulties. See Laverack (2017) for a fuller debate on the challenges of a behavioural change approach.

There are several points to be considered if the aim to change lifestyle is pursued:

- You cannot assume that lay people believe that health professionals know best. Sometimes health experts are proven wrong, and new evidence can contradict existing health messages. For example, over the years, there has been much contradictory advice on what constitutes good nutrition, with some people finding the barrage of information confusing, resulting in a backlash that results in people ignoring advice (see Barnwell et al., 2021 and Delesha et al., 2020 for further discussion on the problems of conflicting health information).
- There is a danger of imposing alien or opposing values. For example, a doctor may perceive that the most important thing for a patient's physical health is to lose weight and cut down on alcohol consumption, but drinking beer in the pub with friends may be far more important in terms of overall wellbeing to the overweight, middle-aged, unemployed patient. Who is right?
- Linked to this, a health promoter advocating lifestyle changes can be seen as making a moral judgement on clients' failure to change, that it is their own fault if, for example, they develop an obesity-related or smoking-related illness.
- Promoting a lifestyle change approach may produce negative and counterproductive feelings in the targeted individual or community, such as guilt for failing to comply or of rebelliousness and anger at being told what to do, resulting in resistance to comply (for examples of resistance to comply, see Mantyselka et al., 2019).
- It cannot be assumed that individual behaviour is the primary cause of ill health. This is a limited view, and there is a danger that focusing on the individual's behaviour distracts attention from the significant and politically sensitive determinants of health, such as the social and economic factors of racism, relative deprivation, poverty, housing, and unemployment as outlined in Chapter 1 in the section 'What affects health?'
- Finally, it also cannot be assumed that individuals have genuine freedom to choose healthy lifestyles. Freedom of choice is often limited by socioeconomic influences. Economic factors may affect the choice of food; for example, fresh fruit, and wholemeal bread are relatively more expensive than biscuits and white bread. Research indicates that the rates of food insecurity in the United Kingdom (UK) have doubled since the COVID-19 pandemic (see Marmot (2020a; 2020b), University of York (2021), and the Food Ethics Council website referenced at the end of the chapter for more details on food poverty).

Social factors are also important. Freedom of choice about smoking for adolescents where both parents smoke, for example, is a complex issue (Department of Health and Social Care, 2021). Also, how much freedom do people really have to change other health-demoting factors such as stressful living or working conditions and unemployment? It is easy to blame an individual for their own ill health or poor lifestyle choices – becoming victim blaming – when they might be the victims of their socio-economic circumstances. In some disadvantaged situations and where resources of time, energy, and income are limited, health choices may become health compromises. What a health promoter or public health practitioner may see as irresponsibility may be what the client sees as the most responsible action in the circumstances. For example, mothers confronted with the day-to-day pressures of parenting may smoke as a way of relieving their stress. Cancer Research UK (2022), in discussing the various factors influencing smoking in various population groups and the reasons for why people smoke if they know it is bad for them or their children, links smoking to the perception of it as a calming activity or something to do in a stressful situation.

Part 3 of this book is about how to promote health in a way that is sensitive to these issues. Chapter 16 looks at what you can do to challenge and change health-related policies.

It is crucially important that everyone engaged in health promotion and public health practice should be aware of these ethical concerns and have an opportunity to consider them in relation to their own work, particularly if they are engaged in interventions that aim to change individual lifestyles. Exercise 4.1 is designed to help you to think through your views on the aims of health promotion and public health practice.

Aiming for Compliance or Informed Choice?

Another key question about the aims of health promotion centres on what you aim to do with or for the client (whether the client is a single individual, a community, or an organisation). Is your aim to ensure that your client complies with your programme and changes behaviour, as is the case with a social marketing approach? Or is it to enable your client to make an informed choice and have the skills and confidence to carry that choice through into action, whatever that choice may be?

EXERCISE 4.1   Analysing Your Philosophical Position on Health Promotion and Public Health Practice

Consider the following statements A and B:

A: The key aim of health promotion and public health practice is behaviour change: To inform people about the ways in which their behaviour and lifestyle can affect their health, to ensure that they understand the information, to help them explore their values and attitudes and (where appropriate) to help them to change their behaviour.

B: The key aim of health promotion and public health practice is to influence the wider determinants of health: To raise awareness of the many socioeconomic policies at a national and local level (such as welfare, employment, housing, food, and transport) that are not conducive to good health and to work actively towards a change in those policies.

1. Taking statement A:
   • List arguments in support of this view.
   • List any points about the limitations of this view and any arguments against it.
2. Do the same with statement B.
3. Do you think that the views in A and B are complementary or incompatible? Why?
4. Imagine these two views at either end of a spectrum:

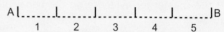

Indicate the two positions on a scale of one to five that most closely reflect (a) what you actually do in practice and (b) what you would like to do if you were free to prioritise work exactly as you would choose.

For example, a health promoter is working with a client whose sexual behaviour is such that there is a serious risk of catching sexually transmitted infections, including HIV. If the aim is compliance, it is more likely that the health promoter will be persuasive, will stress the risks to the client, and will consider the session a failure if the client does not choose to behave differently. If, on the other hand, the health promoter's aim is to enable the client to make an informed choice, the health promoter will ensure that the client understands the facts and the risks, will encourage and support the client and accept that if the client chooses not to change their behaviour, then this choice will be respected. It would not be interpreted as a failure because the client made an informed choice.

The same issues arise with health promotion and public health interventions on a larger scale. For example, is the aim of a campaign to change diets and to promote the consumption of five pieces of fruit or vegetables a day (NHS, 2022) to persuade people to a particular point of view or to give them the information on which to make up their own minds? This is a difficult question. Most health promoters are doing their jobs because they believe that the action they are advocating is in the best interests of individuals and of society as a whole, and their actions are backed by evidence. It raises the question about how far to go in imposing your own values and ideas of what appropriate lifestyle choices are onto other people. In the case of the five a day campaign, there is also the ethical issue of food poverty (see the Food Ethics Council website in the references at the end of the chapter). The persuasive messages concerning the compliance to COVID-19 vaccination uptake were also an example of compliance (James et al., 2021)

ANALYSING AIMS AND VALUES: FIVE APPROACHES

There is no consensus on the appropriate aims for health promotion and public health practice or the right approach. Health promoters need to work out for themselves which aim and which activities they use in accordance with professional codes of conduct (if they exist), professional values and an assessment of the clients' needs.

Different approaches to promoting health are useful tools of analysis, which can help you to clarify your own aims and values. A framework of five approaches is suggested, with the values implicit in any approach identified.

1. The Medical Approach

The aim is freedom from medically defined diseases, illnesses, and disabilities such as infectious diseases, cancers, and heart disease. The approach involves medical intervention to prevent or ameliorate ill health, possibly using a persuasive or paternalistic method: persuading, for example, whole population groups to have the COVID-19 vaccine (James et al., 2021). This approach values preventive medical measures and the medical profession's responsibility to ensure that patients comply with recommended procedures.

2. The Behaviour Change Approach

The aim is to change people's individual attitudes and behaviours so that they adopt what is deemed a healthy lifestyle. Examples include supporting people in stopping smoking through smoking cessation programmes (Black et al., 2020), encouraging people to be more physically active through walking, wheeling, and cycling in the new social prescription schemes (Gov.UK, 2022) and changing people's lifestyle and exercise levels through the Change4Life initiative (see for example, Day et al., 2022). See also the NICE lifestyle and wellbeing website pages referenced at the end of the chapter for evidence on the behavioural change approach.

Health promoters and public health practitioners using this approach will be convinced that a lifestyle change is in the best interests of their clients and will see it as their responsibility to encourage as many people as possible to adopt the healthy lifestyle they advocate. Health-related social marketing fits into this approach when the aim is to change behaviour.

3. The Educational Approach

The aim is to give information, ensure knowledge and understanding of health issues, and enable the skills required to make well-informed decisions. Information about health is presented, and people are helped to explore their values and attitudes, develop appropriate skills, and make their own decisions. Help in carrying out those decisions and adopting new health practices may also be offered. School-sponsored personal, social, economic, and health education (PSHE) programmes in the UK, emphasize helping pupils to learn the skills of healthy living, not merely to acquire knowledge (Department for Education, 2021).

Those favouring this approach will value the educational process, will respect individuals' right to choose, and will see it as their responsibility to raise with clients the health issues which they think will be in the client's best interests.

4. The Client-Centred Approach

The aim is to work in partnership with clients to help them identify what they want to know about and take action on and make their own decisions and choices according to their own interests and values. The health promoter's role is to act as a facilitator, helping people to identify their concerns and gain the knowledge and skills they require to make changes happen. Self-empowerment (or community empowerment) of the client is seen as central. Clients are valued as equals who have knowledge, skills, and abilities to contribute and who have an absolute right to control their own health destinies. See Lindacher et al. (2017)

for an evaluation of empowerment in health promotion interventions.

5. The Societal Change Approach

The aim is to effect changes on the physical, social, and economic environment to make it more conducive to good health. The focus is on changing society, not on changing the behaviour of individuals.

Those using this approach will value their democratic right to activism to change society and will be committed to putting health on the political agenda at all levels and to the importance of shaping the socioeconomic and health environment rather than shaping the individual behaviours of people. See Campbell and Cornish (2021) for interesting international case studies on public health activism).

Table 4.1 summarises and illustrates these five approaches to health promotion and public health practice. An important point to note is that some of these approaches can be used together. For example, a client-centred approach may also use educational processes and a comprehensive health promotion strategy to deal with a public health problem. (See Box 4.1 for examples of using approaches in practice). Exercise 4.2 is designed to enable you to think through the aims and values of your health promotion practice.

ETHICAL DILEMMAS

The following are some of the more common ethical dilemmas that health promoters and others working in public health may encounter.

Bottom Up or Top Down?

There is a key issue of control and power at the heart of health promotion and public health practice: Who decides what health issue to target and how? Who sets the agenda? Is it bottom up, set by people who themselves identify issues they perceive as relevant? Or is it top down, set by health promoters who often have the power (supported by government policy) and the resources to impose strategies? There is a spectrum of possible modes of interventions, from those that eliminate choice and remove freedom, such as those used during the COVID-19 pandemic, to those that just involve information giving (see Fig. 4.1). The interplay and interaction between individuals, communities, and the wider population is important and central to deciding on whether a top down or bottom up approach is used. One of the difficulties in applying ethical principles when promoting health is the tension between the individual and the population. Decisions must be taken about when an individual's rights

TABLE 4.1 Five Approaches to Health Promotion – Summary and Examples Using Smoking Cessation

	Aim	Health Promotion Activity	Important Values	Example – Smoking
Medical	Freedom from medically defined disease and disability	Promotion of medical interventions to prevent or ameliorate ill health	Patient compliance with preventive medical procedures	Aim – freedom from lung disease, heart disease and other smoking-related disorders. Activity – encourage people to seek early detection and treatment of smoking-related disorders
Behaviour change	Individual behaviour conducive to freedom from disease	Attitude and behaviour change to encourage the adoption of a 'healthier' lifestyle	Healthy lifestyle as defined by a health promoter	Aim – behaviour changes from smoking to not smoking. Activity – persuasive education to prevent non-smokers from starting and to persuade smokers to stop
Educational	Individuals with knowledge and understanding enabling well-informed decisions to be made and acted upon	Information about cause and effects of health-demoting factors. Exploration of values and attitudes. Development of skills required for healthy living	Individual right of free choice. Health promoter's responsibility to identify educational content	Aim – clients will have an understanding of the effects of smoking on health. They will make a decision whether or not to smoke and act on the decision. Activity – giving information to clients about the effects of smoking. Helping them to explore their own values and attitudes and come to a decision. Helping them to learn how to stop smoking if they want to
Client-centred	Working with clients on their own terms	Working with health issues, choices and actions that clients identify. Empowering the client	Clients as equals. Client's rights to set agenda. Self-empowerment of clients	Anti-smoking issue is considered only if clients identify it as a concern. Clients identify what, if anything, they want to know and do about it
Societal change	Physical and social environment that enables choice of a healthier lifestyle	Political/social action to change the physical/social/economic environment	Right and need to make environment health enhancing	Aim – make smoking socially unacceptable, so it is easier not to smoke than to smoke. Activity – no smoking policy in all public places. Cigarette sales less accessible, especially to children, promotion of non-smoking as the social norm. Banning tobacco advertising and sports' sponsorship

BOX 4.1   Approaches A and B

Approach A

Jill is a hospital nurse running a programme of rehabilitation for patients who have had heart attacks. She decides that she is working with an educational approach, aiming for her patients to make informed decisions and have knowledge about taking exercise and modifying their diet and other risk factors, such as smoking. She accepts that some patients will choose not to do so. She thinks that sometimes she may be working in a behaviour change model because she sincerely believes that her patients would be better off if they changed their behaviour, and she finds that she sometimes really wants to persuade them. Ultimately, she decides that it is their choice and their life and that she will not pressure them into doing what they do not want to do. Jill is aware, though, that some of her colleagues (who favour the behaviour change approach) think she should be tougher and shock patients into complying with horror stories of what may happen to them if they do not adjust their lifestyles.

Approach B

Terry is a community health worker based in a deprived housing estate. Facilities for recreation, exercise, and buying good food, among other things, are poor. He decides that he is working with a mixture of client-centred and societal change approaches because people in the community have identified that they want a better diet, and he is helping them to set up a food cooperative and to help each other to learn new cooking skills. He is also helping them to lobby their local councillor for better green spaces on the estate where the children can play.

EXERCISE 4.2   Identifying Your Health Promotion and Public Health Practice Aims and Values

This exercise requires you to analyse the aims, values, and ethical issues inherent in two or three specific health promotion interventions you are engaged in (or have been engaged in), such as a group health education programme, a social media campaign, an immunisation programme such as COVID-19, a one-to-one meeting with a client, a community activity. With reference to Table 4.1, identify which approach you are using for each activity (you may find that you will identify more than one approach).

For each activity, define the aim and the important values implicit in your work. You may find it helpful to look at Case studies 4.1 and 4.2.

Discuss your findings with a partner or in a small group.

CASE STUDY 4.1   Ethical Issues Relating to Drug Education In Schools

A group of local people, led by a woman whose son died of a heroin overdose, have got together because they are concerned about drug misuse in the neighbourhood. They are afraid for the safety of their teenagers and younger children: drugs seem to be an established part of the teenage social scene, are easily available in the neighbourhood, and needles and syringes are found in local alleyways.

The group has decided that the best way to combat drugs is to go into local schools and scare the children off drugs with horror stories of bad 'trips' and addiction. They have recruited a former drug addict who is prepared to tell his story. They have asked the school nurse to help by providing supplies of leaflets and supporting them in their approach to the schools.

The school nurse believes that the shock-horror approach the group proposes has been shown by drug education research to be ineffective. At best, it will do no good, and at worst, it could glamorise the drug scene, and a make a hero out of the ex-addict. She believes that the local schools' approach is best: education on the facts of drug taking and how to minimise harm from taking drugs, coupled with building up self-esteem, social skills, and confidence for young people to deal with drug situations. The parents think this is inadequate and believe their idea for a hard-hitting approach will work for their children:

- Identify the ethical issues in this situation.
- What do you think the school nurse should do and why?

CASE STUDY 4.2   **Ethical Issues Relating to Funding Public Health Research**

An environmental health officer (EHO) wants to undertake some research into the impact of air pollution on asthma rates in a neighbourhood that straddles a main road. Town planning colleagues have told the EHO that they expect this road to become even busier soon because it will become the feeder road to a new bypass leading to a massive new out-of-town office development. The EHO has a well worked-out research proposal and the cooperation of local general practitioners (GPs), which will enable him to see if there is any correlation between traffic flow, air pollution levels, and asthma rates. If he can show a correlation, it will help to put health issues on the agenda of the council's planning committee so that the health impact of planning decisions will be considered in future.

He needs to secure a research grant to pay for the additional pollution measurements and traffic flow counts and to collect and process the data from the GPs. If he

does not start within the next month, he will miss the chance to collect vital baseline measurements before the expected increase in traffic when the bypass opens.

Despite applications to many sources, the only offer of research money he has received has come from a research trust which specialises in the impact of environmental pollution on respiratory disease. It is funded primarily by the tobacco industry. The trust assures the EHO that they will not interfere with the research in any way, and the grant will be given with 'no strings attached'. The EHO is unhappy about accepting money from the tobacco industry, but this is now his only chance to get the research underway. Identify the ethical issues in this situation.

• Identify the ethical issues in this situation.

• What do you think the EHO should do and why?

Eliminate choice
Forced lockdowns, face coverings and social distancing during the COVID-19 pandemic
Restrict choice
Banning smoking in public places, industry limits on fat, salt and sugar in processed food
Guide choice through disincentives
Tax on cigarettes/alcohol/sugar, congestion charges and ultra-low emission zones
Guide choice through incentives
eg free fruit to primary school children, social prescribing such as Physical Activity on Prescription Schemes (PARS)
Guide choice through changes in policy
eg school meals, healthy eating standards
Enable and empower choice
eg smoking cessation clinics, cycle lanes, fruit truck shops in school
Provide information
eg sex education in schools, national campaigns such as 5 a day
Do nothing or simply monitor the situation
eg surveillance of population health or behaviour, community profiling

Fig. 4.1 Public health intervention ladder, with examples. (Source: Adjusted form the Nuffield Council on Bioethics (2007) *Full report public health: ethical issues.* http://nuffieldbioethics.org/wp-content/uploads/2014/07/Public-health-ethical-issues.pdf).

should be overridden in the interests of the greater good. Is it ever an ethical choice to initiate public health action that ultimately leads to an infringement of individual liberty to achieve overall health gain within the population, for example, the compulsory lockdowns, mask-wearing, and social distancing imposed on the population during the COVID-19 pandemic?

There is also a danger that local populations are manipulated into changing their agenda to match that of the health promoter or public health practitioner. This was particularly the case during the COVID-19 pandemic. Community development approaches are about empowering the public to work on their own agendas of health issues, even if these are radically different from the priorities of those working for health in a professional capacity (See Popay et al., 2021 for a critical discussion of community empowerment). Health promoters and public health practitioners raise awareness of health issues; they provide information about them and, in doing so, create demand for change. So, where does this process differ from manipulating the community into wanting what the health promoters wanted in the first place? The bottoms-up approach becomes more complex during public health crises such as the pandemic when the priority was to prevent the spread of COVID-19 by, for example, manipulating the population into wanting vaccinations, wearing masks, and socially distancing.

Just Widening the Inequalities?

As discussed in Chapter 1, there are wide differences in the health status of different groups of people; generally, those in poorer social and economic circumstances are the least healthy, with a widening gap between the health status of the rich and poor (Marmot, 2020a).

There is a danger that health promotion and public health activities only reach the people who have the resources and education to make use of health information and take health action. Those who are trapped in poor financial circumstances are often less likely to be able to change their lifestyle, to have the health literacy to fully understand the health messages, to effectively access health services or to have the other competencies necessary to lobby for social or political changes. There is clearly a need to be sensitive to this.

Some ways of working with those most in need, and often hardest to reach, are discussed in Chapter 15.

Efforts to change people's physical environments to improve health may have negative outcomes. An impact assessment of a community regeneration programme highlighted both positive and negative potential health and wellbeing outcomes (McCartney and Collins, 2017).

The Health Promoter and Public Health Practitioner: A Shining Example?

Consider the cases of an overweight dietitian, a public health practitioner who consumes alcohol over the safe limits and a health visitor who smokes. All three are in a position where they need to address these issues as part of their work and may be asked for advice which they clearly do not follow themselves.

Few health promoters would claim that they are perfect examples of healthy living, but we suggest that they have a responsibility to consider their own health and think of ways in which it could be improved and in which they could contribute to a healthier environment. Health promoters are teaching by example, and the examples previously discussed convey silent messages that it is okay to be overweight, to smoke, or to risk health by overconsuming alcohol. It is probably best to be open and honest in situations where health promoters' own lifestyles are at odds with the health-promoting ways they are advocating. Personal experience can also be turned into a good advantage. For example, if the dietitian has a constant struggle to control her own weight, she can use that experience to develop a greater understanding of her client's difficulties.

Facts, Fads, or Fashions?

A concern for the public is that health advice changes. A difficulty is that research continuously turns up new evidence. At what point do you decide that the evidence is sufficiently convincing to begin publicising a new message or to campaign to change an aspect of health policy or legislation? If you have insufficient knowledge or experience to judge or question health information that may be medically or technically complex, on what basis do you make your decision? Is it more ethical to discuss the conflicting views openly and just air the debate more widely?

See Chapter 11 for an overview of the mass media and the social media influence on public health.

Health At Any Cost?

What being healthy means to different people is discussed in Chapter 1.

In their enthusiasm for improving health, there is a danger that health promoters and public health practitioners might lose sight that health means different things to different people and is shaped by their various values and experiences. Health may become a stereotyped image of the health promoter's own idea of perfection, leading to a prescription of what people should and should not do. This is clearly contrary to the concept that health promotion is about enabling people to increase control over their health and improve it in ways they see as appropriate.

Health Information: An Insensitive Blunderbuss?

Health promoters should be sensitive to the social, ethnic, economic, and cultural backgrounds of the individuals and communities with which they work. Health information and large-scale health promotion programmes which portray only white Caucasians, are available only in the English language or assume a common set of values are unethical.

Empower the People?

Health promotion and public health require special competencies, some of which are the subject of this book. It is all or part of the work of very many professions, including health, education, and community work.

Health promoters from this wide range of disciplinary backgrounds, if they are to empower people to take more control over their own health, need to seek to share their knowledge and experience with lay people, to learn from them and to see them and other workers as valued partners in the promotion of health.

Health for Sale?

With a scarcity of resources available for health promotion and public health and in a climate of public service cuts, market economy, and income generation, commercial companies now sponsor some health promotion activities. One pitfall is the issue of perceived endorsement of products. For example, an NHS organisation could be seen as promoting the use of vitamins if it accepted sponsorship of appointment cards printed with the name of the sponsoring vitamin manufacturer.

There is also a move to involve commercial companies in promoting products in a way that also promotes health. For example, food manufacturers may be involved in special promotions for lower-fat products. There are dangers here. The most obvious one being that the interests of the company may not be in harmony with those of the health promoter, who will be perceived as endorsing the product. There is also a possibility that the independent credibility of the health promoter is compromised.

Another pitfall is that promoting individual and population health, which should be a fundamental part of health prevention and promotion services, is seen as a potential money maker. Basic services such as health information materials, health teaching, and giving advice to commercial companies on health for employees become subject to charges.

Individual Freedom or Community Health?

Promoting health can be seen as paternalistic, interfering with personal liberty and freedom. Some might hold the view that doing nothing is the most morally acceptable option as it gives individuals the greatest freedom. However, this does not redress the distribution of power in society, which may limit the ability of individuals (particularly vulnerable groups) to act autonomously. Health promotion principles address this by empowering individuals and communities to increase control over factors that affect their health and wellbeing. However, the interplay and interaction between individuals, communities, and the wider populations are important. One of the difficulties in applying ethical principles in health promotion is the tension between the individual and the population. In what instances should an individual's rights be overridden in the interests of the greater good? Has COVID-19 changed the dynamic between individual choice versus whole population health? When should society step in and save us from ourselves? Our apparently insatiable appetites for smoking, drinking, and over-eating are resulting in a growth in noncommunicable diseases, which are putting a strain on health and social care budgets, and some lifestyle choices may present a health risk to others, such as drinking and driving or smoking in a home where there are children. Where and how should we draw the line between individual freedom and public health? Has COVID-19 changed our position on legislative action for health? When do we reach the point where the

consequences of individual freedom to choose are such a drain on the national purse or put others' lives at risk that we can no longer afford the luxury of letting people have the freedom to make health-damaging lifestyle choices? Is smoking, for example, personal freedom? (OHID, 2022). See also Aliyu Alhaji (2021) for a discussion of a range of ethical issues linked to the public health response to the COVID-19 pandemic and Public Health Ethics (2022) for a range of articles which looks at COVID-19 and ethics around the pandemic response, including questioning whether vaccination passports are a threat to equity (Voigt, 2022).

BEHAVIOUR CHANGE AND NUDGING: AN ETHICAL APPROACH?

Promoting health often focuses on the behavioural change approach previously outlined and discussed again in Chapter 14. Is this ethical, and is nudging ethically more acceptable than other forms of behavioural change interventions? It has been argued that a nudging intervention must not restrict choice. It must be in the interests of the person being nudged; it should involve a change in the architecture or environment of the choice, and it should exploit a mechanism of less than fully deliberative choice. But is nudging manipulation, and is manipulation ethically acceptable? Should governments seek to change the culture of society? Is it legitimate for the government to nudge social norms which were already changing, as in the case of binge drinking? See Jun et al. (2018) for a fuller discussion of the ethical issues in designing public health behaviour change interventions.

MAKING ETHICAL DECISIONS

Areas of ethical concern have been raised that do not present easy resolutions or answers. Beauchamp and Childress (2019) offer four ethical principles which can act as a guide to ethical practice:

Respect for Autonomy: Respecting the decision-making capacities of autonomous persons and enabling individuals to make reasoned, informed choices. Are there groups in society who might be seen as incapable of autonomy, such as people with learning disabilities, young children, or prisoners? And, if so, will this affect your health promotion or public health practice approach? If an individual makes a choice that you consider harmful, the dilemma may be how to respect that person's autonomy whilst doing good and avoiding harm. The key question is: By what right am I intervening, and how do I justify the action I am taking?

Beneficence: This considers the balancing of benefits of an intervention against the risks and costs; the health promoter should act in a way that benefits the client.

Nonmaleficence: To avoid the causation of harm, the health promoter should not harm the client. The harm should not be disproportionate to the benefits of intervention. Victim blaming would be considered harm, as would stigma. It may not always be possible to simultaneously do good and avoid harm. For example, a mass media campaign showing the dangers of drink driving may have the effect of reducing the rates of drink driving but may also impact negatively on those who have been convicted of drink driving by labelling them and/or increasing their feelings of guilt. You will be able to think of other examples.

Justice: This involves distributing benefits, risks, and costs fairly, the notion that clients in similar positions should be treated in a similar manner. Health promotion involves difficult decisions in the dividing of time and resources between individuals and communities and between high-risk groups and whole populations. How do you balance general campaigns on healthy eating for the whole population with targeted interventions such as setting up a food cooperative in a deprived area?

The principles provide a framework for consistent moral decision-making, but health promotion and public health interventions can encapsulate complex and sometimes conflicting choices. Because of this, ethics is a core public health competency, and its importance is being increasingly recognised. Questions regarding the identification and justification of paternalistic interventions (see Plante et al., 2020 for an ethics framework for analysing paternalism in public health policies and interventions), the fair distribution of health, and the overall responsibility for health are prominent (Verweij and Dawson, 2019). Some of the previous examples are taken from Shaping the Future of Health Promotion (SFHP)/Society of Health Education and Promotion Specialists (SHEPS) Cymru (2009). The sets of questions in Box 4.2 draw on the four ethical principles previously outlined and are designed for you to think about intervention ethics.

It is important to also consider how a global pandemic, such as COVID-19, might influence your decision-making in terms of the ethical implications of practice.

Exercises 4.3 and 4.4 (which use Fig. 4.1) are designed to help you to think about intervention ethics. Please also refer to Fig. 4.2, which provides an overview of ethical ways of working that highlight goals and principles.

TOWARDS AN ETHICAL CODE OF PRACTICE

Many professions have codes of practice, which are broad principles and guidelines on how professionals should and should not act. They reflect the values accepted as underpinning ethical practice. Health promoters from different professional backgrounds should ensure they are familiar with the codes of practice of their own professional bodies and be familiar with the ethical standards embedded in the Faculty of Public Health's Good Public Health Practice Framework (Faculty of Public Health, 2016) and Public Health Skills and Knowledge Framework (Gov.UK, 2019). For a more detailed explanation of ethics and the promotion of health, see Solberg (2021)

BOX 4.2   Some Ethical Questions on Health Promotion and Public Health Practice Interventions (Remember to Take Account of the COVID-19 Pandemic Interventions When Drawing on Examples to Support Your Arguments)

1. To what extent can the public good or the public interest justify state interventions that impose limits upon the freedom of individuals in terms of lifestyle choices?
2. What role should the law, both regulatory and fiscal measures, play in regulating health risks?
3. Should governments actively aim to change our preferences about such things as food, smoking, or physical exercise?
4. To what extent do individuals have moral obligations to contribute to protecting the community or the public good?
5. When is it appropriate to concentrate resources on prevention rather than cure?
6. Given the fact that we cannot protect population groups from all harm, what sorts of harm provide a justification for public health action?
7. What limits do we wish to place upon public health activities?
8. How do we ensure that the interests of individuals are not set aside or forgotten in the pursuit of population health benefits?
9. What should be the balance between individual and government responsibility for health?
10. Should medical treatment be refused to those who are morbidly obese?

EXERCISE 4.3   Ethical Decisions in Health Promotion

Look again at Case studies 4.1 and 4.2. You may find it helpful to use the questions in Box 4.2 on making ethical decisions to identify the issues relevant to each situation and to decide what you would do.

EXERCISE 4.4   Ladder of Health Promotion Action

Work in small groups of three or four. Consider the health promotion intervention ladder in Fig. 4.1 and discuss the following:
- The ethical issues that might be relevant to each rung of the ladder.
- Are there modes of intervention that you would reject on ethical grounds?
- Map the differing modes of intervention used during the COVID-19 pandemic and discuss the ethical issues they present.

PRACTICE POINTS

- In choosing approaches to health promotion and public health practice, take account of the different aims and values they reflect.

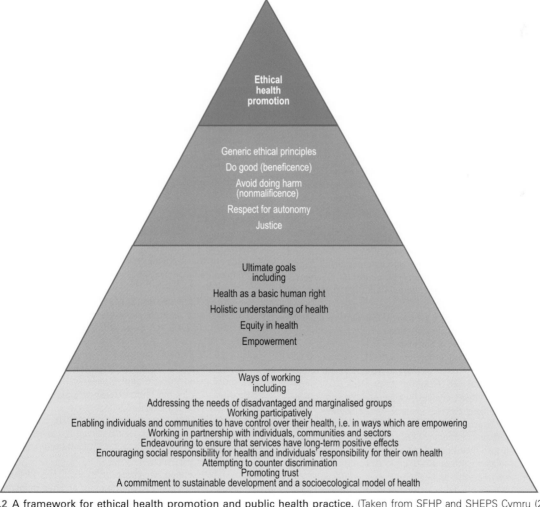

Fig. 4.2 A framework for ethical health promotion and public health practice. (Taken from SFHP and SHEPS Cymru (2009). Reproduced with permission.)

- Remember that ethical issues and dilemmas are inherent in promoting health; think through the process of how you will make ethical decisions.
- Be familiar with the code of professional practice of any profession to which you belong.
- Good practice in health promotion and public health involves working to the specific values and principles of practice.
- COVID-19 public health interventions may have challenged some ethical codes.

References

Aliju Alhaji, A. (2021). Public health ethics and the COVID-19 pandemic. *Annals of African Medicine*, *20*(3), 157–163.

Barnwell, P. V., Fedorenko, E. J., & Contrada, R. J. (2021). Healthy or not? The impact of conflicting health-related information on attentional resources. *Journal of Behavioral Medicine*, *45*, 306–317. https://doi:10.4103/aam.aam_80_20.

Beauchamp, T. L., & Childress, J. F. (2019). *Principles of biomedical ethics* (*8th edition*). Oxford: Oxford University Press.

Black, N., Johnston, M., Michie, S., Hartmann-Boyce, J., West, R., Vietchtbauer, W., Eisma, M. C., Scott, C., & de Bruin, M. (2020). Behavioural change techniques associated with smoking cessation in intervention and comparator groups of randomized control trials: a systematic review and meta regression. *Addiction*, *115*(11), 2008–2020.

Campbell, C., & Cornish, F. (2021). Public health activism in changing times: re-locating collective agency. *Critical Public Health*, *31*(2), 125–133. https://doi:10.1111/add.15056.

Cancer Research UK (2022). *Health inequalities: why do people smoke if they know it's bad for them*? https://news.cancer-researchuk.org/2022/04/01/health-inequalities-why-do-people-smoke-if-they-know-its-bad-for-them/

Day, R. E., Bridge, G., Austin, K., Ensaff, H., Christian, MS. (2022). Parents' awareness and perceptions of the Change4Life 100 cal snack campaign, and perceived impact on snack consumption by children under 11 years. *BMC Public Health*, *22*, 1012. https://doi.org/10.1186/s12889-022-12789-7.

Delesha, M., Carpenter, P., & Han, K. J. (2020). *Conflicting health information*. The Wiley Encyclopedia of Health Psychology New Jersey: John Wiley & Sons Ltd.

Department of Health and Social Care. (2021). *Children whose parents smoke are 4 times as likely to take up smoking themselves*. Press release 28 December 2021. https://www.gov.uk/government/news/children-whose-parents-smoke-are-four-times-as-likely-to-take-up-smoking-themselves

Department for Education. (2021). *Guidance: personal, Social, health and economic (PSHE) education- applies to England*. https://www.gov.uk/government/publications/personal-social-health-and-economic-education-pshe/personal-social-health-and-economic-pshe-education

Faculty of Public Health. (2016). *Good public health practice framework*. http://www.fph.org.uk/uploads/Good%20Public%20Health%20Practice%20Framework_%202016_Final.pdf

Gov.U.K. (2019). *Public health skills and knowledge framework*. https://www.gov.uk/government/publications/public-health-skills-and-knowledge-framework-phskf

Gov.U.K. (2022). *Walking, wheeling and cycling to be offered on prescription in nationwide trial*. Press release. https://www.google.com/search?client=safari&rls=en&q=Gov.UK+2022+Walking%2C+wheeling+and+cycling+to+be+offered+on+prescription+in+nationwide+trial.+Press+release.&ie=UTF-8&oe=UTF-8

James, E. K., Bokemper, S. E., & Huber, G. E. (2021). Persuasive messaging to increase COVID-19 vaccine uptake intentions. *Vaccine*, *39*(49), 7158–7165. https://doi:10.1016/j.vaccine.2021.10.039.

Lavarack, G. (2017). The challenge of behaviour change and health promotion. *Challenges*, *8*(25), 1–4. https://doi:org/10.3390/challe8020025.

Jun, G.T., Carvalho, F., Sinclair, N. (2018). *Ethical issues in designing interventions for behavioural change*. Design Research Society. https://dl.designresearchsociety.org/cgi/viewcontent.cgi?article=1534&context=drs-conference-papers

Lewin, E. (2019). *Victim blaming is an ineffective health tool*. https://www1.racgp.org.au/newsgp/gp-opinion/victim-blaming-is-an-ineffective-health-tool

Lindacher, V., Curbach, J., Warrelmann, B., Brandstelter, S., & Loss, J. (2017). Evaluation of empowerment in health promotion interventions: a systematic review. *Evaluation and the Health Professions*, *41*(3), 351–392. https://doi:10.1177/0163278716688065.

Mantyselka, P., Kautiainen, H., & Miettola, J. (2019). Beliefs and attitudes towards lifestyle change and risks in primary care- a community-based study. *BMC Public Health*, *19*, 1049. https://doi.org/10.1186/s12889-019-7377-x.

Marmot, M. (2020a). *Health equity in England: the Marmot review 10 years on*. London: The Health Foundation.

Marmot, M. (2020b). *Build back fairer: the Covid-19 marmot review: the pandemic, socioeconomic and health inequalities in England*. London: The Health Foundation and The Institute of Health Inequality.

McCartney, G., & Collins, C. (2017). Regeneration and health: a structured, rapid literature review. *Public Health*, *148*, 69–87. https://doi:10.1016/j.puhe.2017.02.022.

OHID. (2022). *Smoking and tobacco: applying all our health*. https://www.gov.uk/government/publications/smoking-and-tobacco-applying-all-our-health.

NHS 2022 Why 5 a day? https://www.nhs.uk/live-well/eat-well/5-a-day/why-5-a-day/

Plante, M., Bellefleur, O., & Keeling, M. (2020). *An ethics framework for analyzing paternalism in public health policies and interventions*. Québec: National Collaborating Centre for Healthy Public Policy.

Popay, J., Whitehead, M., Ponsford, R., Egan, M., & Mead, R. (2021). Power, control, communities and health inequalities: theories, concepts and analytical frameworks. *Health Promotion International*, *36*(5), 1253–1263. https://doi:org/10.1093/heapro/daaa133.

Public Health Ethics Volume 15, Issue 3, November 2022 https:// academic.oup.com/phe/issue/15/3.

Shaping the Future of Health Promotion and Society of Health Education and Promotion Specialists Cymru, (2009). *A framework for ethical health promotion (draft)*. London: Royal Society for Public Health and Society of Health Education and Promotion Specialists Wales.

Solberg, B. (2021). The ethics of health promotion: from public health to health care. In G. G Haugan & M. Eriksson (Eds.), *Health promotion in health care – vital theories and research*. Cham: Springer.

University of York. (2021). *Families have high awareness of healthy eating but low income means many struggle to access food*. https://www.york.ac.uk/news-and-events/news/2021/research/awareness-healthy-eating-struggle-access-good-food/

Verweij, M., & Dawson, A. (2019). Sharing responsibility: responsibility for health is not a zero-sum game. *Public Health Ethics*, *12*(2), 99–102. https://doi:org/10.1093/phe/phz012.

Voight, K. (2022). Covid-19 vaccination passports: are they a threat to equality? *Public Health Ethics*, *15*(1), 51–63. https://doi:org/10.1093/phe/phac006.

Websites

Food Ethics Council for details on food poverty in the UK. https://www.foodethicscouncil.org/issue/food-poverty/

NICE webpages for lifestyle and wellbeing. https://www.nice.org.uk/guidance/lifestyle-and-wellbeing.

Nuffield Council on Bioethics. Exploring ethical issues in biology and medicine. https://www.nuffieldfoundation.org/research/nuffield-council-on-bioethics

BBC Iplayer

BBC (2022) Panorama: obesity: who cares if I'm bigger? Is the prime minister's strategy to help the nation lose weight working? 20 April 2022. https://www.bbc.co.uk/iplayer/episode/m0015082/panorama-obesity-who-cares-if-im-bigger

Blogs

Royal Society of Public Health. *For example- the cost of living crisis will be a protracted public health crisis*. https://www.rsph.org.uk/about-us/news/blog-rsph-ceo-william-roberts-the-cost-of-living-crisis-will-be-a-protracted-public-health-crisis.html

Planning and Managing Health Promotion and Public Health Practice

PART CONTENTS

PART SUMMARY

Part 2 aims to provide guidance on how you can:

- Plan and evaluate your health promotion and public health practice work using a basic framework.
- Identify the views and needs of the clients/users/receivers of health promotion and set priorities for your work.
- Link your work to the efforts of colleagues and to local and national strategies.
- Use an evidence-based approach by using published research, doing your own research when necessary and auditing your work, thus ensuring that your efforts are effective and provide value for money.
- Organise yourself and manage your work to be effective and efficient.
- Develop competencies to work more effectively with colleagues and people from other organisations.

Chapter 5 sets out a planning and evaluation framework, which will help you clarify what you are trying to achieve, what you will do and how you will know whether you are succeeding. The meaning of terms such as aims, objectives and targets are discussed, and there is guidance on how to clearly specify them.

Chapter 6 explains how to identify a need and describes the sources of information you require to establish the needs of a community, a group or an individual. Guidelines are provided on how to gather and apply information to assess needs and set priorities.

Chapter 7 provides an overview of the knowledge and skills required to effectively plan health promotion and public health practice activities, including how to find and use published research. Guidance is included on how you can contribute to national and local public health strategic plans and complement what other people are doing. Evidence-informed practice is discussed, and advice is offered on how to carry out small-scale research, audit your activities and ensure value for money. The chapter includes the key steps required to undertake a health impact assessment.

Chapter 8 focuses on how you can develop the competencies to manage yourself and your work effectively, including managing information, writing reports, using time effectively, planning project work, managing change and working for quality.

Chapter 9 is about how to work with others, including communicating with colleagues, coordination and teamwork, participating in meetings and working in partnerships with other organisations.

Planning and Evaluating Health Promotion and Public Health Interventions

James Woodall

SUMMARY

Recent global events have demonstrated the critical importance of responding and planning effectively to protect and promote public health. This chapter presents an outline of a planning and evaluation cycle for use in the everyday work of public health practitioners and health promoters. It involves seven stages which include the measurement and specification of needs and priorities, the setting of aims and objectives, decisions on the best way of achieving aims, the identification of resources, the planning of evaluation methods, and the establishment of an action plan followed by an intervention. Examples are given of aims, objectives, and action plans, and exercises are provided on setting aims and objectives and using the planning framework to turn ideas into action.

This chapter is about planning and evaluation at the level of your daily work in health promotion and public health practice. It provides a basic framework for you to use to plan and evaluate your projects and activities, whether you work with clients on a one-to-one or group basis or undertake specific projects or programmes.

THE PLANNING PROCESS

Planning is a process that, at its very simplest, should give you the answers to three questions:

1. **What am I trying to achieve?** This question is concerned with identifying needs and priorities, then with being clear about your specific aims and objectives.

2. **What am I going to do?** This can be helpfully broken down into smaller steps:
   - Select the best approach to achieving your aims using evidence.
   - Identify the resources you are going to use.
   - Set a clear action plan of who does what and when.

3. **How will I know whether I have been successful?** This question highlights the importance of evaluation and the integral part it plays in planning health promotion and public health interventions. It should not be an afterthought or left too late to capture the information you need.

Planning is a central part of success, and there are many reasons why we need to plan in health promotion (Woodall and Cross, 2021). At times plans can be delivered as part of a long-term national strategy, but in other cases (such as during the recent pandemic), responses have to be rapid and flexible to adjust, as situations occur. There are many different planning models, but here the planning process has been put together in the seven-stage flowchart in Fig. 5.1. The arrows on the flowchart lead you around in a circle. This is because, as you carry out your plan and evaluation, you will probably find things that make you rethink and change your original ideas. For example, things you might want to change could include working on a need you found you had overlooked; scaling down your objectives because they were too ambitious; changing the intervention or approach because you found that they were not as useful or effective as you had hoped; or, based on new evidence, completely rethinking your strategy. On this latter point, local authorities responsible for public health in England were continually having to adjust their planning and interventions as a result of the increasing risk of COVID-19 during 2020 and 2021.

The direction of the arrows in the flowchart is anti-clockwise, but in reality, planning is not always an orderly process. You may actually start at stage 6 with a basic

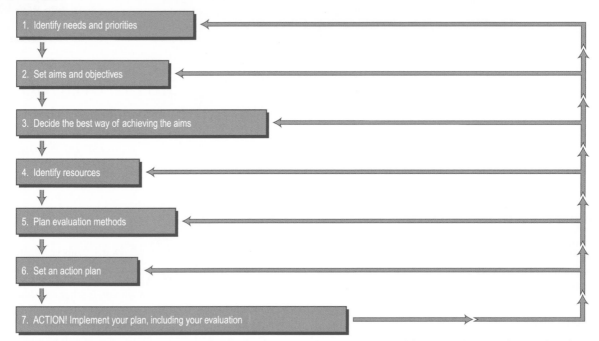

1. Identify needs and priorities

2. Set aims and objectives

3. Decide the best way of achieving the aims

4. Identify resources

5. Plan evaluation methods

6. Set an action plan

7. ACTION! Implement your plan, including your evaluation

Fig. 5.1 A framework for planning and evaluating health promotion and public health practice interventions and projects.

idea of a health promotion intervention. Thinking more about it may lead you to clarify exactly what your aims are (stage 2). Next, you might think about what resources you are going to need (stage 4) and realise that you do not have enough time or money to do what you had in mind, so you go back to stage 2 and modify your aims. Then you think about the best way of achieving your aims (stage 3) and work out an action plan (stage 6) with milestones. After that, you start to think seriously about how you will know whether you are successful (stage 5), and you put your evaluation plans into your action plan (stage 6 again). In effect, you are continually reviewing and improving your plan, using the framework appropriately to help you keep on course.

Planning takes place at many levels. If you are embarking on a major national public health intervention, you will need to take time to plan it in depth and in detail, but that can be a luxury, especially in times of public health emergencies (such as the COVID-19 pandemic). If you are simply planning a short one-to-one session with a client, you will still need to plan and go through all the stages, but the process might be quick and may not even be written down.

For example, a chiropodist seeing a client with a foot care problem may identify that the client needs knowledge and skills in cutting toenails correctly. They decide that their aim is to give the patient basic information

and training. They will know if they have been successful by examining the client's feet and by getting feedback about how they managed the next time they see them. They identify an information leaflet that they can give the patient as reinforcement. They decide on an action plan of explanation and demonstration and then get the patient to practice. They review the patient's toenail cutting skills the next time they see them, reinforcing or correcting them as necessary. All this planning takes place inside the chiropodist's head and is an integral part of their everyday professional practice.

THE PLANNING FRAMEWORK

Stage 1: Identify Needs and Priorities

How do you determine what health promotion is needed? If you think you already know, what are you basing your judgement on? Who has identified the need: you, your clients, the local public health agency, or national policy directives? Identifying needs is a complex process, which is looked at in depth in the next chapter (see Chapter 6).

You may have a long list of public health needs you have to respond to professionally, such as those set out by the Office for Health Improvement & Disparities (HM Government, 2022a) or those set in your local area, so another issue is how to establish your priorities. Again, this is discussed in detail in the next chapter, but the important point is that you must have a clear view of which needs you are responding to and why and what your priorities are.

Stage 2: Set Aims and Objectives

People use a range of words to describe statements about what they are trying to achieve, such as aims, objectives, targets, goals, mission, purpose, result, product, and outcomes. It can be helpful to think of them as forming a hierarchy, as in Fig. 5.2. At the top of the hierarchy are words that tell you why your job exists, such as your job purpose or remit or your overall mission. In the middle of the hierarchy are words that describe what you are trying to do in general terms, such as your goals or aims. At the bottom of the hierarchy are words that describe in specific detail what you are trying to do, such as targets or objectives.

It is worth noting that objectives can be of different kinds. Health objectives are usually expressed as the outcome or end state to be achieved in terms of health status, such as reduced rates of illness or death. However, in health promotion and public health practice, work objectives are often expressed in terms of steps along the way towards an ultimate improvement in the health of individuals, groups, or populations, such as increasing exercise levels or reduction in body mass index or numbers of people who reduce alcohol consumption.

In health education, educational objectives are framed in terms of the knowledge, attitudes, or behaviour to be exhibited by the individual or group. Objectives can also be in terms of other kinds of changes, for example, a change in health policy (introducing a healthy eating policy in the workplace) or health promotion practice (equipping people with skills and capacity to improve community wellbeing). See the following section on setting health education objectives.

The term 'target' is often used in public health and health promotion. Targets usually specify how the achievement of an objective will be measured in terms of quantity, quality, and time (the date by which the objective will be achieved). So a health target can be defined as a measurable improvement in health status by a given date that achieves a health objective. This is the approach used in national strategies for health, such as those targeting oral health promotion and improving the diet and oral hygiene of the population (HM Government, 2022b)

Objectives are framed as health objectives, and the targets are framed as health targets (changes in rates of death or illness by a specific date), behaviour targets (such as changes in sugar consumption or drinking by a specific date) or progress measures (such as the number of people downloading apps to support their behaviour change goals).

When you plan health promotion and public health initiatives, you need to set aims, objectives, and targets or goals and outcomes.

Your aims (or aim, as there does not have to be more than one) are broad statements of what you are trying to achieve. Your objectives are much more specific, and setting these is a critical stage in the planning process.

Objectives are the desired end state (or result or outcome) to be achieved within a specified period. They are not tasks or activities. Objectives should be as follows:

- **Challenging**. The objective should provide you with a health promotion/public health challenge in relation to what needs to be achieved.
- **Attainable**. On the other hand, it should be both realistic and achievable within the constraints of your professional role.
- **Relevant**. It should be consistent with the aims of the organisation and with the overall purpose/remit of your job.
- **Measurable**. You should try to identify objectives that are measurable, for example, specifying quantity, quality, and a time when they will be achieved. For instance (using the example in Exercise 5.1), an objective of 'to improve access to health information through the use of a social media campaign…' can be achieved by assessing how many people access the social media campaign or post and how readily they share this with other people in their social media network.

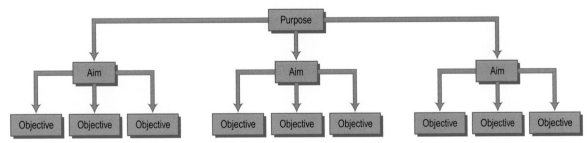

Fig. 5.2 A hierarchy of aims.

EXERCISE 5.1   Clarifying Your Purpose, Aims, and Objectives

Read this example of a health promoter's purpose, aims, and objectives.

Mark is a public health practitioner with a health promotion role working for a local authority (LA). His *purpose/remit* is to reduce inequalities in health in the population living and working in the area covered by the LA. To do this, one of his *aims* is to improve the levels of health knowledge of marginalised groups in the community. One of his *objectives* is to improve access to health information through the use of a social media campaign. He sets a target of developing social media posts focusing on five different health topics in three languages available on all of the social media sites (Instagram, Twitter, Facebook) within a six month period.

Now:

1. Thinking of your own job, write down what you believe to be its remit or purpose.
2. Then, give an example of one of your health promotion public health aims.
3. Finally, give an example of an objective you are trying to achieve in fulfilment of the aim you selected.

If you cannot find an example from your practice, make up an example of what you would like to do if you had the opportunity.

It is sometimes difficult to distinguish between aims, objectives, and action plans. For example, a dietician who wants to improve the information they give to obese patients may describe their aim as 'to produce an information leaflet', but this is also their objective and action plan. The answer is to think it through further and ask: Why produce a leaflet? What am I aiming to achieve by producing the leaflet? It then becomes clearer that the aim is to improve patient compliance with dietary treatment, and one of the objectives is to improve patients' understanding of their dietary instructions. The action is to produce the leaflet. The importance of actually thinking through your aims and objectives in this way is that it helps you to be absolutely clear about *why* you are doing something, not just *what* you are doing. Failure to think through this stage means that health promoters waste time and energy (and indeed public resources that often fund their activities) proceeding with what seems like a good idea only to realise, too late, that what they are doing is not actually achieving what they want. This is obviously very inefficient and ineffective.

Setting Health Educational Objectives

If your health promotion activity is based on a health education approach (for example, if you are working in schools or with communities whereby health awareness and consciousness might be low), it is useful to plan in terms of *educational* objectives. Educationalists traditionally think of objectives (sometimes called learning outcomes) in terms of what the clients will gain. Furthermore, the objectives are considered to be of three kinds: what the health educator would like the clients to *know*, *feel*, and *do* as a result of the education. In the language of the educationalist, these may be referred to as cognitive, affective, and behavioural objectives.

Objectives about 'knowing'. These are concerned with giving information, explaining it, and ensuring that the client understands it, thus increasing the client's knowledge, for example, explaining the weight loss advantages of increasing exercise levels to someone who is obese; or the importance of good hand washing and hand hygiene. Here, the objective would be to develop an understanding of the issues to enable them to make informed choices in terms of their health and wellbeing.

Objectives about 'feeling'. These objectives are concerned with attitudes, beliefs, values, and opinions. These are complex psychological concepts, but the important feature to note is that they are all concerned with how people feel. Objectives about feelings are about clarifying, forming, or changing attitudes, beliefs, values, or opinions. In the previous example, when the health promoter is educating a client about exercise and mental health, in addition to the knowledge objective, there could be an objective about helping the client to explore their attitude towards exercise and any values, beliefs, or opinions that might be forming a barrier to increasing exercise levels.

Objectives about 'doing'. These objectives are concerned with a client's skills and actions. For example, teaching a routine of aerobic or yoga exercises has the objective that clients acquire practical skills and are able to do exercise-related specific tasks.

- In the health education approach to health promotion and public health, a combination of the knowing, feeling, or doing educational objectives is usually required. For example, when a health visitor is advising a parent about feeding their toddler, they may be planning to achieve the following objectives within three home visits: the objective of ensuring that the parent knows which foods constitute a healthy eating programme for their child and which are best given in restricted amounts.

- The objective of relieving the parents' anxiety that their healthy child's food fads may cause serious ill health.

- The objective is that the parent learns what to do at mealtimes when the child has a tantrum about eating.
- To summarise the key points about setting aims and objectives: the focus is on what you are trying to achieve.
- Be as specific as possible. Avoid vague or subjective notions of what you want to achieve.
- Express your objectives in ways that can be measured. How much? How many? When?
- Do not get bogged down in terminology. It does not matter whether you talk about goals, aims, objectives, targets, or outcomes. The key principle is to be very clear about what you are trying to achieve.

To practise setting aims and objectives, undertake Exercises 5.1 and 5.2.

Stage 3: Decide the Best Way of Achieving the Aims

Occasionally, there might be only one possible way of accomplishing your aims and objectives. Usually, however, there will be a range of options. In Case study 5.1, Jim has a number of options about how to achieve his objective of increasing the sun safety measures being taken by the school and the children. He could write to the schools or

---

EXERCISE 5.2 Setting Aims and Objectives

Yewtree Scheme
The three practices at Yewtree Health Centre have agreed to establish physical activity assessment sessions, backed up by a display in the shared waiting area, with the long-term aim of reducing the incidence of coronary heart disease in the practice populations.

The detailed objectives are:
1. To raise the users' awareness of the link between inadequate exercise and coronary heart disease and the part that individuals can play in reducing their own vulnerability to the disease.
2. To assess and advise about individuals' physical fitness levels and help them to prepare an appropriate exercise action programme based on those results.
3. To monitor and evaluate, on a continuing basis, the effectiveness of the fitness testing in respect of the resources involved and the reduction in vulnerability to heart disease.

Ask yourself the following questions:
1. Do the objectives match the characteristics of the objectives previously described? Are they challenging, attainable, as measurable as possible and relevant?
2. How would you suggest changing the objectives?

CASE STUDY 5.1

Jim is an environmental health officer. His project is to tackle sun safety in schools. This fits in with the overall purpose of his job, which is to ensure safer environments. Jim works out that his *aim* is to work with local schools to set up a scheme that will result in sun safety measures being taken by the school and the children. He researches the subject in detail, looking at the results achieved from similar projects and working out how much time and money it is likely to take. He then decided that it was reasonable to set his *objective* as follows:

- Within 6 months to have raised awareness of the feasibility and advantages of developing shaded play areas with 10 primary schools and worked with at least 5 to set up shaded areas.

Health promoters such as Jim in this case study and Sue in Case study 5.2 are faced with the problem of how to identify the best strategy for achieving their objectives.

Factors to consider include:

- Which methods are the most appropriate and effective in meeting your aims and objectives?
- Which methods will be most acceptable to the individual or population group?
- Which methods will be easiest?
- Which methods are the cheapest?
- Which methods do you find comfortable to use?

---

parents of school-age children; he could hand out leaflets at school gates; he could lobby parents to take up the cause; he could find out if there are any school governors' meetings and ask to speak at them; he could conduct a sun safety campaign in the local media; he could write an article on the issue of sun safety in school playgrounds for the education journals that teachers read; or he could try to meet each Head Teacher face-to-face. Or he could do two or more of these together.

There is more about evidence for success, cost-effectiveness, and value for money in Chapter 7, and part 3 of this book covers how to use these methods to develop the necessary competency.

Looking at the first of these questions about which methods are most appropriate and effective for your aims, there is an accumulated body of evidence that helps identify effective methods for particular aims at the National Institute for Health and Care Excellence (NICE, 2022) and the Cochrane Database of Systematic Reviews or the Cochrane Library (see website references at the end of the chapter). Table 5.1 identifies the range of aims, grouped into categories, and the appropriate and

CASE STUDY 5.2

Sue is a nurse specialising in coronary care. Her project is to run patient education programmes so that discharged patients know how to look after themselves. This fits in with the overall purpose of her job, which is to care for patients while they are in the hospital and maximise their chances of a healthy life following discharge.

Sue decides that her *aim* is that patients will have participated in a cardiac rehabilitation programme for post-heart attack patients. Her *objectives* are:

- That every patient, before leaving the hospital, knows what they are advised to do about diet, exercise, smoking, and stress control.
- That every patient will be confident and competent to put this advice into practice.
- That every patient and their carers and relatives will have had an opportunity to discuss questions and anxieties with a qualified member of the staff.

Sue's programme is a continuous course of group sessions each week, with each session focusing on a specific issue. So each individual session also has a set of objectives. Objectives for the session on 'Eating well when you go home', for example, include the following:

- Patients will understand the basic principles of a healthy diet: low fat, low salt, low sugar, and high fibre.
- Patients will know which foods they can eat in unlimited amounts, which they should restrict, and which they should avoid.
- Patients will know what their ideal weight should be.
- Patients who are overweight will have devised a personal weight loss plan.

TABLE 5.1   Aims and Methods in Health Promotion and Public Health Practice

Aim	Appropriate Method
Health awareness goal Raising awareness, or consciousness, of health issues	Talks Group work Mass media and social media Displays and exhibitions Campaigns (which could include mass media and social media)
Improving knowledge Providing information	One-to-one teaching Displays and exhibitions Written materials Mass media and social media Campaigns Group teaching
Self-empowering Improving self-awareness, self-esteem, decision making	Group work Practising decision making Values clarification Social skills training Simulation, gaming, and role play Assertiveness training Counselling
Changing attitudes and behaviour Changing the lifestyles of individuals	Group work Skills training Self-help groups and peer support One-to-one advice and instruction Group or individual therapy Nudging Written material, social media, YouTube Social marketing approach
Societal/ environmental change Changing the physical or social environment	Positive action for under-served groups Lobbying for fiscal and legislative change Pressure and campaign groups, e.g. 38 degrees Community development Community-based work Advocacy schemes Environmental and social measures Planning and policy making Organisational change Enforcement of laws and regulations

effective methods for achieving them. This provides a general guideline which may have exceptions.

You may have decided on more than one of these categories of aims. For example, the inputs that contribute towards changing the behaviour of individuals can be complemented by societal changes so that, together, they are more effective than either intervention alone by creating synergy. So, for example, to reduce the overconsumption of alcohol by young people, you could:

- Provide health education about alcohol as part of schools' personal, social, health, and economic education programmes.
- Provide educational rehabilitation programmes for young drink-drive offenders.
- Work with young people to promote the social acceptability of consuming non-alcoholic drinks.

- Lobby for an increase in alcohol taxation (a unit price) or for increasing the age at which young people can buy alcohol or for changes to the labelling of alcoholic drinks.

- Work with alcohol companies in terms of promoting sensible drinking.

  The example in Fig. 5.3 shows a range of aims and methods that might be used to promote healthy eating.

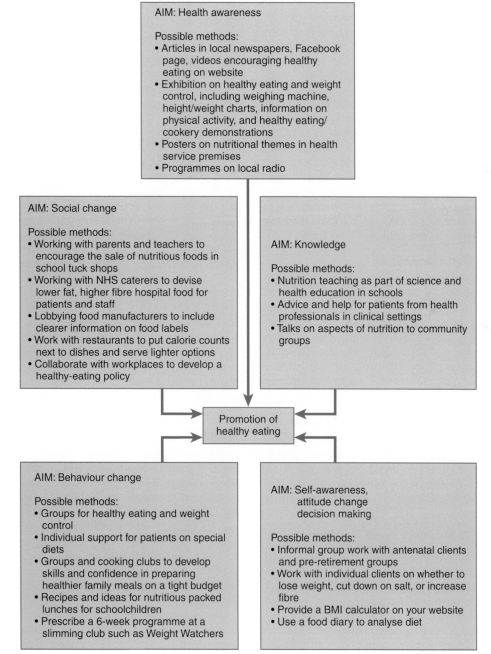

Fig. 5.3 Aims and methods for the promotion of healthy eating.

A health promoter or public health practitioner may not use all these at any one time, but they are given here to illustrate the range of possibilities.

Stage 4: Identify Resources

What resources are you going to use? You have to establish what resources you are going to need and what are already available, what additional resources you are going to have to acquire and whether you will need extra funding. A number of different kinds of resources can be identified.

Professional Input

Your experience, knowledge, skills, time, enthusiasm, and energy are vital resources. It helps identify all the other professional and lay people with something to offer. This may include colleagues and others in your professional networks (see Exercise 3.2 in Chapter 3) with relevant expertise who can advise and help you make your plans; clerical and secretarial staff who can help with administration; and technicians, graphic designers, and web designers, artists who can help with exhibitions, displays, teaching/publicity materials, and internet-based resources.

Your Client or Client/Target Group

These are another key resource. Clients may have knowledge, skills, enthusiasm, energy, and time, which can be used and built upon. In a group, clients can share their knowledge and previous experience and, in this way, help each other to learn and change. An ex-client can be a very valuable resource too. For example, someone who has successfully lost weight or has increased their physical activity levels can be a great help to clients who are grappling with similar problems and experiences.

People Who Influence Your Client or Client Group

These may include clients' relatives, friends, volunteers, patients' associations, and self-help groups. It may also be possible to harness the help of significant people in the community who are regarded as opinion leaders or trendsetters, such as political figures, religious leaders, or media celebrities.

Existing Policies and Public Health Strategies

National and local policies and strategies for public health are useful to locate in terms of the work that you are planning. If, for example, you are planning to develop an intervention to educate young people about substance misuse, find out if there is already a strategy on alcohol and drug misuse in your area. Also, find out whether your work fits into wider Government policy drivers – in this instance, it would be advisable to consult the UK Government's ten year drugs plan to cut crime and save lives (HM Government, 2021).

Existing Facilities and Services

Find out what relevant local facilities already exist and whether they are fully utilised, for example, sports centres offering facilities for exercise and local classes or groups on cooking for healthy eating.

Material Resources

These might include leaflets, posters, and display/publicity materials, or if you are planning health promotion involving group work, you need resources such as rooms, space, seats, audio-visual equipment, and teaching/learning materials.

Media Resources

Multimedia resources can include Facebook, blogs, Twitter, Instagram, and YouTube on a wide range of health-related topics, including those provided by statutory public health agencies such as the Department for Health and Social Care and the Office for Health Improvement and Disparities. There is a wide assortment of media resources available on the internet, but it might be that your public health project would lend itself to the development of a new social media presence.

Stage 5: Plan Evaluation Methods

How will you measure success and know whether your health promotion and public health practice is successful? Sophisticated methods are required to evaluate large-scale health promotion interventions. However, this should not deter health promoters; less complex methods of evaluating the everyday practice of health promotion can, and should, be used routinely.

What Is Meant by Evaluation?

Evaluation is about making a judgement about the value of a public health or health promotion intervention, whether it is, for example, a health education programme, a community project or an awareness-raising campaign to change local policy. Evaluation is crucial for ongoing quality improvement in your practice and involves the process of assessing *what* has been achieved and *how* it has been achieved. It means looking critically at the activity or programme, working out what were its strengths and its weaknesses, and how it could be improved.

The judgement can be about the *outcome* (what has been achieved) and whether you achieved the objectives which you set. So, for example, you should judge whether people understood the recommended limits for alcohol consumption as a result of your sensible drinking education, whether people in a particular community became more articulate about their health needs as a result of your community empowerment work or whether you achieved media coverage for your health campaign.

Judgements should also be about the *process* (how it has been achieved) and the cost benefit, for example, whether the most appropriate methods were used, whether they were used in the most effective way and whether they gave value for money. So, for example, you could consider whether the vlog-based discussion you used in your teaching programme was the best teaching method to use, whether the community development approach you chose was the most appropriate one in the circumstances, or whether you would have achieved more public awareness with less money if you had opted for a media stunt with possible free news coverage rather than an expensive advertising and leaflet campaign (see Hubley et al., 2020 and Woodall and Cross, 2021) for chapters with in depth discussion on the complexities of public health practice evaluation).

Key terms often used in discussions about evaluation are defined in the Glossary at the end of this book.

Why Evaluate?

You need to be clear about why you are evaluating your work because this will affect the way you do it and the amount of effort you put in. Some reasons could be the following:

- To improve your own practice: next time you deliver a similar intervention, you will build on your successes and learn from any mistakes.
- To help other people to improve their public health practice: if you disseminate your evaluation, it can help others improve their practice as well. It is vital to publicise failures as well as successes.
- To build broader evidence for public health and health promotion.
- To justify the use of the resources that went into the intervention and to provide evidence to support the case for doing this type of health-promoting intervention in the future.
- To give you the satisfaction of knowing how useful or effective your work has been, in other words, for your own job satisfaction.
- To identify any unplanned or unexpected outcomes that could be important. For example, a publicity campaign to deter young people from taking drugs could have the opposite effect by unwittingly glamorising drug-taking and making it appear to be a more common activity than it really is.

Who Is the Evaluation For?

Who will be using your evaluation data? The answer to this affects what questions you ask, how much depth and detail you go into and how you present the information.

If you are solely assessing how well a health promotion intervention went for your own benefit so you can change it appropriately next time you run a similar session, you will simply make a judgement on how you think it went based on your observation and the clients' reactions and make a few notes. But if you are writing a report for your manager or for a body that you want to fund the work, you need to think through what questions those people will expect to be answered and how much detail they will want.

For example, a group of health visitors evaluating a pilot scheme for a telephone advisory service at evenings and weekends need an evaluation report after six months for their manager who is funding the service. What will the manager need to know? At the very least, they will probably need a clear indication of the use made of the service. This might include how many people used it, the characteristics of the users (for example, whether they were first-time parents), how much it was used, what sort of issues people rang about, what the clients gained from it and how much it cost. It would be helpful for the health visitors to ask their manager what evaluation data will be required at the planning stage of the project so that the appropriate data can be collected from the start.

Assessing the Outcome

Looking first at outcome measures, which are called summative evaluation, you need to go back to the objectives you set and plan how you are going to determine whether you have achieved the objectives. Objectives are about the changes the intervention was designed to achieve and might have included changes in people's knowledge or behaviour or changes in policies or ways of working. Long-term health promotion projects may also have objectives about changes in health status. The following lists indicate the kinds of changes that may be reflected in your objectives and what methods you might use to assess or measure those changes.

Changes in health awareness can be assessed by:
- Measuring the interest shown by consumers, for example, how many people took up offers of leaflets, how many people enquired about preventive services, or how many people visited a website, friended or shared a Facebook page, or retweeted.
- Monitoring changes in demand for health-related services such as breastfeeding support groups.

- Analysis of media coverage of the public health issue if it is a national campaign.
- Questionnaires, interviews, focus group discussions, or observation with individuals or groups.

Changes in knowledge or attitude can be assessed by:
- Observing changes in what clients say and do: does this show a change in understanding and attitude?
- Interviews and discussions involving question-and-answer between health promoters and clients.
- Discussion and observation on how clients apply knowledge to real-life situations and how they solve problems.
- Observing how clients demonstrate their knowledge of newly acquired skills.
- Written tests or questionnaires that require clients to answer questions about what they know. The results can be compared with those of tests taken before the health intervention or from a comparable group that has not received the health promotion.

Behaviour change can be assessed by:
- Observing clients' behaviour.
- Recording behaviour. This could be based on records such as numbers attending an intervention to improve levels of physical activity or clients keeping a diary which is used at the end to assess behaviour change. It could be a periodic inventory, such as a follow-up questionnaire or interview, to check on physical activity levels six and 12 months after attending the intervention. Records of client behaviour can be compared with those of comparable groups in other areas or with national average figures.

Policy changes can be assessed by:
- Policy statements and implementation, such as the increased introduction of healthy eating choices in workplaces and schools.
- Legislative changes such as the sugar tax or minimum alcohol pricing.
- Increases in the availability of health-promoting products, facilities, and services such as social prescribing schemes.
- Changes in procedures or organisation, such as more time being given to patient education or GP brief interventions.

Changes to the physical environment can be assessed by:
- Measuring changes in such things as air quality, traffic or pedestrian flows, the number of bike lanes, or the amount of open green space available to the public within a defined area.

Changes in health status can be assessed by:
- Keeping records of simple health indicators such as weight, blood pressure rates, pulse rates on standard exercise or cholesterol levels.
- Health surveys to identify larger scale changes in health behaviour or self-reported health status.
- Analysis of trends in routine health statistics such as infant mortality rates or hospital admission rates.

It will be seen from this list that common evaluative methods are the generation of data from observation, holding discussions, and distributing questionnaires and data analysis of health and other records.

Assessing the Process

Assessing intervention processes, often referred to as process formative evaluation, is an important but complex aspect of a comprehensive evaluation of health promotion and public health activities. For example, efforts to understand how to improve fruit and vegetable consumption in children require an understanding of the processes as well as the actual outcomes (Ismail et al., 2021). These types of interventions require a systematic approach to designing and conducting the process evaluations, drawing on clear descriptions and identification of key process questions. This involves examining what went on during the process of implementation and making judgements about effectiveness and efficiency. Was it done as cheaply and quickly as possible? Was the quality as good as you wished? Were the appropriate methods and materials used? You may, for instance, achieve your objectives but in a time-consuming, costly, or inefficient way. So it is important to evaluate the process and identify whether you have achieved your desired outcome. Formative evaluation can be ongoing so that changes can be made to the intervention if it is found not to be working while it is in the process of delivery.

How are you going to assess the process? There are key aspects to process evaluation which involve measuring the input, self-evaluation by asking yourself questions and getting feedback from other people.

Measuring the input. This is essential if you are going to make judgements about whether the outcome was worthwhile. You need to record everything that went into your health promotion or public health intervention in terms of time, money, and materials. Then, you can make an informed judgement about the cost benefit and whether the outcome justified the cost.

Self-evaluation. Ask yourself, 'What did I do well?', 'What would I like to change?' and 'How could I improve that next time?' All kinds of health promotion and public health interventions can be subjected to process evaluation, whether it is a one-to-one health education intervention with a client, facilitating a self-help group, undertaking community empowerment work, developing and implementing a health policy, or lobbying for organisational and structural changes.

An important point to note about self-evaluation is the need for a balanced, objective critique which highlights both the positive and the negative aspects. Identify the things that have worked and look for constructive ways of moving forward with things that could be improved.

Feedback from other people. Giving and receiving feedback is an essential skill for every health promoter. Getting feedback from a trusted colleague on your intervention is a valuable form of peer evaluation. Asking for and getting feedback from your manager should be part of the regular monitoring of your performance. See the section in Chapter 10 on asking questions and getting feedback.

Obtaining feedback from the clients or users themselves should also be part of assessing the process of every intervention. The important thing is to encourage a non-judgemental atmosphere of openness and honesty. It can be done in many ways; simply observing clients and users accurately is an important tool. Do they look anxious or relaxed? Do they look interested and alert or bored and detached? You can also ask for feedback in such ways as a suggestions box, through noting any spontaneous verbal feedback you receive or through asking questions.

Stage 6: Set an Action Plan

Now that you know:
- What you are trying to achieve and have identified the best way to go about it,
- How to evaluate it,
- What resources you need,

you can get down to planning in detail exactly what you are going to do. This means writing a detailed statement of who will do what, with what resources, and by when.

It is helpful, especially if you are tackling a large project, to break down your plan into smaller, manageable elements. One way of doing this is by thinking in terms of *key events*. Draw up a schedule showing the key events that are planned to happen at particular points in time. The schedule should specify deadlines that must be met by the people involved. Another way of breaking down a large project is by *milestone* planning. This is different from key events planning: instead of listing events, it lists a series of significant dates at fixed intervals (the milestones) and shows what must have happened by each of them. Box 5.1 illustrates both types of action plans.

For more discussion about the skills of project management, see Chapter 8, the section on managing project work.

BOX 5.1   Action Plans

A **key events plan** drawn up by a public health practitioner who plans to set up an interactive multimedia health stall in a local supermarket to promote sensible drinking over the Christmas period could look like this:
1. *Discuss with my manager* at the June meeting.
2. *Identify support from colleagues* by July.
3. *Approach the supermarket manager* by August and agree to space and times.
4. *Convene a planning group* of colleagues in August to sort out who will do what and when to evaluate plans and identify the resources required.
5. Planning phase, September to November, including resource development.
6. *Set up the first stall* in late November.

A brief **milestone plan** for the early stages of setting up a community health project could be like this in a framework of three monthly 'milestones':

January to March 2023	The steering group agrees on the job description for the community health worker. Job advertised.
By the end of June 2023	Interviews; appointment made. Community worker takes up post.
By the end of September 2023	Community worker induction programme completed.
By the end of December 2023	First progress report to the steering group.

Stage 7: Action!

This is the stage in which you deliver your health-promoting intervention, remembering to evaluate the process as you go along.

Exercise 5.3 gives you the opportunity to apply this planning framework.

Be aware that when you are thinking about one section of the planning framework, it may have implications for the others, so you may find yourself going back to modify and refine what you have already written.

To summarise, the planning process consists of a series of stages which enable you to more systematically organise your health promotion and public health practice work by focusing on key questions around What? Why? When? Who? Where? and How?

Useful additional reading to support planning is Eldredge et al., 2016, who propose an intervention mapping approach, and for some theoretical and practice

EXERCISE 5.3   Ideas Into Action: Planning a Health Promotion and Public Health Practice Intervention

Work alone or in a small group.

Think of an area of health promotion or public health practice where there is an identified need and within the remit of your job to meet that need. It could be an established area of work, such as antenatal education, teaching food hygiene, or an area of new work you would like to tackle, such as an intervention to prevent obesity in children. If you are not currently in a job which involves health promotion or public health, think of a health-related project you would like to tackle in your personal life or a project for any voluntary/community group you are associated with, or just imagine what you would like to do if you had the opportunity (see the WHO website in the following references for programme and project ideas).

Work through the following stages of the planning cycle. Start by writing each of the following headings at the top of a separate large sheet of paper or word document, and then work through them:

1. **Aims and objectives**
   Ask yourself, 'What am I trying to achieve?' Identify your broad aim or aims, then be more specific and identify your objectives.

2. **The best way of achieving my aims**
   Think of all the ways in which you could achieve your aims and identify the best way.

3. **Resources**
   Identify the resources you already have available and any extra ones you will need.

4. **Evaluation**
   Ask yourself, 'How will I know if I am succeeding?' Identify how you will evaluate both the process and outcome of your work.

5. **Action plan**
   Identify who will do what, with what resources, and by when. Set milestones, if appropriate.

insights into the evaluation of complex health interventions, see Bell and Aggleton (2016). NICE provides excellent guidance on planning for behavioural change interventions based on a series of principles. The social context principle is an important one for those planning behavioural change interventions (refer to the website reference at the end of the chapter). Finally, the National Social Marketing Centre also provides a planning model and tools for planning behavioural change interventions. Their website is also referenced at the end of this chapter.

PRACTICE POINTS

- Health promotion and public health practice interventions benefit from being planned and evaluated in a systematic way.
- A planning cycle should ensure that needs and priorities are identified, aims and objectives are clearly set, and methods for achieving aims and objectives are carefully considered in the context of available resources.
- Evaluation is an important component of the planning process, and evaluation methods should be formative, measuring the process, and summative, measuring the outcome of the intervention.

References

Bell, S., & Aggleton, P. (2016). *Monitoring and evaluation in health and social development: Interpretive and ethnographic perspectives*. Oxford: Routledge.

Eldredge, L. K. B., Markham, C. M., Reiter, R. A. C. E., Fernandez, M. E., Kook, G., & Parcel, G. A. S. (2016). *Planning health promotion programs: an intervention mapping approach* (4th edition). Jossey-Bass Public Health.

Ismail, M. R., Seabrook, J. A., & Gilliland, J. A. (2021). Process evaluation of fruit and vegetables distribution interventions in school-based settings: a systematic review. *Preventive Medicine Reports, 21*, 1–10. California.

NICE. (2022). *Guidance, NICE advice and quality standards*. https://www.nice.org.uk/guidance/published?ngt=NICE%20guidelines

HM Government, (2021). *From harm to hope: a 10-year drugs plan to cut crime and save lives*. London: Crown.

HM Government. (2022a). Latest from the office for health improvement and disparities. https://www.gov.uk/government/organisations/office-for-health-improvement-and-disparities

HM Government. (2022b). Delivering better oral health: an evidence-based toolkit for prevention. https://www.gov.uk/government/publications/delivering-better-oral-health-an-evidence-based-toolkit-for-prevention

Hubley, J., Copeman, J., & Woodall, J. (2020). *Practical health promotion* (3rd edition). Cambridge: Polity Press.

Woodall, J., & Cross, R. (2021). *Essentials of health promotion*. London: Sage.

Websites

Cochrane Library. To inform the planning of interventions. https://www.cochranelibrary.com/

For social marketing planning models and tools. https://www.thensmc.com/

NICE. For their guidance and quality standards. https://www.nice.org.uk/guidance/published?ngt=NICE%20guidelines

HM Government. Guidance on evaluation in health and wellbeing. https://www.gov.uk/government/collections/evaluation-in-health-and-wellbeing

Twitter

Institute for Health Metrics and Evaluation (IHME) https://twitter.com/IHME_UW

Office for Health Improvement and Disparities Twitter profile to follow key developments. https://twitter.com/OHID

Identifying Health Promotion and Public Health Practice Needs and Priorities

James Woodall

CHAPTER OUTLINE

SUMMARY

This chapter begins with an analysis of the concept of need. This is accompanied by an overview of essential factors for you to consider when identifying health promotion and public health needs. These include the scope and boundaries of professional remits, the difference between reactive and proactive choices, and the importance of placing the people who are the targets and users of health promotion at the centre of the needs identification process. This discussion is supplemented with an exercise on the user-friendliness of services. In the next section on finding and using health information, types and sources of information are identified, and exercises are included on gathering and applying information. This is followed by a framework for assessing health promotion needs with a case study and an exercise. In the final section, there is a focus on priority setting with exercises on analysing the reasons for and the setting of health promotion and public health practice priorities and on setting priorities.

Many organisations at different levels have a role in identifying public health needs, including those needs that can be addressed by health promotion and public health practice interventions. These range from international agencies such as the World Health Organisation (WHO) and national organisations such as government departments to organisations at the local level such as local authorities, clinical commissioning groups or National Health Service (NHS) Trusts.

See Chapter 3 for information on the range of agencies with a public health and health promotion role, Chapters 3 and 16 for national and local health strategies, and Chapter 16 for making and implementing national and local health policies.

The focus of this chapter is on the need for interventions undertaken by health promoters and public health practitioners working with individual clients, families, groups, and communities.

Identifying the people or target group who are intended to benefit from health promotion activities is a complex process. These people may be referred to as *users*, which implies they use health promotion services such as smoking cessation groups. In some cases, people receive help that they may or may not use, for example, receiving advice and information leaflets. Alternatively, people may be called *consumers*, *customers*, *clients* or *patients* if they are receiving their health promotion via medical services such as a coronary rehabilitation service. Positive action may be necessary to ensure that everyone has equal access to services and can benefit from them.

Going one stage further and identifying and prioritising people's needs is also a complex and difficult process. Needs may exceed the finite resources available to meet them, so difficult choices may have to be made.

Before looking further at how the needs of the users and receivers of health promotion can be met, it is worth considering what is understood as a need.

CONCEPTS OF NEED

It is useful to think of need in terms of:
- The kinds of health problems that people experience or are at risk from.
- The requirements for a particular kind of health promotion response.

- The relationship between health problems and the health promotion responses available.

Bradshaw's (1972) taxonomy of need was established many years ago, but it is still very useful in distinguishing between four different kinds of need.

1. Normative Need – Defined by the Expert

Normative need is a need defined by experts or professionals according to their own standards; falling short of those standards means that there is a need. For example, a dietitian may identify a certain level of nutritional knowledge as the desirable standard for her client and defines a need for nutrition education if her client's knowledge does not reach that standard. This normative need is based on the judgements of professional experts, which may lead to problems. One is that expert opinion may vary over what is the acceptable standard (debate exists over how many 'portions' of fruit or vegetables is ideal, for instance), and the values and standards of the experts may be different from those of their clients.

Some normative needs are strongly advised by government or healthcare agencies (and can even be mandated for some activities), such as vaccination, to protect against COVID-19 (UK Health Security Agency, 2022).

2. Felt Need – Wants

Felt need is the need that people feel; it is what they *want*. For example, a pregnant woman may feel the need for (and want) information about childbirth. Felt needs may be limited or inflated by people's awareness and knowledge about what could be available; for example, people will not feel the need to know their blood cholesterol level if they have never heard that such a thing is possible or know about the potential risk of high blood cholesterol levels to health.

3. Expressed Need – Demands

Expressed need is what people say they need; it is felt need that has been turned into an expressed request or demand. Commercial weight-control groups and exercise classes are examples of expressed need; they are provided in response to demand.

Not all felt need is turned into expressed need or demand. Lack of opportunity, motivation, or assertiveness could all prevent the expression of a felt need. Lack of demand, therefore, should not be equated with a lack of felt need.

Expressed needs may conflict with a professional's normative needs. For example, a patient may express a need for a course of individual professional counselling as a result of experiencing a mental health problem, but

the resources may not be available for this type of health-promoting service, and normative needs and priorities may be focused on other types of interventions to promote mental health.

4. Comparative Need

Comparative need for health promotion is defined by comparison between similar groups of clients, some in receipt of health promotion and some not. Those who are not are then defined as being in need. For example, if Company A has an employee health policy covering stress at work and the provision of healthy food choices in the staff canteen and Company B does not, it could be said that there is a comparative need for health promotion in Company B. This assumes that the health promotion in Company A is desirable and ideal, which of course it may not be.

NEED, DEMAND AND SUPPLY

Over time, there has been debate over need, demand, supply, and quality of health services and other public sector services that relate to health, such as education. Levels and quality of service vary nationally and internationally (see Dorling 2019) and in the United Kingdom (UK) between service provision in the UK, resulting in what has been termed as a postcode lottery Ashby et al., 2019. The need for services may be similar or different, but supply is unevenly distributed, and this results in significant health inequalities (see for example Stephenson, 2016 reporting variation in specialist children's care provision, and De Camargo, 2021 discussing access to personal protective equipment for police officers during the COVID-19 pandemic).

If demand outstrips supply, it means that people do not always get the access or the quality of the health provision they want or that health professionals believe they need. This issue of uneven provision also applies to health promotion and public health services, with an early survey showing different levels of health promotion provision in different geographical areas in the UK (Scriven, 2002). The problem of uneven provision arises because the health services and other public bodies have a finite pot of money to spend, so they have to prioritise. This results in rationing, as seen during the COVID-19 pandemic (Srinivas et al., 2021). In some situations, and to overcome some of the problems associated with rationing, adults receiving NHS Continuing Healthcare and children in receipt of continuing care have had a right to have a personal health budget. A personal health budget is an amount of money to support personally identified health and wellbeing needs, planned and agreed upon between the person and their local NHS team. The aim is to give people with long-term conditions and disabilities greater choice and control over the health care and support they receive if they desire this (NHS Choices, 2020). Measures to address the uneven supply and quality of health services have also included the development of national standards. The National Institute for Health and Care Excellence (NICE) provides the standards not only for clinical and healthcare practice but also for public health and health promotion. Quality standards set out the priority areas for quality improvement. Quality standards cover:

- Areas where there is variation in care.
- Topics across health and social care.

Each standard contains a set of statements to help you improve quality. It also tells you how to measure progress against the statement.

The standards are developed independently in collaboration with health and social care professionals, practitioners, and service users. They are based on NICE guidance and other NICE-accredited sources.

Example of a Quality Statement

Older people using home care services have a home care plan that identifies how their personal priorities and outcomes will be met, *Home care for older people, NICE quality standard* (NICE, 2016).

- Anyone wanting to improve the quality of health and care services should consult the standards. For example, commissioners – Use the quality standards to ensure that high-quality care or services are being commissioned.
- Service providers – Use the quality standards to monitor service improvements, to show that high-quality care or services are being provided, and highlight areas for improvement.
- Health, public health, and social care practitioners – Use audit and governance reports to demonstrate the quality of care, as described in a quality standard or in professional development and validation.
- Regulators – For example, the Care Quality Commission.

Quality standards are not mandatory. They support the UK government's vision for a health and care system focused on delivering the best possible health outcomes and are therefore important for all professionals with a public health remit.

IDENTIFYING HEALTH PROMOTION NEEDS

How do health promoters and public health practitioners set about identifying individual and/or group needs? There are three key areas that are useful to think about

first: the scope and boundaries of your job, the balance between being reactive and proactive in your work, and the extent to which you are putting your clients first. Each of these is addressed in turn.

The Scope

For some public health practitioners and health promoters, the task of identifying needs has already taken place. For example, dental hygienists working in dental surgery with individual patients already have the clearly identified task of educating patients in oral hygiene. But they may want to think carefully about how they can make their service as person-centred and user friendly as possible, and they will certainly have to identify and respond to the individual needs of each patient.

Some professionals with a public health remit, however, have more choice and scope in the range of health promotion activities they can undertake. Health visitors and community workers may have a considerable scope, but the degree of autonomy they have will vary according to the policy of their managers and the resources available. All health promoters will need some competency in being responsive to the health promotion needs of their clients and will need to be clear about the boundaries of their work: Which health promotion activities are within their remit to undertake, and which are not (however desirable they may be)? For example, a family planning nurse may be asked to undertake sex education with young people in schools, but is this within the boundaries of her job?

Reactive or Proactive?

It is useful to make an initial distinction between being *reactive* and being *proactive* when identifying needs. Being reactive means responding or reacting to the needs and demands that other people make. Pressure from vested interest groups and the media may introduce bias into how needs are perceived and produce pressure to react. Being proactive means taking the initiative and deciding on the area of work to be done. It may include rejecting the demands of other people if these do not fit existing policies and priorities. (See Chapter 4, the section on analysing your aims and values: five approaches.)

Being reactive or proactive can be related to the approaches to health promotion, which were discussed in Chapter 4. Using a client-directed approach means being reactive to consumers' expressed needs, whereas using a medical or behaviour change approach probably means being proactive. This is particularly true of preventive medical interventions such as immunisation campaigns. In practice, there is usually a balance to be struck between being reactive and proactive.

Putting Users' Needs First

It is important to ask questions about whose needs should come first, the users or the providers of health promotion. There may be conflict between the two: for example, users may want a family planning service to be open on Saturdays to improve access, but providers are unable to supply this service because of difficulties in getting staff to work on weekends. However, numerous international policy directives such as the seminal *Ottawa Charter* (WHO, 1986) and national public health policy papers such as *The future of public health* (Department for Health and Social Care, 2020) have emphasised the need for more people-centred health promotion and being responsive to the health needs of local communities. For example, the UK government's view of the future of public health, positions communities at the forefront using a 'local first' approach that reacts quickly to the needs of local people. The implications of these values are clear. People have the right to participate in making decisions about their health and should be enabled to do so. The needs, wants, and expectations of individuals, families, and communities should be respected by health promoters and public health practitioners and influence priority setting and the delivery of health promotion services. You can measure how user friendly your services are by undertaking Exercise 6.1.

Let us now return to the central question: How are the needs for health promotion and public health practice identified?

EXERCISE 6.1   Using Services That Promote Health or Prevent Ill Health: User Views

Find out about some services available locally, designed for the public, which aim to promote health and wellbeing or prevent ill health. The public library, NHS trust, or local council, for example, may be able to provide information about what services are available. These could include swimming facilities, exercise classes, weight support, or smoking cessation classes or be part of the services, campaigns, or activities of your local public health departments.

Select one of these that are appropriate and acceptable to you and visit it. Make notes about what happens and how the service was responsive to its users.

See also the section on working for quality in Chapter 8 for information on quality in health promotion and public health services.

- Is it easy to find out that the service exists?
- Is it easy to locate with clear signposting where needed?
- Is public transport easily available? Is there easy access for parking your car?
- Are the times convenient to you?
- If there is a charge for the service? Is it affordable and a good value for money?
- How are you welcomed? Are you given all the information you need? Do you feel at ease? Are the health promoters or public health practitioners friendly?
- What do you think about the environment? Is it safe, clean, and comfortable?
- What do you think about the quality of the service you received? Do you have any ideas about how it could be improved? Will you use this service again?
- What have you learned as a service user which you can now apply to health promotion and public health practice?

These values suggest that key characteristics of people-centred health promotion and public health practice might include the following:

For individuals, communities, and population groups:
- Access to clear, concise, and intelligible health information and education that increase health literacy and enable needs to be expressed.
- Equitable access to health, including treatments and psychosocial support.
- Development of personal skills which allow control over health and engagement with healthcare systems: Communication, mutual collaboration and respect, goal setting, decision making, problem solving, and self-care.
- Supported involvement in health decision making, including health policy.

For health promotion and public health practitioners and specialists:
- Holistic understanding and approach to health improvement.
- Respect for people and their decisions.
- Recognition of the needs of people seeking to improve their health.
- Professional and personal skills to meet these needs: competence in promoting health, communication, mutual collaboration and respect, empathy, responsiveness, and sensitivity.
- Commitment and adherence to quality, evidence-informed decision making, and practice and ethical practice.
- Teamwork, collaboration, and partnership across organisations and professional disciplines and with clients.

FINDING AND USING INFORMATION

The starting point for defining health promotion and public health practice needs is information of various kinds from a range of sources. If you are gathering information on a local area for the first time, it would be helpful to share the work and the findings with colleagues. For example, health visitors may have done a neighbourhood profile as part of their training; the public health department in the local authority (LA) will probably have health data on the local population. Gathering and updating all these different kinds of information is an ongoing project for every health promoter, and sharing the task is a more efficient use of time. Working with colleagues needs to be done in conjunction with establishing links with local people to ensure the active participation of users and receivers.

There are a number of different kinds of information you can access when identifying need.

Epidemiological Data

Epidemiology is the key quantitative discipline that underpins public health. It is the study of the distribution and determinants of disease in communities. Epidemiological data indicate how many people are affected by a health problem, how many people die from a particular health problem, and who are most at risk within sex, age, ethnic, socioeconomic, occupational or geographical groupings or perhaps by taking account of lifestyle factors such as smoking or physical activity levels or personal characteristics such as weight.

Detailed discussion of the sources and limitations of epidemiological data is outside the scope of this book, but for texts on epidemiology, see for example, Stewart (2022). The important point to make here is that epidemiological data provide essential information on the health of the population, the causes and risk factors related to ill health, and, in doing this, highlights the potential for prevention and health promotion.

Mortality and morbidity data are collected nationally, and some data are also available on a regional and local basis. Mortality data are concerned with causes of death, whereas morbidity data are concerned with types of illness and disability. Mortality data are derived from death certificates; morbidity data are derived from a wide range of sources, including medical records, sickness absence certificates, child health records, returns of notifiable diseases, disability registers, and many others. In addition, the Office for National Statistics (ONS) is the UK's largest independent producer of official statistics and the recognised national statistical institute for the UK. It is responsible for collecting and publishing statistics related to the economy, population (and population health), and society at national, regional, and local levels (see Office for National Statistics, 2022 for specific data on wellbeing). Other health surveys carried out for research purposes by, for example, university research centres provide a considerable amount of health statistics and information (see the Global Health & Development Group, Imperial College London, 2022).

- Your local NHS organisation, such as a trust, and the LA will have information about the local population, including mortality and morbidity data (such as hospital admission rates for particular conditions). This may be broken down to the level of the population of smaller areas such as electoral wards. It might be helpful to compare data for the whole population and electoral ward data (for a neighbourhood) on, for example the major causes of mortality.
- The key causes of childhood admission to hospital.
- The main conditions for which adults are admitted to hospital.

In England, local government organisations will also have assessed the health and wellbeing needs of people in their geographical scope (adults, young people, and children) through a Joint Strategic Needs Assessment process. The data from this will have been used to produce a Joint Health and Wellbeing Strategy, which will have set out the priorities for action based on the health and wellbeing needs identified.

Exercise 6.2 is designed to enable you to find out about local health information.

Lifestyle Data

An increasing amount of information about people's health-related behaviour and lifestyles, such as physical activity, sexual behaviour, smoking, and drinking, is available on a national basis from survey data. See for example, the Schools and Students Health Education Unit surveys (http://www.sheu.org.uk) which have up to date data on the lifestyle of young people at school. There are active surveys that date back to 1977 and therefore act as valuable benchmarks. You may also find that a LA or regional NHS organisation has done a lifestyle survey of your local population and published the findings (see for a good example, NHS Digital, 2021).

Socioeconomic Data

The planning or information departments of local government departments should be able to help with information about housing, employment, social class, and social/leisure/recreation/shopping facilities. Many produce

---

EXERCISE 6.2   Gathering Local Public Health Information

Undertake an internet search of your local NHS organisations, such as your local trust and LA (or equivalent in Scotland, Wales, and Northern Ireland), for reports or data on the health status of your local population. Some local data may also be available on national websites such as fingertips (see web address at the end of the chapter). Browse through the data and see if you can find out the following for your local population:

- What are the major causes of death?
- What are the major reasons for people to be admitted to hospital?
- What are the major risk factors for ill health? For example, is there information on what percentage of people smoke in your local population or are living in poverty?
- How many people have had communicable diseases (diseases caught from other people), such as measles or sexually transmitted infections?
- Which neighbourhoods or communities have the poorest health? How is health being measured?
- What steps are being taken to achieve the local health and wellbeing strategy and prevent ill health and promote good health?

Can you find information on anything else to help you in your health promotion and public health work?

---

summaries of census data. It might be helpful to compare district/borough/city and electoral ward data on social and economic factors such as:

- Unemployment
- Household amenities
- Income
- Ethnicity

It is advisable to ask for figures that are as full and recent as possible. Much information is obtained from the national census, which takes place every ten years. Information from the analysis of public health data is also available at the government resource called 'fingertips' (https://fingertips.phe.org.uk/), which organises data usefully into thematic areas of interest to public health professionals.

By setting illness data alongside social and economic data, you may be able to see patterns that might inform your needs identification and priority setting process. You may want, for example, to determine if areas where people with less financial and other resources live are also likely to be the areas of the poorest health. For international

comparisons, statistics can be gleaned from, for example, the World Health Organisation's global observatory (WHO, 2021).

Professional Views

The views of the wider public health workforce reflect experiences and perceptions accumulated over the years, which would be foolish to ignore. What do other professionals in your geographical area, such as teachers, youth workers, social workers, general practitioners (GPs), health visitors, district nurses, environmental health officers, police officers, community workers, and religious leaders, consider the major health concerns?

Public Views

Public sector organisations are now charged with the responsibility of seeking the views of the communities that they serve, but some organisations have developed good practice in this area over a number of years. Try contacting the local government in your area for information on this type of work, such as Citizens' Panels, which are representative samples of residents who give their views on local services, priorities, and plans (for an example of the work of Citizens' Panels, see Subica and Brown, 2020 or perhaps look at your own local council website).

There is more about research methods for finding out people's views in Chapter 7, section on doing your own small scale research.

There are several methods of obtaining the views of the public, from informal discussions/interviews to large-scale surveys using questionnaires or in-depth interview techniques. Identifying priority groups and thinking clearly about them will influence the choice of methods used to contact and involve them.

It is best to start with the characteristics of the groups and then design the best approach. For instance, how large are the relevant groups? Do they have particular age, class or ethnic structures? What makes it a group (geography, membership, current use of services and facilities)? Are the members of the group mobile? Do they have easy access to transport? What times of day are they likely to be available for meetings? Be absolutely clear about what sort of relationship you are proposing to have with local groups and individuals. For example, if you plan simply to establish consultation mechanisms, there may be hostility if local people have played a much stronger partnership role in the past. Public consultation and involvement are discussed in detail in Chapter 15.

The groups involved may include local Health Watch (see Healthwatch England, 2021 and Case study 6.1) – an organisation which seeks to support more people to have

CASE STUDY 6.1   Big Leeds Chat

The aim of the Big Leeds Chat was to tour the city and to hear what people think about living in Leeds, and to show the communities that the health and care system is working together and taking note of their concerns. The Big Leeds Chat is a 'conversation' about what matters to local people. People were asked three questions:

- What do you love about living in Leeds?
- What do you do to stay healthy?
- What would you like to see change to make Leeds an even better city to live in?

The conversations highlighted how much people enjoyed living in the city of Leeds, but there were some concerns about public transport infrastructure, and not everyone knew what was happening in their local places. Often the cost of healthy activities was a barrier to health and wellbeing for people. The recommendations from the Big Leeds Chat are being taken forward and discussed with strategic leaders in the city.

Source: Healthwatch Leeds (2022).

their say and provide clear information and advice to help them take control of their health and care. Other groups involved could comprise of local voluntary organisations and community groups such as self-help groups, black and minority ethnic groups, pensioners' clubs, tenants' associations, and a variety of local advisory groups or planning subcommittees, in addition to groups of key clients such as parents. Gathering views informally is useful, but there are problems in ensuring accuracy, and that subjective information is representative. However, these subjective data can usefully feed into the wider picture.

You might want to consider undertaking some first-hand research but first think about how much time and money it will take. Will the results justify the costs? If you still think it is worth doing, who could do it? If it is very small scale, you could perhaps undertake it yourself, maybe in collaboration with some colleagues.

Local and National Media and Social Media

The opinions and data collected from local and national media will provide you with a picture at a particular point in time. Monitoring radio, TV, newspapers, webpages, Twitter, and Facebook pages (particularly those focusing on specific community issues) will give a view of any major needs in the community. All this adds to the profile of needs you are building up, providing a basis for planning health promotion and public health action.

ASSESSING HEALTH PROMOTION AND PUBLIC HEALTH PRACTICE NEEDS

The assessment of health promotion and public health needs can be approached systematically by asking a series of key questions. The answers will help you to decide whether you should respond to a particular need and, if so, how.

1. What Type of Need Is It?

Is this a normative, felt, expressed, or comparative health need?

In a sex education class in a school, for example, what kind of need is being met: the **normative needs** decided by the school nurse or the personal, social, health, and citizenship education (PSHCE) teaching team or the school governors; or the **felt or expressed needs** of the school pupils or their parents; or the **comparative needs** decided after comparing the PSHCE curriculum in other schools; or for example, when teenage pregnancy rates in a local area are compared to national figures and suggest a need for more work on contraception?

2. Who Decided That There Is a Need?

Whose decision is it: The health promoter/public health practitioner, the individual or target group, or both?

Sometimes the answer to this question is not immediately obvious because the need has emerged after a discussion between the health promoter/public health practitioner and their clients. People do not always know what they need or want because their awareness and knowledge of the possibilities are limited. The health promoter may help by raising awareness and knowledge of health issues; in this way, they may create a demand (an expressed need) for health promotion. For example, the public's demand for non-smoking in restaurants came only after health promoters had raised awareness of the hazards of passive smoking, which motivated people to express their need for a smoke-free environment in eateries. An ideal situation is when there is a synergy between the client's, health promoter's and public health practitioner's needs.

3. What are the Grounds for Deciding That There Is a Need?

Is there any evidence of need in the form of objective data? If local data are not available, has the information been collected in other localities and is it reasonable to assume that the same conditions will apply? Be aware that gathering data can be a delaying tactic to avoid doing something about an obvious problem. For example, surveys have shown that elderly people without cars find it difficult to get to hospitals if public transport is poor. It is reasonable to assume that this applies in most localities with poor public transport. So, collect information only if the answer to a question is really not known. Have the views of the clients been sought? Do they see this as a need?

4. What are the Aims and the Appropriate Response to the Need?

See the section on setting aims and objectives in Chapter 5 for a more detailed look at setting aims and objectives and identifying appropriate ways of achieving them.

Health promotion and public health cannot solve all problems or meet all health needs. You should be clear on what the need is, then what your aims are for meeting that need, then the appropriate way to meet it. For example, there may be an identified normative need to increase the uptake of immunisation and aim to achieve an 80% uptake rate. You then have to decide the appropriate way to achieve your aim. It would be all too easy in this case to say that there is a need for a health education campaign to get parents to have their children immunised because messages about attending immunisation clinics may be seen to be the answer. But this may make no difference because the appropriate response is to educate the health professionals who are being too cautious and withholding immunisation wrongly when a child has only a mild contraindication or to move the time and/or location of the clinics so that working parents, and those without cars, are able to bring their children.

Case study 6.2 is an example of how the need for health promotion and public health practice is assessed, applying the four assessment questions.

CASE STUDY 6.2   Eat 4 Health

Background
The levels of obesity in Western Berkshire are higher than the national average and are a cause for concern as a number of severe and chronic medical conditions are associated with being overweight and obesity, including type 2 diabetes, hypertension, coronary heart disease, stroke, osteoarthritis, and some cancers (West Berkshire JSNA [Joint Strategic Needs Assessment], 2015).

Body mass index (BMI) is a strong predictor of premature mortality among adults. Overall moderate obesity (BMI 30 to 35 kg/m^2) was found to reduce life expectancy by an average of three years. While morbid obesity (40 to 50 kg/m^2) reduces life expectancy by eight to ten years, research shows that 19% of adults in Reading (Reading JSNA, 2016), 18.5% of adults in West Berkshire (West Berkshire JSNA, 2015), and 19.7% of adults in Wokingham (Wokingham JSNA, 2012) are obese, whereas 55.3% of adults in Reading, 65.5% of adults in West Berkshire and 57.4% of adults in Wokingham are overweight.

Levels of physical activity are closely linked to the prevalence of obesity, with fewer people taking enough exercise to maintain a healthy weight. Research shows that 56.6% of adults in Reading, 55.4% of adults in West Berkshire and 62.3% of adults in Wokingham are physically active.

What Type of Need Is It?
Assist residents of West Berkshire to access a community-based weight management programme and achieve long-term weight loss. The underlying principles of the programme are based on NICE guidelines, including the principle of behavioural change and self-management.

Who Decided There Is a Need?
- The local public health specialists and practitioners acting on national policy directives decided there was a need for this initiative. The main aims and outcomes of national policy directives were to decrease the percentage of adults who are overweight or obese in West Berkshire.
- To help adults who have a BMI > 25 to decrease their weight to become a healthy weight and maintain their weight.
- To increase the percentage of adults eating a healthy diet.
- To increase the percentage of adults being moderately physically active for 30 min per day on most days of the week.
- To decrease the rates of coronary heart disease, stroke, diabetes, hypertension, osteoarthritis and some cancers in West Berkshire.

What are the Grounds for Deciding there is a Need?
The grounds for deciding that there was a need to provide weight management programmes across West Berkshire was the above average overweight and obesity levels across the area and low uptake of physical activity.

CASE STUDY 6.2 Eat 4 Health—Cont'd

What are the Aims and Appropriate Response to the Need?

The aim and appropriate response is to provide an accessible tier two lifestyle adult weight management programme service for overweight and obese adults aged 16 and over within the locality, which forms an integral part of the weight management care pathway.

The Eat 4 Health programme is adapted to ensure it is appropriate for different cultures. Courses are delivered in many different languages, including English, Urdu, Hindi, and Nepalese, ensuring the service is provided to groups that are usually hard to reach. Eat 4 Health has also developed different resources, including recipes, snacking and cooking guidance specific to different cultures and traditions to support participants in making changes towards a healthier diet. Eat 4 Health targets local high footfall events, including local Caribbean and Diwali events, to increase accessibility for hard to reach groups.

The team have been active in taking the Eat 4 Health programme into the heart of the community through the provision of sessions and outreach in some of the most deprived areas in West Berkshire.

Courses are held in a range of different locations, including evenings to increase accessibility.

Target outreach has been held in a number of different surgery waiting rooms across GP surgeries in West Berkshire. This is a great opportunity to engage with patients at a time when they are receptive to bettering their health.

Training is delivered to local GP surgery staff to ensure they have appropriate knowledge of Eat 4 Health services in their local area. The training session also equips practice staff with the skills to raise the issue of weight with patients and motivate them to join a local service.

Monthly newsletters are distributed to GP practices across Berkshire to increase interest and maintain engagement.

Case study prepared by Leena Sankla, Solutions4Health, Reading, Berkshire, UK.

SETTING HEALTH PROMOTION AND PUBLIC HEALTH PRIORITIES

You may have a large number of needs that you feel should be met, but there are always constraints on resources such as time and finance. Concentrating effort on priority areas is essential to ensure quality and effectiveness.

Before attempting to set priorities, it is helpful to analyse current practice and recognise the wide range of criteria that will affect decisions about health promotion interventions. Undertaking Exercises 6.3 and 6.4 enables you to focus on these factors.

The need to prioritise is vital, but one difficult issue to consider is how to approach work with people whose health experience is poor.

It is automatic to consider that these people should be a top priority, but it is important to consider whether focusing all health promotion efforts on those most at risk will, in the end, be of greatest benefit.

When reducing the incidence of coronary heart disease, for example, two broad approaches can be used: the *high-risk* and the *whole population* approaches. The high-risk approach identifies people particularly at risk, such as smokers, people who are obese or who have high blood pressure and develops interventions with these people to change lifestyle factors and treat their raised blood pressure, for example. But there may be poor return for effort, as these groups could include addictive smokers with poor diets who have no intention of changing or people so overwhelmed with social and/or psychological issues in their lives that tackling smoking and eating habits is too difficult, even if they would like to make changes.

The whole population approach works at the community rather than individual level, with, for example, strategies to improve access to cheap healthy food, increase skills and confidence in producing healthy meals for families, and community development approaches to build up social support. At the same time, supporting changes at a wider population level, such as reducing the underage sales of cigarettes, and lobbying for increased income support, could result in better health gain across whole populations.

Generally, both approaches need to be taken (not necessarily by the same health promoters), as they complement each other. This is why developing partnership working is so important, as it allows different aspects of the same issue to be addressed by the health promoters who are best placed to tackle a particular aspect at a particular time, thus achieving a greater impact.

There can be no exact method for setting priorities because they ultimately depend upon the normative judgements and the available resources of the health

---

EXERCISE 6.3   Analysing the Reasons for Health Promotion and Public Health Practitioner Priorities

Identify a health promotion activity that has a high priority in your work. This could be work that you undertake with a number of clients (such as a social prescribing programme) or just one (for example, a health visitor talking to a mother about maintaining breastfeeding); it could be part of your usual work or a special event such as a campaign. It will be especially helpful for the purposes of this exercise if you can identify an area of work that has recently become a priority.

Now work through the following tasks.

1. Identify who it was who decided that this work should take priority (e.g. You? Your manager(s)? Your clients? All three?).

2. List all the possible reasons why this work has priority; include the reasons that you are sure about, as well as any that are speculation.

Your reasons could include any of the following and probably many more:

- I feel that it is an important public health issue.
- It is the established public health priority of senior managers.

- We have always had it as a priority and see no reason to change.
- There was pressure from the public.
- It was in response to a public health crisis.
- There is new evidence of need.
- There is evidence that the work has been effective in a similar area.
- It was the current national/local theme (e.g. World Mental Health Day).
- We had a new staff member with special expertise, which we wanted to use.
- We had to economise and be more efficient.
- It was politically expedient.
- There was a change in national public health policy or local public health strategy.

3. Identify what you think the most important reasons are. Do you think that they are sound reasons for setting priorities?

EXERCISE 6.4   Setting Priorities For Health Promotion and Public Health Practice

1. Health promotion issues, approaches, and activities

Do you define your priorities in terms of:

- Issues that have an influence on health (the wider determinants such as poverty, unemployment, racism, ageism, and inequalities)?
- Health promotion approaches (such as medical, behaviour change, social marketing, educational, client-centred, societal/environmental change)?
- Health promotion activities (preventive health services, community-based work, organisational development, economic and regulatory activities, environmental measures, health education programmes, healthy public policies)?
- Health problems (such as heart disease, food poisoning, cancers, HIV/AIDS, obesity, mental illness)? Why?

2. Consumer/target groups

Who are the people your health promotion/public health practice is aimed at?

- Policy makers and planners?
- Individual clients or service users?

- Families?
- Selected target groups?
- The whole community? If so, how do you define your community? Why?

3. Age groups

Do you define your target groups further in terms of age: children, young people, older people? Why?

4. At risk groups

- Do you define your target groups further in terms of high-risk categories such as smokers, people with high blood pressure, the unemployed, or those living on low incomes? If so, why? Have you examined the evidence leading to the identification of these at risk groups?
- If your group includes people with the highest health needs, for example, people living in areas of social deprivation with many health and social needs, do you know whether there is evidence that work focusing on specific issues will be successful? Would you get more health gain for your effort if you focused on whole populations rather than those most in need?

EXERCISE 6.4   Setting Priorities For Health Promotion and Public Health Practice—Cont'd

5. Effectiveness
- Have you any evidence that health promotion in your priority areas is likely to be effective?

See Chapter 7 for information on how to collect evidence.
- Have you any evidence that it will provide value for money?
- How could such evidence be collected?

6. Feasibility
- Is it feasible for you to spend time with your priority groups?
- Do you have access to these groups?
- Do you have credibility with these groups?
- Do you have the skills and resources to work with these groups?

7. Working with others
- Do you know what work is already being done with your target groups by other health promoters/public health practitioners, community groups, and voluntary organisations?

- Are you sure that your work will complement other public health activities that are going on and not be seen as duplication or interference?
- Does your work fit in with existing local and national public health strategies and plans for health promotion?
- Are there any local partnership groups already set up to address the needs of your target group?

8. Ethics
- Are there ethical aspects to your work which you need to consider?
- Is your work ethically acceptable to you?
- Will it be acceptable to your consumer groups?
- Will it be congruent with their values?
- How may the desired outcome affect their lives?

9. Add anything else you feel is important to consider
Now identify your top priority and add any other priorities.

---

promoters involved. But it may be helpful to work through the checklist in Exercise 6.4.

PRACTICE POINTS

- You will have some scope for making choices about the range of health promotion and public health activities you undertake. These choices must be based on a careful assessment of public health needs. The starting point is to undertake a needs identification process.
- The views of users and receivers of services are paramount; therefore, developing skills in gathering information directly from them is especially important.
- You can assess public health needs systematically by asking four key questions: What kind of need is it? Who decided that there was a need? What is the evidence for deciding that there is a need? What is the appropriate response to the need?
- Health promoters and public health practitioners have a duty to reassess priorities regularly by analysing whether your activities are targeted effectively, are feasible, complement the work of other practitioners and are acceptable to local people.
- Priorities depend ultimately on the normative judgements of those involved. Best practice involves in-depth discussion on priority setting with other health promotion and public health practitioners and local people.

References

Ashby, J., Ahmed, N., & Goldmeier, D. (2019). Sexual difficulties service provision within sexual health services in the UK: a casualty of postcode lottery and commissioning? *Sexually Transmitted Infections*, *95*(6). 397–397. http://dx.doi.org/10.1136/sextrans-2019-054186.

Bradshaw, J. R. (1972). A taxonomy of social need. In G. McLachlan (Ed.), *Problems and progress in medical care*. Oxford: Oxford University Press.

De Camargo, C. (2021). The postcode lottery of safety: COVID-19 guidance and shortages of personal protective equipment (PPE) for UK police officers. *The Police Journal*, 1–25.

Department of Health and Social Care, (2020). *The future of public health: the National Institute for Health Protection and other public health functions*. London: Crown.

Dorling, D. (2019). *Inequality and the 1%*. London: Verso Books.

Healthwatch, (2021). *Our strategy 2021-2026*. London: Healthwatch.

Healthwatch Leeds (2022). https://healthwatchleeds.co.uk

Imperial College London. (2022). *Global health & development group*. https://www.imperial.ac.uk/mrc-global-infectious-disease-analysis/hosted-initiatives-and-groups/global-health-development-group/

NHS Choices. (2020). *Personal health budgets*. http://www.nhs.uk/choiceintheNHS/Yourchoices/personal-health-budgets/Pages/about-personal-health-budgets.aspx

NHS Digital. (2021). *Lifestyles*. https://digital.nhs.uk/data-and-information/areas-of-interest/public-health/lifestyles

NICE. (2016). *Home care for older people, NICE quality standard [QS123] June 2016*. https://www.nice.org.uk/guidance/qs123

Office for National Statistics. (2022). *Personal well-being in the UK, quarterly: April 2011 to September 2021*. https://www.ons.gov.uk/peoplepopulationandcommunity/wellbeing/bulletins/personalwellbeingintheukquarterly/april2011toseptember20212013-01-30

Reading Borough Council. (2016). Reading Joint Strategic Needs Assessment. https://www.reading.gov.uk/about-reading/joint-strategic-needs-assessment-jsna/

Scriven, A. (2002). *Report of the survey into the impact of recent national health policies on specialist health promotion services in England*. London: Brunel University.

Srinivas, G., Maanasa, R., Meenakshi, M., Adaikalam, J. M., Seshayyan, S., & Muthuvel, T. (2021). Ethical rationing of healthcare resources during COVID-19 outbreak. *Ethics, Medicine and Public Health*, *16*, 100633.

Stephenson, J. (2016). *Charity nurses warn of 'postcode lottery' in specialist children's care*. Nursing Times. http://www.nursingtimes.net/news/workforce/specialist-childrens-nurses-warn-of-postcode-lottery/7004943.article?blocktitle=Today%27s-headlines&contentID=19152

Stewart, A. (2022). *Basic statistics and epidemiology: a practical guide*. London: CRC Press.

Subica, A. M., & Brown, B. J. (2020). Addressing health disparities through deliberative methods: citizens' panels for health equity. *American Journal of Public Health*, *110*(2), 166–173.

UK Health Security Agency. (2022). *COVID-19 vaccination programme*. https://www.gov.uk/government/collections/covid-19-vaccination-programme

West Berkshire Council. (2015). West Berkshire Joint Strategic Needs Assessment. https://www.westberks.gov.uk/article/40912/Joint-Strategic-Needs-Assessment-JSNA

Wokingham Borough Coucil. (2012) Wokingham Joint Strategic Needs Assessment. (2012). http://jsna.wokingham.gov.uk/living-and-working-well/overweight-and-obese-adults/

World Health Organisation, (1986). *The Ottawa charter for health promotion*. Geneva: World Health Organisation.

World Health Organisation, (2021). *World health statistics 2021: monitoring health for the SDGs*. Geneva: World Health Organisation.

Websites

NICE. For evidence and advice on what interventions works. http://www.nice.org.uk

Office of National StatisticsFor a wide range of people, population and community data. https://www.ons.gov.uk/peoplepopulationandcommunity

SHEU Lifestyle survey results. http://sheu.org.uk/content/page/lifestyle-surveys

For local health and social statistics. http://www.neighbourhood.statistics.gov.uk

WHO Global Health Observatory For international comparison data. http://www.who.int/gho/en/

For UK public health profiles. https://fingertips.phe.org.uk/

Facebook

ONS For up-to-date notifications on national health and wellbeing statistics. https://www.facebook.com/ONS

The Local Government Association. https://www.facebook.com/LocalGovAssoc/

Twitter

ONSNotification of data and discussion of national (England and Wales) health statistics. https://twitter.com/ONS

Healthwatch England. https://twitter.com/HealthwatchE

Evidence and Research for Health Promotion and Public Health Practice

Gareth Morgan, Angela Scriven

CHAPTER OUTLINE

SUMMARY

This chapter covers several aspects of knowledge and skills relating to evidence and research. This will help equip and enable you to draw appropriately on evidence, undertake research, and use various techniques to inform and prioritise your health promotion and public health practice work. This will include basing your work on the evidence of effectiveness, using published research, doing your own small-scale research within your professional setting, getting value for money from the programme budget, conducting audits, and doing a health impact assessment (HIA).

EVIDENCE-INFORMED HEALTH PROMOTION AND PUBLIC HEALTH PRACTICE

Evidence is essential to underpin robust international, national and local public health strategies and policies that practitioners act on in the course of their professional duties. Many of these policies charge those with a responsibility for promoting health to adopt an evidence-informed approach to their work. The opposite also clearly applies, namely, delivering a project without supporting evidence is inappropriate, counterfactual and may even have the potential to be harmful, at least by using resources that would have other beneficial uses.

As an example of being evidence-informed, the Public Health England five-year strategy 2020-25 sets out several interventions that are supported by evidence, such as a smoke-free society, healthier diets and weight, clean air and better mental health (PHE, 2019). Therefore, it is essential for health promoters and public health practitioners to know how to access, assess and apply the evidence to practice. It is also important to be able to identify circumstances where a project lacks an evidence base and to introduce corrective measures as appropriate. This might include, for example, highlighting concerns and making recommendations to modify or improve the delivery of the work being done.

There are some key competencies required to deliver evidence-informed practice, including:
- Knowledge of the hierarchy of evidence and an ability to recognise different types of evidence.
- Understanding and critically appraising primary and secondary research.
- Critically assessing the robustness of evidence relating to the effectiveness of services, programmes and interventions which impact upon health.
- Conducting a literature search and producing a review, which includes the i) use of electronic databases, ii) defining a search strategy and iii) summarising and applying the results to practice.
- Applying research evidence, evidence of effectiveness, outcome measures, evaluation and audit to influence a variety of situations, including public health programme interventions, services or development of practice guidelines.

- Interpreting and balancing evidence of effectiveness from a range of sources to inform decision-making.
- Delineate conflicting and contested evidence.

An evidence-informed approach provides a framework to guard against the indiscriminate use of practices in situations which have no research based legitimacy. Evidence-based health promotion and public health practice is also predicated on a culture where you openly share your experience. This includes writing up and publishing or producing a report on your work, which enables others to learn from your successes and failures. It uses the skills of reflective practice, thinking about what you do and questioning whether it is the right approach as well as whether it also offers value for money. This is important in regard to accountability, and there are several practical ways of undertaking reflective practice within a busy work environment (Health and Care Professions Council [HCPC], 2022).

What Health Promotion and Public Health Interventions Work?

There can be a gap between evidence and practice. The research on a particular topic may need to evolve quickly, such as during the COVID-19 pandemic. Therefore, it may be challenging for health promoters and public health practitioners to keep updated with new research findings or apply them in their own situation. Sometimes, research is incomplete and may need to evolve over time; for example, we may continue to have gaps in knowledge on long COVID for many years to come as in this situation, there will need to be longer term follow-up, such as cohort studies, which follow populations over time. As the name suggests, long COVID refers to the ongoing effects of the viral Infection, which may not become clear until years of research have been accumulated. Indeed, an urgent need for more research on long COVID has been highlighted (Michelen et al., 2021).

Attention, therefore, needs to be given to how research findings can best influence and emerge from practice, as well as the processes of disseminating and implementing health promotion and public health research. There are many published research studies, and there are organisations that provide summaries of which health promotion interventions work best, as shown in Box 7.1.

In addition to online evidence websites, there are also many tools and models online to help you engage in an evidence-informed approach. The National Collaborating Centre for Methods and Tools (NCCMT, 2021) offers a range of excellent models, tools, and resources (see the website at the end of the chapter). For an example of one model, see Fig. 7.1 along with the explanatory notes and then undertake Exercise 7.1 to research further models.

BOX 7.1   Sources of Published Research on Health Promotion Interventions

Cochrane Library is a collection of high-quality, independent evidence to inform healthcare decision-making.

The National Institute for Health and Care Excellence (NICE) offers guidance, advice, and information service for health, public health, and social care professionals.

Strategic Health Asset Planning and Evaluation (SHAPE) is a web enabled, evidence-based application that informs and supports the strategic planning of services.

The King's Fund is an English health charity that shapes health and social care policy and practice.

The Health Foundation is an independent charity committed to bringing about better health and healthcare for people in the United Kingdom (UK).

The Joseph Rowntree Foundation is an independent social change organisation working to solve UK poverty.

The websites for these organisations are listed at the end of the chapter.

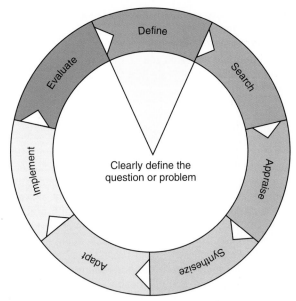

Fig 7.1 Model of the steps in evidence-informed health promotion and public health practice. Source: NCCMT. (2021). Evidence-informed decision-making in public health.

Notes on Fig. 7.1 – The seven-stage model of evidence-informed health promotion and public health practice
Stage 1. Define – Clearly define the issue or problem.
'Who is my target group? What is the issue we are dealing with? What interventions are we considering?

What specifically are we trying to change or understand?'

The more specific you are in framing the question, the easier it will be to search for relevant information. Quantitative questions about the effectiveness of a possible intervention should include four elements population, intervention, comparison and outcome. Quantitative questions about exposure should include population, exposure, comparison and outcome. Qualitative questions should identify the population and situation.

Stage 2. Search – Efficiently search for research evidence.
'Where should I look to find the best available research evidence to address the issue?'

Your search strategy should first aim to locate the strongest quality and most relevant evidence. When searching for quantitative evidence (e.g. effectiveness of an intervention, health effects, cost-effectiveness), some study designs (such as randomised trials or cohort studies) are considered stronger than others. It is important that the research design is the most appropriate to answer the question being asked.

Stage 3. Appraise – Critically and efficiently appraise the research sources.
'Were the methods used in this study good enough for me to be confident in the findings?'

Different types of public health questions will require distinct research designs. Critical appraisal tools can be applied to assess the quality and relevance of each type of research question.

Stage 4. Synthesize – Interpret information and/or form recommendations for practice based on the relevant literature found.
'What does the research evidence tell me about the issue?'

Decipher the 'actionable messages' (i.e. clear recommendations or actions for practice) from the research evidence that you have reviewed. Base recommendations on the highest quality and most synthesized research evidence available.

Stage 5. Adapt – Adapt the information to a local context.
'Can I use this research with my client, community or population?'

Having developed 'actionable messages', you can now tailor those messages to ensure their relevance and suitability for the local community.

Stage 6. Implement – Decide whether (and plan how) to implement the adapted evidence in practice or policy.
'How will I use the research evidence in my practice?'

The implementation plan uses the adapted research evidence to create a tangible plan of action to create a change in practice, policy or to deliver a new programme.

This step focuses on identifying how to use the adapted evidence in your local setting.

Stage 7. Evaluate – Assess the effectiveness of the implementation efforts.
'Did we do what we planned to do? Did we achieve what we expected?'

Evaluate the intervention (programme evaluation), if applicable and the implementation strategies (the knowledge translation strategy).

Source: NCCMT, 2021

Promoting health is complex, and it is sometimes difficult to provide evidence of effectiveness for single interventions. This is because it is often not one intervention that produces results but a combination of public health activities of which you may be involved in just one. An example of this complexity is the UK Government's range of strategies targeting COVID-19 as an endemic infection (HM Government, 2022). Endemic means that the virus and ongoing infection will continue to remain in the community. The strategies encompass:

- Living with COVID-19 by encouraging safer behaviours.
- Protecting the most vulnerable, such as those with a chronic illness.
- Maintaining resilience, including ongoing monitoring.
- Securing innovations and opportunities from the response.

Safer behaviours might include wearing a face covering in crowded or enclosed spaces, whereas protecting the most vulnerable includes a national vaccination programme, trying to boost 'herd immunity' and build sufficient resistance to break chains of transmission. It may be difficult to isolate and evaluate what each element makes to reducing COVID-19 numbers. In practice, many health promotion interventions require a combination of approaches, and you may be asked to contribute to a single element or perhaps several parts of a project.

EXERCISE 7.1

Consider the model and the explanatory notes of the steps in evidence-informed health promotion and public health practice outlined in Fig. 7.1. Is this a suitable model for use in your health-promoting practice? Undertake a search of the internet for other evidence-informed practice models and compare the one in Fig. 7.1 to these and the planning model, Fig. 5.1, in Chapter 5. What are the similarities? What are the differences? Which is the best for your practice?

To take another example of the complexity in promoting health, reducing health inequalities requires action at many levels. The World Health Organisation recognises numerous social determinants which require a comprehensive and integrated intervention (WHO, 2022a). Strategies require action from all sectors and civil society, plus changes to such things as the environment as well as legislative and fiscal policies.

Evidence may also not exist or may be unclear. The piece of work you plan to undertake may not have been done before, or perhaps the specific set of circumstances in which you are working may be unique. In such circumstances, it is important to be aware of what the published research in related areas of work tells you and to reflect critically on how this might apply to your circumstances. If evidence is not available, it is vital to ensure that you evaluate your work to add to the evidence base by organising the evidence from your practice and disseminating the results. Work-based evaluation and research can offer a vital contribution to knowledge and is a worthwhile undertaking (Black et al., 2019). Whilst the focus has often been on the translation of evidence into practice, the reverse is also important.

It also helps to think carefully about what constitutes evidence in public health. Public health evidence often derives from a variety of sources, including cross-sectional studies, quasi-experimental studies and intervention evaluations, rather than the gold standard of randomised controlled trials that are often used in clinical medicine. Study designs in public health sometimes lack a comparison group, so the interpretation of study results may have to account for different types of variables, such as the local demographics of the community, which might include whether this is in a rural or urban setting. All these factors might need to be considered as part of the interpretation of a study.

As already highlighted, public health interventions are seldom a single intervention and are often alongside large-scale environmental or policy changes, such as disease prevention in urban environments (D'Allesandra, 2020). As was seen in the COVID-19 pandemic, there are also often competing priorities and political judgements that need to balance both the scientific and non-scientific considerations that influence public health, such as the economy (Basu, 2021).

Evidence can also be drawn informally, with the views of local people and your own experience also constituting a valid source of evidence. Gathering this into a useful summary can help generate ideas or further research. Your job as a health promoter or public health practitioner is to use your judgement to decide whether the evidence available applies to your project and, if so, how. For example,

GPs may quote several factors which they believe provide evidence that health promotion is effective, including changes in the health or health behaviour of their patients over time. This may be based on individual perceptions and experience of working with individual patients, which can still be valuable information.

However, formal sources of evidence are generally regarded as the most reliable, so you should plan carefully and evaluate or audit what you do. In this way, you will be building up your own body of knowledge about what is effective. Replication is also a key consideration, so repeating work can be helpful, and this could also be undertaken via audit, which is covered later in this chapter.

Finally, it is also important to bear in mind that your decision about whether to do a particular piece of health promotion work should also be based on ethical considerations. You could decide that it is your responsibility to intervene, even though you have little or no information about what might work. If you are part of a team, then raising this at a meeting could be helpful in determining the course of action. Health promotion is driven by both values and evidence, which are often intertwined. So, there are two key questions: 'Do we think this ought to be done?' and 'Will it work?'

It is also important to act within the constraints of your job role and competency, which should be a part of regular supervision with your line manager. As an interesting example of how health promotion activities can be embedded within our programmes, see 'Making Every Contact Count', which provides a video of a health check and health promotion at a COVID vaccination centre.

See Chapter 4 for more about values and ethics in health promotion.

JUDGING THE COST-EFFECTIVENESS OF PUBLIC HEALTH INTERVENTIONS

In addition to assessing the evidence, it is important to judge cost-effectiveness. The funds available for prevention are limited and finite, plus the budget will also have an alternative use which is sometimes given a health economic term of an opportunity cost. As an example, local authorities in England are given a ring-fenced public health budget (HM Government, 2021). Detailed conditions for this grant are set out, along with reporting requirements, as well as the main objectives of the central funding, including tackling inequalities in health and improving drug and alcohol treatment.

Therefore, spending in this area needs to be clearly justified on cost-effectiveness grounds, possibly underpinned by a business case. This requires investment in public health to be based on the best available evidence of effectiveness from a range of sources. As a health promoter and public health practitioner, therefore, you need to think not only about evidence but also about the question of whether you are getting value for money and how you can demonstrate this. Using robust methods to identify and interpret evidence, along with clear and transparent processes, will enable you to provide effective and cost-effective health promotion and public health interventions and services. Public Health Scotland (2021) provides an informative discussion on the cost-effectiveness of health inequalities interventions, arguing that there is increasing evidence that taxation or other policies affecting prices, regulations and legislation to change behaviours are likely to be both cost-effective and efficient in reducing health inequalities. Sohn et al., 2020 also argue that failing to account for the resources required to successfully implement public health interventions can lead to an underestimation of costs and budget impact, optimistic cost-effectiveness estimates and ultimately a disconnect between published evidence and public health decision-making. They offer a useful conceptual framework for costing public health interventions in resource-limited settings.

Cost-Utility Analysis

NICE, (2016) use several ways of assessing the cost-effectiveness of public health promotion interventions and to determine the effectiveness of a public health intervention (NICE, 2009). Cost-utility analysis is one method of determining the cost-effectiveness of public health interventions (NICE, 2009). This method considers someone's quality of life and the length of life they will gain due to an intervention. The health benefits are expressed in units such as quality-adjusted life years (QALYs).

Generally, NICE considers that interventions costing the National Health System (NHS) less than £20,000 per QALY gained are cost-effective. Those costing between £20,000 and £30,000 per QALY gained may also be deemed cost-effective if certain conditions are satisfied (for further details of this, see NICE, 2012). NICE does not accept or reject interventions on cost-effectiveness grounds alone but assessing effectiveness, and cost-effectiveness is an integral part of the way they develop guidance. Indeed, the NHS receives public funding through taxation, and NICE are therefore safeguarding a prudent use of this resource.

Health promoters and public health practitioners are recommended to use the NICE guidance when planning interventions. The UK Government (HM Government, 2020) have also published guidance on cost-utility analysis and offer an interesting example, which is given in Case study 7.1.

NICE now places more emphasis on cost-consequences and cost-benefit analyses when assessing public

---

CASE STUDY 7.1 Cost-Effectiveness and Cost-Utility of Internet-Based Computer Tailoring for Smoking Cessation

Background

Although effective smoking cessation interventions exist, information is limited about their cost-effectiveness and cost-utility.

Objective

To assess the cost-effectiveness and cost-utility of an internet-based multiple computer-tailored smoking cessation programme and tailored counselling by practice nurses working in Dutch general practices compared with an internet-based multiple computer-tailored programme only and care as usual.

Methods

The economic evaluation was embedded in a randomised controlled trial, for which 91 practice nurses recruited 414 eligible smokers. Smokers were randomised to receive multiple tailoring and counselling (n=163), multiple tailoring only (n=132), or usual care (n=119). Self-reported

cost and quality of life were assessed during a 12-month follow-up period. Prolonged abstinence and 24-hour and 7-day point prevalence abstinence were assessed at the 12-month follow-up. The trial-based economic evaluation was conducted from a societal perspective. Uncertainty was accounted for by bootstrapping (1000 times) and sensitivity analyses.

Results

No significant differences were found between the intervention arms with regard to baseline characteristics or effects on abstinence, quality of life and addiction level. However, participants in the multiple tailoring and counselling group reported significantly more annual healthcare-related costs than participants in the usual care group. Cost-effectiveness analysis, using prolonged abstinence as the outcome measure, showed that the mere multiple computer-tailored programmes had the highest probability of being cost-effective. Compared with usual care,

(Continued)

CASE STUDY 7.1   Cost-Effectiveness and Cost-Utility of Internet-Based Computer Tailoring for Smoking Cessation—Cont'd

in this group €5100 had to be paid for each additional abstinent participant. With regard to cost-utility analyses, using quality of life as the outcome measure, usual care was probably the most efficient.

Conclusion

To our knowledge, this was the first study to determine the cost-effectiveness and cost-utility of an internet-based smoking cessation programme with and without counselling by a practice nurse. Although the internet-based multiple computer-tailored programme seemed to be the most cost-effective treatment, the cost-utility was probably highest for care as usual. However, to ease the interpretation of cost-effectiveness results, future research should aim at identifying an acceptable cutoff point for the willingness to pay per abstinent participant.

Keywords: randomised controlled trial, economic evaluation, smoking cessation, internet, computer tailoring, general practice

Reference

Smit, E. S., Evers, S. M., de Vries, H., & Hoving, C. (2013). Cost-effectiveness and cost-utility of internet-based computer tailoring for smoking cessation. *Journal of Medical Internet Research, 15*(3), e57. https://doi.org/10.2196/jmir.2059.

---

health interventions (NICE, 2012). This dual approach aims to ensure all relevant outcomes, such as health improvement and community benefits, are considered. The idea is to help local authorities, as well as other organisations interested in improving people's health, better judge whether a public health intervention represents value for money. Cost-utility analysis is also used, when needed, to make comparisons with previous economic analyses, as well as to compare prevention programmes. Such analyses can be broadly considered to be 'return on investment', which implies added value. An informative article published by the King's Fund provides more detail on this (Buck, 2018).

It is important to note that it may take several years before the health benefits of some public health interventions start to have an impact, although the costs may need to be incurred in advance. This is because there may be a delay for the intervention to show benefit. Such interventions may be cost-effective or even cost-saving over the medium to long term and so would be recommended for funding on that basis, using the cost-effectiveness threshold. However, they may not be deemed to be value for money in the short term in a simple return on investment analysis, which is cost savings minus the cost of intervention.

Where possible, NICE will report on costs and benefits over the short, medium, and long term (NICE, 2016). This highlights the professional difficulties in balancing investment now versus return on investment later in situations where there are competing needs. See Case study 7.2 for an example of cost-effectiveness applied to a smoking cessation intervention.

AUDIT

Results of audits provide valuable evidence of 'real-time and real world' impacts. Audit is the systematic examination of the operations of a service, followed by the implementation of recommendations to improve quality. Basically, an audit will scrutinise how the service carries out each stage of the planning/evaluation cycle, which are described in Chapter 5. Such audits will also often use readily available data, so-called 'natural evidence', to assess an impact. For example, the quality outcome framework (QoF) is one tool used to measure the effectiveness of primary care services in general medical practices. For a more recent consideration of the QoF, see NHS Digital (2021).

Within an audit, strengths and weaknesses will be revealed, and this will help identify ways of overcoming difficulties. An audit can involve either an internal review by the people responsible for delivering a service or scrutiny by an independent external auditor. For examples of audits relevant to health promotion and public health practice, such as the national audit of cardiac rehabilitation, see NHS Digital (2019).

It may be helpful for you to undertake your own audit of the service or intervention you are providing. The example of an audit cycle in Fig. 7.2 starts with the specification of standards or criteria, followed by the collection of data, the assessment of performance and the identification of the need for change and implementing the improvements. It is important to note that this is a circular process, allowing it to be repeated, which might be good practice to monitor any subsequent impacts.

CASE STUDY 7.2   Cost-Effectiveness of Facilitated Access to a Self-Management Website, Compared to Usual Care, for Patients With Type 2 Diabetes (Help-Diabetes): Randomised Controlled Trial

Background

Type 2 DM is one of the most common long term conditions and costs health services approximately 10% of their total budget. Active self-management by patients improves outcomes and reduces health service costs. Whilst the existing evidence suggested that uptake of self-management education was low, the development of internet-based technology might improve the situation.

Objective

To establish the cost-effectiveness of a web-based self-management programme for people with type 2 diabetes (HeLP-Diabetes) compared to usual care.

Methods

An incremental cost-effectiveness analysis was conducted, from a National Health Service and personal and social services perspective, based on data collected from a multi-centre, two-arm, individually randomised controlled trial over 12 months. Adults aged 18 or over with a diagnosis of type 2 diabetes and registered with the 21 participating general practices (primary care) in England, UK, were approached. People who were unable to provide informed consent or to use the intervention, were terminally ill, or currently participating in a trial of an alternative self-management intervention were excluded. The participants were then randomised to either usual care plus HeLP-Diabetes, an interactive, theoretically informed web-based self-management programme, or to usual care plus access to a comparator website containing basic information only. The participants' intervention costs and wider healthcare resource use were collected, as well as two health-related quality of life measures: the problem areas in diabetes (PAID) scale and EQ-5D-3L. EQ-5D-3L was then used to calculate QALYs. The primary analysis was based on intention-to-treat, using multiple imputations to handle the missing data.

Results

In total, 374 participants were randomised, with 185 in the intervention group and 189 in the control group. The primary analysis showed incremental cost-effectiveness ratios of £58 (95% CI -411 to 587) per unit improvement on the PAID scale and £5550 (95% CI -21,077 to 52,356) per QALY gained by HeLP-Diabetes, compared to the control. The complete case analysis showed less cost-effectiveness and higher uncertainty with incremental cost-effectiveness ratios of £116 (95% CI -1299 to 1690) per unit improvement on the PAID scale and £18,500 (95% CI -203,949 to 190,267) per QALY. The cost-effectiveness acceptability curve showed an 87% probability of cost-effectiveness at £20,000 per QALY willingness to pay threshold. The one-way sensitivity analyses estimated 363 users would be needed to use the intervention for it to become less costly than usual care.

Conclusion

Facilitated access to HeLP-Diabetes is cost-effective, compared to usual care, under the recommended threshold of £20,000 to £30,000 per QALY by the National Institute of Health and Care Excellence.

Trial registration: International Standard Randomised Controlled Trial Number (ISRCTN) 02123133; http://www.controlled-trials.com/ISRCTN02123133 (Archived by Web Cite at http://www.webcitation.org/6zqjhmn00).

Keywords: cost-effectiveness; internet; self-management; type 2 diabetes mellitus.

Reference

Li J., Parrott S., Sweeting M., et al. (2018). Cost-effectiveness of facilitated access to a self-management website, compared to usual care, for patients with type 2 diabetes (HeLP-Diabetes): randomized controlled trial. *Journal of Medical Internet Research*, *20*(6), e201. https://doi.org/10.2196/jmir.9256

It is also in the nature of cycles that you can, in practice, start anywhere. So you might start with collecting data on performance, assessing performance and recommending the need to specify standards pending that

the audit findings support this conclusion. The difficulty with auditing health promotion in practice is that it is often embedded in other work. For example, an audit of health promotion in clinical settings, such as cardiac

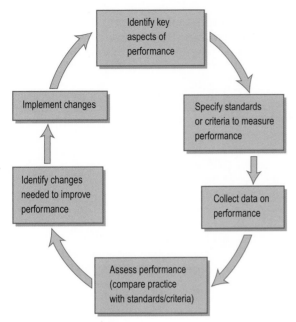

Fig. 7.2 An audit cycle.

rehabilitation, may involve exploring issues about relationships and communication. This may further involve exploring related issues such as organisational culture and dignity in care for patients.

All of these are vital to the quality of health promotion work but may not relate specifically to clinical audits. It is important to note that in the specifying of standards to measure performance, these may be specified in legislation, such as those currently in England, with standards published as per Health and Social Care (2012). For further reading on quality standards, see Chapter 8, a section on working for quality.

Many of the tools described in the section on research in this chapter can also be used in audits. So, for example, you could engage with patients outside of a healthcare setting to gather their views about service provision. This could be done in a variety of ways, including by telephone or via a focus group. Patients would need to be reassured their contribution is voluntary and comments will be confidential. This means that the views received are non-attributable to an individual, often presented anonymously or grouped in a thematic analysis.

An example of this in practice is discussions with a group of visually impaired patients in mid-Wales (Morgan, 2015) regarding the health services they access and how these could be improved. As a public health practitioner, it is important to gather such information and be inclusive of the stakeholders consulted.

Audit, Research and Evaluation

Audit, research and evaluation are complementary activities. Research is concerned with generating new knowledge and approaches which can be applied beyond the specific context of the research study. Evaluation involves making a judgement of about one specific intervention, campaign or project and the value it has. An audit seeks to improve the performance of a continuing service, such as an environmental health service or a midwifery service, by reviewing its practice. All three elements of audit, research, and evaluation are crucial to the pursuit of evidence-informed health promotion and public health practice. As suggested in Fig. 7.3, they can co-exist and inform one another.

You should not need to do a detailed evaluation of everything you do because you may be basing what you do on techniques and materials that have already been evaluated by others and form part of the published evidence. Of course, this will also be impractical in terms of time commitments. What you should do is audit your health promotion practices regularly to check whether what you have planned and the techniques you have chosen are working effectively and efficiently. If you need further training in how to carry out an audit of your health promotion practice, it would be worth finding out about local opportunities for training in clinical audit, as the basic concepts can be applied to health promotion and public health. The alternative to this is to find colleagues locally with an interest and experience in auditing that can potentially mentor you.

Another area to pursue could be training related to measuring and improving quality or quality assurance. Quality and audit cycles are very closely related, so you could also discuss local arrangements for performance appraisal with your manager through your annual professional development plans and supervision.

See the section on working for quality in Chapter 8.

HEALTH IMPACT ASSESSMENT (HIA) TOOLS AND METHODS

HIA is a practical approach used to judge the potential health effects of a policy, programme or project on a population, for example on vulnerable or disadvantaged groups. Recommendations are produced for decision-makers and stakeholders, with the aim of maximising the proposal's positive health effects and minimising any possible negative health effects. The approach can be applied in diverse economic sectors and uses quantitative, qualitative and participatory techniques.

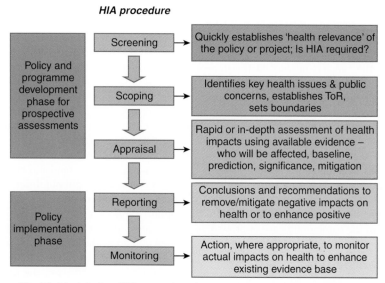

HIA procedure

Fig. 7.3 Model of an HIA procedure from the World Health Organisation.

Screening
The screening stage selects an intervention, a policy or a project for which an HIA would be beneficial. Potential effects on the determinants of health, health outcome and population groups are identified. Screening results in three types of decisions 1) HIA is needed; 2) HIA is not needed, as the effects are already known; 3) HIA is not needed, as the effects are negligible.

Scoping
The second step is the planning of the HIA and identifying what health risks and benefits to consider. A steering group is created to develop and adopt the terms of reference for the HIA. Scoping involves bringing together the major stakeholders of the proposal by creating a steering group and developing and adopting terms of reference for the HIA. It is important to be systematic in the development of the HIA to reduce the risk of presenting only one side of the evidence.

Appraisal
An appraisal is the core of any HIA activity. All the data and evidence are gathered and analysed, affected populations are identified, and health impacts are estimated. The impact estimates allow giving suggestions and recommendations for actions that promote positive health effects and minimise negative health effects. Depending on the context, an HIA can be conducted with a rapid appraisal or with a comprehensive appraisal.

Reporting
Presenting clear results to communities and decision-makers is an important step in HIA. The contents of the report should include a description of the scope, the priorities identified at the beginning of the process, the views expressed by the stakeholders, the evidence available from the various sources, the overall findings and any recommendations.

Monitoring
Monitoring is the final step in the HIA process and allows the process and the effectiveness of the HIA to be evaluated.
Source WHO (2022b).

HIA provides a way to engage with members of the public affected by a particular proposal. It also helps decision-makers make choices about alternatives and improvements to prevent disease or injury and to actively promote health. It is based on the four interlinked values of democracy (promoting stakeholder participation), equity (considering the impact on the whole population), sustainable development, and the ethical use of evidence. HIA is also a diverse and versatile tool. WHO (2022b)

provides both tools and methods in HIA, some of which are set out in the following section.

HOW TO UNDERTAKE AN HIA

HIA provides decision-makers and stakeholders with comprehensive information about the consequences on the health of interventions, policies and projects. Guidance documents often break HIA into four, five or six stages.

Despite the differing number of stages, it is important to note that there are no significant differences between the methods, which usually include screening, scoping, appraisal, reporting and monitoring activities.

Evaluating whether the HIA has influenced the decision-making process (and the subsequent proposal) is an important component of HIA. As with any intervention, evaluation is required to see if it has worked.

Monitoring the implementation of the proposal is critical to ensure that any recommendations that decision-makers agreed on are actually achieved. Longer term monitoring of the health of populations is sometimes a component of larger proposals. This long term monitoring can be used to see if the predictions made during the appraisal were accurate and to see if the health, or health-promoting behaviours, of the community have improved.

USING PUBLISHED RESEARCH

Health promoters and public health practitioners need to be well informed about health research and also how to both interpret and apply their knowledge of research findings to improve their practice. One such tool is the realist review, which is driven by questions including what works, for whom and in what circumstance. This takes account of the locally sensitive context and circumstances, for example how people with long term health conditions face their individual challenges across different healthcare settings (Brown et al., 2019). The realist review is a useful tool to use in practice as it naturally draws from the local context and experience of delivering interventions in the community.

Familiarity with research findings can also give you arguments on which to base a case for more, different or better health promotion. Keeping abreast of current research evidence should be part of your everyday working practice. Local library departments within NHS and other public sector organisations may produce the latest current awareness bulletin. This is worth exploring in your professional role or perhaps working collaboratively with others to prepare such as a bulletin.

How to Search the Literature

You may sometimes need to find out about research on a particular topic, perhaps because you are proposing to introduce new health promotion work and want to know what has been shown to be most effective. For example, imagine you are a nurse working in a hospital, and you are considering introducing a counselling service for patients presenting with alcohol-related illnesses, such as liver disease. You want to know if research shows what the health promotion needs of these patients are and how best to meet them. Where do you start?

First, you need to establish a research question. It pays to take time to discuss this with colleagues, and you could also discuss it with someone who has recently been treated for an alcohol-related illness. What did they find helpful?

Once you are clear about what you want to find out, list no more than six key words that feature in your question. The nurse might include the words 'alcohol', 'needs' and 'counselling' in their list. Then write words that mean the same thing or are similar in meaning by each keyword. For example, you might put 'brief intervention', which is a short, structured conversation with signposting to alcohol support services, as an alternative to 'counselling'. These key words and their alternative synonym will be helpful when you go to the library or search on the internet. For an excellent guide to doing your literature search and finding information online, see the British Geriatrics Society (2018). This guide also provides recommendations for search engines, such as the PubMed database, to source the literature.

In addition, many journal articles include a list of key words after the title, which will help you to know whether the article is likely to be of interest to you. The title of the article itself should also often be a rapid way to determine if the article is likely to be relevant to the situation. When you have found a few references, you can start by reading the most recent one. This may also provide you with more references.

Once you are underway, the next problem is to avoid being swamped by peripheral information. Here again, your key words should be useful in stopping you from being side-tracked and in keeping your research question in mind.

It is important to keep records of what you read. There are many reference management software packages designed to help you store and retrieve references, such as EndNote20 (EndNote, 2022)

- Author's (or editor's) surname and initials.
- Year published.
- Title and subtitle.
- Edition, if not the first.
- Chapter, or number of pages, if you are only going to refer to the part of the book.
- Place of publication.
- Publisher.

For articles in journals, you need to record the following:

- Author's surname and initials.
- Year of publication.
- Title and subtitles of an article.

- Journal title.
- Volume and part numbers.
- The inclusive page numbers of the article.
- Date of publication.

If you are gathering research evidence that will be used to inform a health promotion decision or action, then the first thing you need to know when reading an article is whether it is a report of actual research or just a knowledgeable account of facts and opinions. The former is usually described as original research, whilst the latter is often called a commentary or editorial. The abstract, the summary paragraph at the start of an article, will quickly inform you why a study was done and the main findings. Research reports usually have the following format:

- Introduction – background to the study.
- Literature review – critical summary of previous and related research.
- Method – a description of how the study was carried out.
- Results – the findings of the study.
- Discussion – a discussion of the findings.
- Conclusions – the implications of the findings.
- References – all the studies and books referred to in the article.

You need to read research articles critically, so the following questions might be helpful. When was the research carried out? Although the article is recent, it could be reporting on research that was carried out some years previously and has been superseded by more up-to-date research. This is particularly important in a rapidly evolving situation, for example as was seen with the COVID-19 pandemic, where the evidence base evolved rapidly.

Why was the research undertaken? Do you see the need for this research? Will it contribute new knowledge on the subject? Will this knowledge be useful in practice? It is important to differentiate between a contribution to knowledge that is of interest or perhaps generates more questions and new research findings that can be quickly translated into practice.

How was the research carried out? Did it use methods and tools that were likely to provide answers to the questions posed by the researchers? What type of research was carried out? For example, if the researchers wanted to find out what works in changing the behaviour of sedentary people with type 2 diabetes mellitus (DM) to cause them to do more exercise, then experimental research would be required. This is research that establishes a relationship between cause and effect, often through studying subgroups of people, where the experimental subgroup experiences the intervention under consideration, and the control subgroup does not. This may sometimes be called a randomised controlled trial where one group of individuals receive the active intervention, and the control group receives standard treatment. The diagram below shows a trial design for where exercise could help improve outcomes for patients with type 2 DM, a condition which is sometimes related to being sedentary.

The Centre for Evidence-Based Medicine suggests four questions:

- Does the study address a clearly defined question?
- Did the study use valid methods to address this question?
- Are the valid results of this study important?
- Are these valid, important results applicable?

(Adapted from Centre for Evidence Based Medicine [CEBM], 2022)

Another type of research is action research. This is used to find out exactly how to implement changes, or solve problems, in a specific situation through watching and documenting in a systematic manner how the changes are introduced. Action research is a highly versatile tool that has been widely used around the world to help knowledge build knowledge (Cordeiro and Soares, 2018).

Does the researcher draw reasonable conclusions from the results? This can be a difficult question to answer, especially if, for example, it is quantitative research and you are unfamiliar with statistics. If you are not sure that you understand, it is important that you read more on critiquing research, particularly if you are going to be implementing the findings (see (RCN, 2022) for more detail on critiquing research articles).

In a clinical setting, critical appraisal has been suggested as being essential to combat information overload, identify papers that are relevant and for continuing professional development (Al-Jundi and Sakka, 2017). These considerations are also relevant for health promotion and public health practitioners.

How could or should research affect health promotion practice or policy? Even if the research was not carried out in your specialty or area of work, it could still have implications. For example, findings about how best to communicate with patients who are experiencing anxiety after a serious health risk, such as a heart attack, could be used to help improve communication with patients who have other serious illnesses, such as cancer. For example, skills of empathic communication might be relevant in both situations.

Through asking these, as well as other, questions you should be able to come to a judgement about whether a piece of research is reliable. Most journals will publish reliable research based on a peer-review process, where other experts in the field review the findings. Good practice, however, still requires being critical about the research. A checklist to consider the robustness of it should consider:

- The credibility and skills of the researchers.
- Whether an appropriate research design was used.
- The research contained valid baseline data.
- Used a recognised research instrument, such as a questionnaire.
- Evidence that has been piloted, that is tried and tested first to identify and correct any problems.
- Evidence the instrument was validated, that is tested to show that it really does measure what it was supposed to measure.

Some articles will have already critiqued the research for you in the form of 1) systematic reviews (see for example, Patnode (2021) for a systematic review of smoking cessation interventions for adults, including pregnant persons) or 2) meta-analysis (see Stjepanović et al., 2022, for a meta-analysis of the efficacy of smokeless tobacco in smoking cessation). A systematic review answers a defined research question by collecting and summarising all empirical evidence that fits pre-specified eligibility criteria. A meta-analysis is the use of statistical methods to summarise the results of these studies. In both cases, articles that present systematic reviews or meta-analysis provide excellent sources of evidence on which to base public health practice and health promotion interventions.

More recently, it has been suggested that public health systematic reviews are enhanced if a visual diagram is presented to summarise the findings. This could be particularly helpful in improving the translation of the findings into practice. The suggested steps to achieve this include starting simply and improving the diagram iteratively through stages of development (Rohwer et al., 2021).

DOING YOUR OWN SMALL-SCALE RESEARCH

Whilst you can improve your effectiveness by examining research findings and considering whether and how they apply to your work, in certain situations, you may wish to carry out research yourself. For example, you and a group of colleagues may have uncovered an unmet public health promotion need, and you have agreed on funding for a study to look in more detail at the need and how it could best be met. This illustrates the more general point that the evidence base evolves and new questions arise.

What is defined as research here is a planned, systematic gathering of information for the purpose of increasing the total body of knowledge. If you are inexperienced, it is important for you to read extensively and try to elicit help from an experienced researcher, either within your organisation or from a local University department. The following information should help to guide you in your

reading and introduce you to the process of undertaking small-scale research.

The research process involves carrying out some specific tasks, which are set out in Box 7.2. Although the tasks tend to be carried out in the sequence set out in the box, this is not always the case; for example, you may write parts of the research report incrementally as you go through each research task. You may have a much clearer idea about the purpose of the research after you have read the literature on other investigations in your area of interest.

The most important task in this list is the first one, as the kind of question you want to answer will form the basis of the whole project. For example, suppose you set the question, 'What is the best way to encourage ethnic minority communities to be confident in accessing the COVID-19 vaccine?'. The National Institute for Health and Care Excellence has set out an evidence base on this (NICE, 2021), including engaging with communities and informing and educating the target groups about COVID-19 vaccines using multi-platform approaches, including social media, print and press.

Your own small-scale research could include defining the local demographic, using population data held in your area or from national sources such as the UK Census. This could then be represented in a geographical form, either in the form of a map or by presenting the data in a table to demonstrate where members of the community reside. You might undertake some research to identify if there are networks locally, for example community groups. Local health records might be available to work out, on an anonymous basis, the uptake of the COVID-19 vaccine. This research could help prepare a report to set out recommendations to improve ethnic minority community uptake of the vaccine whilst also drawing in research evidence about what works best. This could then help inform an evidence-based response to improve rates of community vaccination for COVID-19, and further research could then be undertaken to monitor the impact.

BOX 7.2   Research Tasks

- Define the purpose of the research (and set a research question, if appropriate).
- Review the literature.
- Plan the study and the method(s) of investigation.
- Test the method by carrying out a pilot study.
- Collect the information or data.
- Analyse the information or data.
- Draw objective conclusions based on the findings of the analysis.
- Compile the research report.

Such a research project might be sufficiently strong to also inform practice in other areas and potentially be published in a journal or conference abstract. Furthermore, there could be scope to involve a range of colleagues in this work, including those delivering the vaccination, partnership managers who work with ethnic minority communities, medical records staff, and colleagues working in communication, including the use of social media channels. The importance of partnership working is covered in other chapters.

The planning phase of the research is an essential investment and should be conducted thoroughly. If you are going to apply for funding, your planning must include investigating sources of funding and the particular interests of different potential funders. This background reading may also help identify if similar research is ongoing or, indeed, if there are other researchers working on this topic.

It is also worth noting that many tasks can take longer than the initial estimate, and you will need to allow plenty of time for consulting people; for example, to arrange interviews if this is part of the research. Ethical issues and the need to apply for permission from ethical committees must also be considered. Ethics committees in the NHS will evaluate the research proposal and will require additional information about issues such as confidentiality (for an example of an ethical framework and toolkit for research, see the NHS Health Research Authority, 2022).

You will also need to consider ways of collecting the information you need. Any information collected needs to be valid and reliable. Validity means measuring what you purport to measure. For example, if you are attempting to measure the success of health education in encouraging a group of people to reduce their intake of alcohol, a valid measure would be to measure their consumption patterns. Asking them to complete a written questionnaire may not give valid responses because people might respond to questions and questionnaires in ways they think the experts want. In the case of alcohol intake, this may be particularly true as people may be reluctant to accurately disclose their true drinking levels due to social stigma associated with this or fear of being judged by a healthcare professional. Alcohol misuse itself is associated with denial, where those who drink to excess may minimise their intake or may not accurately recall it due to the effects that alcohol can have on memory.

Reliability means that if the research is repeated using the same research instruments, it will give the same results. If the research is sufficiently robust, then it can potentially be generalised to other areas. For details on the different types of reliability and validity in social and health sciences research, see Middleton (2022).

Basic Tools Of Research

There are several basic tools used in health promotion research that will be discussed below.

Questionnaires

These are useful when you want to collect information from relatively large numbers of people. An example of this is the Health Survey for England which is an important annual survey looking at changes in the health and lifestyle of people all over the country (see NHS Digital, 2022) which covers about 10,000 individuals, about 80% are adults and the remaining sample from children.

Questionnaires should be kept as simple as possible and to a minimum so that non-relevant information is excluded. However, this does not mean that they are easy to design, and much care is needed in the formulation of questions to ensure that valid conclusions can be drawn from the answers. Questionnaires are most useful for collecting information that is quantifiable, such as factual knowledge.

Advantages of questionnaires include:
- They can be answered anonymously, and respondents may therefore be more truthful.
- They can also be given to a whole group of people at the same time, thereby using the respondents' and researcher's time effectively. As a general rule, the bigger the sample size then the more likely the information collected is to be valid as a true representation of the community.

The questionnaire should always first be piloted on a small sample of people from the group for which it is intended. You will then be able to identify and redesign any questions that have been misinterpreted, potentially changing the wording or flow if required. It will also give practice in collecting the data and how this can be analysed.

The response rate to questionnaires can be low, and you may need to think about the implications of this; for example, will the results really reflect the views of the target population? When the response rate is low, it may be worth initiating a follow-up approach, for example resending the questionnaire or perhaps offering it in a different format, for example as an email attachment, so that it can be completed electronically. Also, some people may not want to complete the questionnaire, and even if they fill one in, they may do so casually without giving it careful thought. Having some quality assurance on the accuracy of the returns is worth considering, for example contacting some respondents to confirm their answers and whether they wish to amend any of their answers.

You need to consider right from the start how the information collected will be analysed. An overly complex analysis might be time consuming, so try to have in mind some basic but effective methods, such as a trend analysis over time or a geographical representation to show a cluster of illness in a particular region. Decisions about which computer software programmes, such as SPSS, will be needed to analyse the information. This may influence the design of the questionnaire. Consultation with a statistician and/or an experienced researcher may be helpful at this point, to gain their advice on the questions posed and the potential analytical techniques that could be used.

It is always helpful to put a lot of thought into the design of quantitative questionnaires by clarifying closed questions with defined ways of responding (such as tick boxes) so that they will give accurate results. Qualitative questionnaires with open questions can be more complicated to analyse. The general rule with qualitative questionnaires is to undertake a thematic analysis that draws out key themes from the information collected from the respondents. It might be helpful to have some ideas on how to group data ahead of the study.

Using online survey tools speeds up the process of generating data from questionnaires. For examples of online tools, see Stanjevic (2021).

See Chapter 10, a section on asking questions and getting feedback, for more about open and closed questions.

Personal Interviews

With face-to-face interviews, you can develop rapport and encourage people to talk more openly. You may find out things that you did not think to ask about but which are very relevant.

The main advantage of personal interviews is that there is more scope for initiative by the interviewee. For example, the interviewee can seek clarification and may be able to express views and opinions more easily verbally than in writing. The disadvantage is that, unless you are very skilled, you may bias the response; that is, you may get the responses you want to get or expect to get. For example, asking 'You do feel better, don't you?' biases the answer towards 'Yes', whereas 'Do you feel better?' removes some of this bias. It is therefore important to ask neutral questions and also to give an option of 'prefer not to say'.

Interviews can be one-to-one or with groups, face-to-face or by telephone. They can be organised by using pre-prepared questions (a structured interview) or allowed to flow more freely. At one extreme, you could design an interview schedule that looks like a questionnaire; at the other extreme, you might simply have three or four broad headings which you wish to discuss (a semi-structured interview). During the COVID-19 pandemic, telephone

---

> ### BOX 7.3   Client Satisfaction With a Smoking Cessation Programme: Telephone Survey Schedule
>
> - Did the brochure on quitting smoking provide the information you were seeking?
> - Do you now feel you have sufficient information to enable you to quit smoking?
> - Were you able to discuss the barriers you feel will inhibit you from quitting?
> - Who did you prefer to discuss things with? Prompt: was it the smoking cessation adviser or members of the group?

interviews had to be used for research purposes. For an interesting telephone-administered research questionnaire on the impact of lockdown on elderly people, see Brown et al., 2021.

Box 7.3 is an example of a telephone interview schedule. Special interview groups, such as focus groups, concentrate on a particular issue by focusing on pre-determined questions (see Walden, 2019 for step-by-step guidance on conducting focus groups).

What else might the smoking cessation programme have offered that would have supported you in your efforts to quit smoking? Prompt: nicotine patches?

Participant and Non-Participant Observation

This can include observing behaviour, such as how well a person performs an exercise routine, and physiological observations, such as monitoring weight. Participant observation happens when the researcher is also actively involved in what is being observed, such as actively contributing to discussions in a meeting. Non-participant observation means the researcher takes no part in what is being observed.

The advantages of participant observation are that the researcher may be more aware of what is going on, including less tangible things such as the mood of a group of people. However, the researcher could have difficulty in making objective observations and may find it difficult to record what is happening, so that information could be lost. The non-participant researcher may find it easier to make objective observations and may be able to plan and record observations more easily. On the other hand, having an observer who does not participate can seem threatening as people might not open up or may not behave as they normally do. This could have a big effect on what is observed and invalidate the research (see Pope and Allen, 2019) for more details on observational methods in health research).

Sampling

If it is too expensive or time consuming to collect information from the whole population or group you are interested in, then you need to select individuals so that you avoid getting a biased response. There are a number of sampling techniques which can be used to ensure that the sample is representative of the whole population (for examples of different sampling methods, see McCoombes, 2022).

Random sampling

This involves identifying people at random from the whole group. For example, imagine you are a practice nurse. Using the practice register, you could decide at random on a number between 1 and 10 (say 5) and send out questionnaires to the 5th, 15th, 25th, 35th (and so on) person on the list. In this case, the sampling level has also been set at 10%.

Quota Sampling

This uses your knowledge of a particular group to help set criteria about who to include in the sample. Criteria you might use include age, gender and ethnicity. Once the group has been divided into segments, using your criteria, you can use a proportion from each segment for your sample. This also ensures that people with certain characteristics are proportionately represented.

Convenience Sampling

This means that researchers question the people they can get hold of at the time. This is biased; although accepting that it is very difficult to avoid bias altogether, it is important to decide whether the particular bias that has been introduced is acceptable. Bias should be discussed in any dissemination of the research.

Case studies 7.1, 7.2 and 7.3 provide examples of public health research projects.

The Research Report

See also the section on report writing in Chapter 8 and the section on written communication in Chapter 10.

The final stage of your research will be to produce a written report, which will disseminate your findings. People who read the report may be interested in the following:

- Assessing the validity of the findings for themselves.
- In repeating the research in similar circumstances and avoiding any pitfalls, or

---

CASE STUDY 7.3   The Uptake of Harm Reduction Services in West Wales: Estimates of the Negative Impact of the SARS-CoV-2 Pandemic

The severe acute respiratory syndrome coronavirus 2 (SARS-CoV-2) pandemic, often abbreviated to COVID-19, has been a significant global public health challenge. This challenge has required healthcare services to not only respond to the pandemic but also to maintain other services, such as those provided in primary care and hospital. In practice, this dual challenge has been considerable, given resources are finite, and a large study across 20 counties found health provision decreased by one-third (1).

It is, therefore, possible that the pandemic might have led to reductions in other services, whether due to the need to prioritise COVID-19 related services or the result of social restrictions. The COVID-19 pandemic might have impacted negatively on harm reduction services for individuals with substance misuse problems. The analysis of service activity data could help investigate this further.

The West Wales Context

Wales is one of the constituent countries of the UK, with a population of about 3 million individuals. The West Wales area with the historical name of Dyfed covers three local authority areas and one large NHS provider, with a resident population of nearly 400,000 individuals. Dyfed is a large geographical area, covering about one-third the land mass of Wales, and many of the communities are rural.

There are two large towns with good transport links within the area. Llanelli is located in the southern end of the area, whilst Aberystwyth is a coastal town located in the northern part. Dyfed Drug and Alcohol Service, a consortium of specialist substance misuse agencies, provides a needle exchange harm reduction programme in these two towns. Given there are considerable gaps in knowledge about the impact of the pandemic on substance misuse (2), this reports offers a perspective in practice on the situation.

Did the Pandemic Impact the Uptake of the Harm Reduction Programme?

This is a very important question for the provision of services and policymakers. Indeed, substance misusers also appear to have worse outcomes from COVID-19 compared to the general population (3). The relationship between mental health, substance misuse, and COVID-19 seems a particularly important research avenue (4).

(Continued)

CASE STUDY 7.3   The Uptake of Harm Reduction Services in West Wales: Estimates of the Negative Impact of the SARS-CoV-2 Pandemic—Cont'd

Table 7.1 provides a summary of the key data and shows a marked reduction in the uptake of harm reduction in Dyfed. To expand on Table 7.1, annual data were analysed using the records from Dyfed Drug and Alcohol Service. This data was collected from two needle exchange sites in West Wales over a two-year time interval from April 1, 2019 to March 31, 2021. Data were collected regarding the number of transactions, new registrations and items dispensed. The years were split into 2019/20 and 2020/21, divided into pre-COVID and lockdown. In the UK, the national lockdown started on March 23, 2020 and continued, with intervals of ease of restrictions, into the summer of 2021. The data, therefore, offers a good approximation of the impact of COVID-19 lockdown restrictions on harm reduction services provided.

As can be seen from Table 7.1, there was a substantial fall in the uptake of harm reduction services delivered by Dyfed Drug and Alcohol Service. Across all measures, there was a substantial reduction of more than one-third in the uptake of harm reduction services. The number of transactions, that is, the number of exchanges undertaken, fell by 39% and per month, this dropped from an average of 70 pre-COVID to 42 post-COVID. Similarly, the number of new people registered per month dropped from an average of about 14 pre-COVID to about nine people post-COVID. Further to this data, the biggest reduction related to the number of items dispensed. This measure is related to the provision of a harm reduction kit, such as clean needles and syringes.

There was a fall from nearly 7000 items per month pre-COVID to just over 4000 items post-COVID. There was also a fall in the number of items dispensed per transaction, although this was small. This suggests that substance misuse practice for those engaged in the service continued in a similar way pre-COVID and post-COVID.

Implications For Practice

Based on a quantitative analysis of the data, it appears that COVID-19 was associated with a significant reduction in the uptake of harm reduction services. Given the nature of substance misuse, it is unlikely that the need for these services has reduced during COVID-19, and possibly, the psychological stress from the lockdown may have exacerbated the situation. From a public health perspective, efforts to boost harm reduction are urgently needed as this data suggests the pandemic has negatively impacted an already hard to reach group. The hidden harm of this is unknown as there might have been compensatory practice associated with increased health risk. For example,

lower uptake might have resulted in high-risk sharing of used needles, given that the target population had accessed considerably fewer clean supplies.

Many questions remain unanswered by this data. Firstly, what drove the reduction in uptake? One possibility might be that the lockdown might have created a fear of attending due to the perceived risk of being exposed to and acquiring COVID-19. Another possibility is that the economic consequences of the lockdown resulted in a loss of income for some individuals to create a financial barrier to being able to travel to the services.

A second question relates to what health impacts will be seen from the reduced uptake. For example, might there be more blood-borne viruses within the community? A third question relates to the future provision and how best to deliver the service going forward. Outreach might be one option worth consideration, especially in areas where there are rural communities, such as in the area of West Wales reported on.

In closing, it appears that the COVID-19 pandemic will continue to impact the field of substance misuse, and there remain major gaps in knowledge (5). Lessons also need to be learned to ensure future readiness for service disruptions going forward.

Acknowledgement: This is based on work from Dyfed Drug and Alcohol Service.

References

Moynihan, R., Sanders, S., Michaleff, Z. A., et al. (2021). Impact of COVID-19 pandemic on utilisation of health services: a systematic review. *BMJ Open, 11,* e045343. https://doi.org/10.1136/bmjopen-2020-045343.

Kumar, N., Janmohamed, K., Nyhan, K., et al. (2021). Substance use and substance use disorder, in relation to COVID-19: protocol for a scoping review. *Systematic Reviews, 10,* 48. https://doi.org/10.1186/s13643-021-01605-9.

Baillargeon, J., Polychronopoulou, E., Kuo, Y. F., & Raj, M. (2021). The impact of substance use disorder on COVID-19 outcomes. *Psychiatric Services, 72*(5), 578–581.

Kim, Y. J., Qian, L., & Aslam, M. S. (2020). The impact of substance use disorder on the mental health among COVID-19 patients: A protocol for systematic review and meta-analysis. *Medicine (Baltimore), 99*(46), e23203. https://doi.org/10.1097/MD.0000000000023203.

Wilkinson, R., Hines, L., Holland, A., Mandal, S., Phipps, E. (2020). Rapid evidence review of harm reduction interventions and messaging for people who inject drugs during pandemic events: implications for the ongoing COVID-19 response. *Harm Reduction Journal, 17,* 95. https://doi.org/10.1186/s12954-020-00445-5.

TABLE 7.1   Summary of Harm Reduction Service Uptake in West Wales 2019-21

Measure	2019/20 (Pre-COVID)	2020/21 (Post-COVID)	% reduction
Number of transactions	833	509	39%
New people registered	166	110	34%
Number items dispensed	83,453	49,161	41%
Average per transaction	100.2	96.6	3.6%

BOX 7.4   Checklist of the Contents of a Research Report

- **Abstract** (concise summary of the research including key results and conclusions).
- **Background** (statement about the purpose of the research, the background, the reasons for carrying out the research and the questions to be answered).
- **Literature review** (critiquing other research in the field).
- **Methods**:
  - A description of the methods used for collecting the information and the reasons for selecting these methods.
  - A description of the population sample studied plus the sampling methods and response rates.
  - A discussion of the ethical implications.
  - Data analysis methods and the reasons for selecting these methods.
  - A description of the pilot study and any changes that were made as a result.
- **Results** (all appropriate data displayed clearly).
- **Discussion** (analysis of the findings, stating clearly the limitations of the study).
- **Conclusion** (with recommendations for further research).
- **References** (listing source material).

- In applying the research findings in the context of commissioning or providing health promotion services.

So the report should be written with the objective of helping readers to use it in these ways. You may need to consider producing more than one version of the report for different groups of readers: for example, a two-page summary for community groups and a full report for your health promotion professional and managers.

The contents of your research report may include the information set out in Box 7.4, although not every point will be applicable to a particular report, which should be written with the needs of the readers in mind.

Finally, in a field like health promotion and public health practice, the interpretation of research data is a complex matter, often because of the multifaceted determinants of health and wellbeing. It is extremely important that any health promotion and public health research is methodologically sound, ethically conducted, and unbiased and objective in its interpretation. Poor research is worse than no research because it wastes resources and has the potential to mislead.

PRACTICE POINTS

- Good practice requires you to identify how your health promotion and public health work helps to deliver to local and national strategies. Your effectiveness relates to your professional practice and how well this complements that of other colleagues working alongside you.
- It is essential, indeed a duty, to properly appraise evidence and to deliver programmes of work that are underpinned by evidence of effectiveness where it exists.
- Conducting research involves a skill set, and it is important to achieve the appropriate competencies that the particular type of research requires. Equally important is to only act within your level of competency.
- Given that resources always have a competing use, demonstrating value for money is important, and this often draws on health economics.
- Good professional practice should involve a regularly undertaken audit to take stock of the current situation and reflect on how things can be improved.
- The HIA is a useful and versatile tool that should be undertaken as part of the delivery of health promotion and public health programmes.

References

Al-Jundi, A., Sakka S. (2017). Critical appraisal of clinical research. *Journal of Clinical and Diagnostic Research*, *11*(5), JE01–JE05. https://doi:10.7860/JCDR/2017/26047.9942

Basu, S. (2021). Evidence-based health policies and its discontent – comparative global and Indian perspectives with a focus on the COVID-19 pandemic. *Indian Journal of Community Medicine*, *46*(3), 363–366. https://doi:10.4103/ijcm.ijcm_622_21

Black, A. T., Ali, S., Baumbusch, J., McNamee, K., & Mackay, M. (2019). Practice-based nursing research: Evaluation of clinical and professional impacts from a research training programme. *Journal of Clinical Nursing*, *28*(13-14), 2681–2687. https://doi.org/10.1111/jocn.14861.

British Geriatrics Society. (2018). Guide to literature searching. https://bgs.org.uk/resources/guides-to-literature-searching

Brown, S., Lhussier, M., Dalkin, S. M., & Eaton, S. (2019). Care planning: what works, for whom and in what circumstances? A rapid realist review. *Qualitative Health Research*, *28*(14), 2250–2266. https://doi.org/10.1177/1049732318768807

Brown, L., Mossibir, R., Harrison, N., Bundle, C., Smithe, J., & Clegg, A. (2021). Life in lockdown: a telephone survey to investigate the impact of COVID-19 lockdown measures on the lives of older people (≥75 years). *Age and Ageing*, *50*(2), 341–346. https://doi:10.1093/ageing/afaa255

Buck, D. (2018). Talking about the 'return on investment of public health': why it's important to get it right. https://www.kingsfund.org.uk/blog/2018/04/return-investment-public-health

Centre for Evidence Based Medicine (CEBM). (2022). *Critical appraisal tools*. https://www.cebm.ox.ac.uk/resources/ebm-tools/critical-appraisal-tools

Cordeiro, L., & Soares, C. B. (2018). Action research in the healthcare field: a scoping review. *JBI Database of Systematic Reviews and Implementation Reports*, *16*(4), 1003–1047. https://doi.org/10.11124/jbisrir-2016-003200

D'Alessandro, D. (2020). Urban public health, a multidisciplinary approach. *Urban Health*, 1–8. https://doi.org/10.1007/978-3-030-49446-9_1.

EndNotes. (2022). *Accelerate your research*. https://endnote.com

Health and Social Care. (2012). *Section 250*. http://www.legislation.gov.uk/ukpga/2012/7/contents

Health and Care Professions Council [HCPC] (2022). *Recognise, reflect, resolve: the benefits of reflecting on your practice*. https://www.hcpc-uk.org/standards/meeting-our-standards/reflective-practice/

HM Government. (2020). *Cost utility analysis: health economic studies*. https://www.gov.uk/guidance/cost-utility-analysis-health-economic-studies

HM Government. (2021). *Public health ring-fenced grant 2021 to 2022: local authority circular*. https://ww.gov.uk/government/publications/public-health-grants-to-local-authorities-2021-to-2022/public-health-ring-fenced

HM Government. (2022). *COVID-19 response. Living with COVID-19*. https://www.gov.uk/government/publications/covid019-response-living-with-covid-19

McCoombes, S. (2022). *Sampling methods | types, techniques, & examples*. https://www.scribbr.co.uk/research-methods/sampling/

Michelen, M., Manoharan, L., Elkheir, N., et al. (2021). Characterising long COVID: a living systematic review. *BMJ Global Health*, *6*, e005427. https://doi:10.1136/bmjgh-2021-005427

Middleton, F. (2022). *Reliability vs validity in research | differences, types & examples*. https://www.scribbr.co.uk/research-methods/reliability-or-validity/

Morgan, G. (2015). Quality of primary care for visually impaired patients in mid-Wales. *Quality in Primary Care*, *23*(4), 259–261.

National Collaborating Centre for Methods and Tools. McMasters University. (2021). Evidence-informed public health. http://www.nccmt.ca/professional-development/eiph

NHS Digital. (2019). *National audit of cardiac rehabilitation*. https://digital.nhs.uk/data-and-information/clinical-audits-and-registries/national-audit-of-clinical-rehabilitation

NHS Digital. (2021). *Quality and outcome framework, 2020-21*. https://digital.nhs.uk/data-and-information/publications/statistical/quality-and-outcomes-framework-achievement-prevalence-and-exceptions-data/2020-21

NHS Digital. (2022). Health Survey for England - Health, social care and lifestyles. https://digital.nhs.uk/data-and-information/areas-of-interest/public-health/health-survey-for-england---health-social-care-and-lifestyles

NHS Health Research Authority. (2022). *Student research toolkit*. https://www.hra.nhs.uk/planning-and-improving-research/research-planning/student-research/student-research-toolkit/

NICE. (2009). *Methods for the development of NICE public health guidance* (2nd edition). London: NICE.

NICE. (2012). *Methods for the development of NICE public health guidance* (3rd edition). London: NICE.

NICE. (2016). *NICE's approach to assessing public health interventions*. https://www.nice.org.uk/advice/lgb10/chapter/judging-the-cost-effectiveness-of-public-health-activities

NICE. (2021). COVID-19 vaccine hesitancy – debunking the myths using a community engagement approach underpinned by NICE guidance. https://www.nice.org.uk/sharedlearning/covid-19-vaccine-hesitancy-debunking-the-myths-using-a-community-engagement-approach-underpinned-by-nice-guidance

Patnode, C. D., Henderson, J. T., Coppola, E. L., Melnikow, J., Durbin, S., & Thomas, R. G. (2021). Interventions for tobacco cessation in adults, including pregnant persons: updated evidence report and systematic review for the US preventive services task force. *JAMA*, *325*(3), 280–298. https://doi.org/10.1036/0268-6133.24.2.226.

Public Health England. (2019). *Public Health England strategy 2020 to 2025*. https://www.gov.uk/government/publications/phe-strategy-2020-to-2025

Public Health Scotland. (2021). *Cost effective actions overview*. https://www.healthscotland.scot/reducing-health-inequalities/take-cost-effective-action/cost-effective-actions-overview

Pope, C., & Allen, D. (2019). Chapter 6 observational studies. In C. Pope & N. Mays (Eds.), *Qualitative research in health care* (3rd edition). New Jersey: Wiley.

RCN. (2022). *Critical appraisal*. https://www.rcn.org.uk/library/Subject-Guides/critical-appraisal

Rohwer, A., Taylor, M., Ryan, R., Garner, P., & Oliver, S. (2021). Enhancing public health systematic reviews with diagram visualization. *American Journal of Public Health*, 111(6), 1029–1034. https://doi.org/10.2105/AJPH.2021.306225.

Sohn, H., Tucker, A., Ferguson, O., Gomes, I., Dowdy, D. (2020). Costing the implementation of public health interventions in resource-limited settings: a conceptual framework. *Implementation Science*, 15, 86. https://doi.org/10.1186/s13012-020-01047-2.

Stanjevic, M. (2021). *5 best survey software for academic research*. Windowsreport.com/survey-software-academic-research/

Stjepanović, D., Phartiyal, P., Leung, J., et al. (2022). Efficacy of smokeless tobacco for smoking cessation: a systematic review and meta-analysis. *Tobacco Control, Feb*. https://doi.org/10.1136/tobaccocontrol-2021-057019.

Walden, V. (2019). *Conducting focus groups- Oxfam digital repository*. https://oxfamilibrary.openrepository.com/bitstream/handle/10546/578994/ml-conducting-focus-groups.pdf;jsessionid=DC74CA1CDA86A72B78D457C5CC1AF516?sequence=6

WHO. (2022a). *Social determinants of health*. www.who.int/health-topics/social-determinants-of-health#tab=tab_1

WHO. (2022b). *Health impact assessment (HIA) tools and methods*. https://www.who.int/tools/health-impact-assessments.

YouTube

EIA Study. Health impact assessment. https://www.youtube.com/watch?v=ETH6xWN_fd4

Chartered Institute for Personnel and Development (CIPD). Introduction to reflective practice. https://www.youtube.com/watch?v=M9hyWVEG2x0 Introduction to statistics. https://www.youtube.com/watch?v=kyjlxsLW1ls (additional resource)

Chartered Institute for Personnel and Development (CIPD) YouTube video on reflective practice.

Let's Learn Public Health. https://www.youtube.com/watch?v=8PH4JYfF4Ns

Making Every Contact Count. Health checks and health promotion at a COVID vaccination centre. https://www.youtube.com/watch?v=JhipfCAYWo8

National Collaborating Centre for Healthy Public Policy. https://www.youtube.com/watch?v=3xnyvynoaxY

University of Derby. Work-based learning. https://www.youtube.com/watch?v=u1Gs3_TdY98

Types of Sampling Method. https://www.youtube.com/watch?v=pTuj57uXWlk

Webpages

Cochrane. Trusted evidence, informed decisions, better health. https://www.cochrane.org.

Health Foundation. Data analytics for better health. https://www.health.org.uk/what-we-do/data-analytics

Joseph Rowntree Foundation. Main focus is research on UK poverty. https://www.jrf.org.uk.

The Kings Fund. Publication spanning a wide range of public health evidence resources. https://www.kingsfund.org.uk

National Collaborating Centre for Methods and Tools (NCCMT). Your journey to evidence-informed decision making in public health. https://www.nccmt.ca

NICE. Evidence-based recommendations developed by independent committees, including professionals and lay members, and consulted on by stakeholders. https://www.nice.org.uk/about/what-we-do/our-programmes/nice-guidance/nice-guidelines

Strategic Health Asset Planning and Evaluation (SHAPE). A web enabled, evidence-based application that informs and supports the strategic planning of services and assets across a whole health economy. https://shapeatlas.net

Skills of Personal Effectiveness

Gareth Morgan, Angela Scriven

CHAPTER OUTLINE

SUMMARY

In this chapter, the skills to effectively manage your health promotion and public health practice work are developed. The skills covered are varied and include the following:

- Managing information.
- Report writing.
- Time management.
- Project management.
- Change management.
- Working for quality.

To both illustrate and give the context in which health promotion and public health practice skills are applied, case studies and practical exercises are included. Effective professional practice in health promotion and public health requires clarity of aims and plans and the necessary management competencies to implement your projects and goals.

Further details on planning for health promotion and public health practice can be found in Chapters 5, 6, and 7.

MANAGEMENT SKILLS IN HEALTH PROMOTION AND PUBLIC HEALTH PRACTICE

Whilst management may not be easy or simple to define, in general terms, it is about adopting practices which ensure effectiveness and efficiency in the work to be delivered. *Effectiveness* can be considered to be producing effects or impacts and accomplishing your goals. *Efficiency* means producing results with little wasted effort or resources, essentially a ratio of input to output. This might also include the ability to carry out actions quickly if there are time constraints. Sometimes there may be a trade-off between being effective and efficient, so it is important to establish the correct balance.

Although a comprehensive introduction to management and project management is beyond the scope of this book, for further details, you could consult Horine (2022) for a beginner's guide to project management and Broddy (2017) for a general introduction to management.

- Previously in this book, aspects of management have been covered, such as setting priorities and planning. Several other managerial skills that will help you be an effective and efficient health promoter and public health practitioner are outlined in this chapter.
- It is important to clarify that possessing these skills is only a part of being effective and efficient. Other factors are also important, for example how well you integrate ethical principles into your basic everyday work. In addition, how you exercise your *responsibility* as a health promoter is also key.
- 'Response-ability' can be considered to be your ability to choose your response, and this is a product of your conscious choice, based on values, rather than a reaction to your circumstances. For further reading on ethics and values in health promotion and public health, see Chapter 4.
- Another key factor is the people you work with. Your effectiveness and efficiency are influenced, potentially

BOX 8.1   The Core Values That Underpin the NHS in Wales

Putting quality and safety above all else. Providing high value evidence-based care for our patients at all times.

Integrating improvement into everyday working and eliminating harm, variation and waste.

Focusing on prevention, health improvement and inequality as a key to sustainable development, wellness and wellbeing for future generations of the people of Wales.

Working in true partnership with partners and organisations and with our staff.

Investing in our staff through training and development, enabling them to influence decisions and providing them with the tools, systems and environment to work safely and effectively.

Source NHS Wales. *Values and standards of behaviour framework*. https://nwssp.nhs.wales/a-wp/governance-e-manual/living-public-service-values/values-and-standards-of-behaviour-framework/.

EXERCISE 8.1   What Information Is Essential for You to Store?

Start a personal journal and list of all the types of information you collect at present. This might include, for example, project documents, patient records, and minutes of meetings. Reflect on this by asking yourself the following questions about each one:

1. Do I need to keep this information? Is this essential?
2. How easy is it for me to retrieve information when I need it? Ask this for all the information systems you manage, both hardcopy and electronic.
3. Could someone else, or another information system, keep the information for me? If yes, how might this be achieved? Are there any risks?
4. Who else might need access to this information? What are their needs, and how could they be met? Would it be easy and quick for them to find it?
5. What would be the best way for this information to be stored? An example might include the organisations website or in a shared electronic file.

Revisit your journal list after 3 to 6 months and reflect on the situation. Has anything changed? Does something need to be changed?

both positively and negatively, by the competencies and motivation of those you work with. This might include receptionists, secretaries, colleagues and others within and outside your organisation.

- The values in your organisation are also important; see Box 8.1 below for an example from the National Health Society (NHS) Wales on how these underpin service delivery and staff development. These will guide the actions of health promoters working in the NHS in Wales.
- Both the structure and culture of your organisation will influence what you are able to achieve.
- The wider world is also crucial; for example, as was experienced during the COVID-19 pandemic, economic factors, government legislation, local government and social trends are examples of factors outside your organisation that influence your effectiveness.

This chapter is intended to help increase your awareness of these wider influences on your work and give you learning opportunities to develop your own competencies. In this chapter, some key aspects of personal effectiveness are covered to help you to manage health promotion and public health practice.

MANAGING INFORMATION

Information exists both in digital and hardcopy formats. Whether you keep information electronically or in a manual filing system, keep only what is required and only what you need. It might be worth considering sharing systems with colleagues to avoid duplication if this is appropriate.

Reflect on who else holds information within your work situation and their storage systems. For example, is there a central system accessible to several work colleagues? Is this fit for purpose? What information is best held centrally? Exercise 8.1 might help you identify what information you need to store.

Principles of Effective Information Systems

When reviewing or setting up your information system, it is useful to keep reminding yourself of three basic principles:

Firstly, do not overcomplicate. Systems are only as effective as the people who put in and take out the information. The simpler the system, the more likely it is that busy people will use it correctly.

Secondly, do not devise any more systems than are absolutely necessary.

Thirdly, organise systems so that anyone who might want to use them can easily understand them.

Basic principles of information systems are also informed by various legislation, such as the Data Protection Act (UK Government, 2018). Whilst a comprehensive review of information governance falls outside of the scope of this book, further reading is advised.

WRITING REPORTS

Important information is often conveyed through written reports, such as a project initiation document that sets out plans for health promotion or an evaluation report on a specific programme of work. You may need to write reports for your colleagues or manager or prepare formal reports for committees. Written reports might be read and considered when you are not there, in which case there is no immediate feedback about whether the key points have been understood. To reduce the potential of being misunderstood, good skills in preparing and writing reports are essential, including writing clearly, concisely with a logical flow and no repetition. (See Chapter 10, a section on written communication skills.)

Fig. 8.1 offers a quick visual guide to report writing.

Stage 1: Define the Purpose

It might help to clarify the purpose by completing the following sentence: 'As a result of reading this report, the reader/audience/committee will …'.

The answer could include being informed on a situation, being better able to make a decision, agreeing to release a budget for a course of action or persuading finance colleagues to fund a project. Whatever the answer, it is essential to keep the purpose in mind throughout all the subsequent stages of writing the report.

Stage 2: Define the Readers

Know your audience and consider them at all stages. Ensure that the report addresses the needs and interests of the readers. You might want to ask or find out what they already know about the subject. How much time do they have for reading, which will help determine if this is to be a long or short report or one that contains an executive summary? Also, consider what kind of style is appropriate, formal or informal? It is also important to consider whether there are any particular communication needs, for example for stakeholders with sensory loss who might need an alternative format, such as large print or braille.

Stage 3: Prepare the Structure

Decide on the structure of the report, which is appropriate for the process and audience. A report normally contains the following sections:

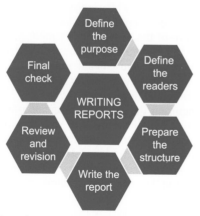

Fig. 8.1 Steps in report writing.

- Title – this should accurately describe what the report is about; ideally, this should be self-explanatory.
- Origins and affiliations – for example, the author's name, occupation, work base and date.
- Distribution list – it is a great help to readers if they know who else has seen the report. It is important to consider all relevant stakeholders and circulate appropriately.
- Contents list – a long report will need a contents list showing the main sections of the report and the pages on which the reader can find them. Sometimes readers may have different interests; for example, a finance manager may want to focus on the budgetary elements. A contents list may not be necessary for short reports.
- Summary – this is vital for all except the very shortest of reports of less than a page or two. It helps the reader if the summary is easy to find at the beginning of the report.
- Introduction, main body of the report, conclusion, recommendations, references, appendices. Please see Box 8.2 for more details on the structure.

Stage 4: Write the Report

Develop the various sections of the report in the order that makes it easiest. For example, it may be easiest to start by writing the detailed body of the report first, then summarise the information, then discuss the information, draw your conclusions, set out your recommendations, then write the summary of the report and lastly, finish it off with the title, contents list, origin, distribution list and other essential details. Sometimes it may be necessary to repeat certain sections, and report writing can be iterative.

Stage 5: Review and Revision

After the draft report has been produced, review it and revise it as necessary. Make sure pages are numbered and check that sections and subsections are correctly numbered. It is a good idea to get a colleague to proofread the report, someone with good report writing skills who will give constructive comments. It may also be helpful to ask for a colleague to review this who has no prior knowledge of the situation. Are they able to quickly understand the key messages?

Stage 6: Final Check

It is good practice to do a final check for writing and typing errors, spelling and other mistakes. It can be helpful to ask someone who has not seen the report before to check it for typing and layout errors. For ideas on how to prepare, write and present reports, see Reid (2018). There are also many examples of reports on health, health promotion and public health practice projects on the internet.

BOX 8.2   Report Structure

- Busy people may have limited time and will often read only the summary and perhaps the conclusions and recommendations. So the summary needs to set out the essence of the report clearly and concisely. It is sometimes referred to as the executive summary.
- Introduction – this sets the context for the report, for example, why the work was undertaken. Again, it is important to ensure the introduction engages the audience.
- The main body of the report – this will be the bulk of the report. You need to break up the content into sections and subsections, all with clear headings. Headings should be signposts to help the reader to see a route through the document and have an overview just by skimming through the headings. Sections need to be ordered in a way which will be logical for the reader. It may help to organise material into sections by writing all the possible headings and subheadings down, then move them around until you are satisfied that they are in the most logical order. You could use a numbering system for each section, heading and subheading (e.g. 1, 1.1, 1.1.1).
- Conclusion – summarises the conclusion which can be drawn from the information in the report.
- Recommendations – these relate to the future and summarise any changes needed.
- References – putting any references at the end makes the report easier to read.
- Appendices – a misused feature of some reports, to be avoided unless really necessary. Appendices might include additional information readers might wish to refer to as they read the report. If the information is crucial, it should be in the main body of the report.

USING TIME EFFECTIVELY

It is important to be organised and effective at work. In the following sections, there are some ideas about how to improve your effectiveness by focusing on how you use your time. Time is an expensive resource and has an opportunity cost, namely that using time for one activity means then it cannot be spent on something else. For some people, time is the one resource that they may find the hardest to manage; understanding how this is used via a baseline exercise may be helpful. Exercises 8.2 and 8.3 and the next section are intended to help analyse and improve the use of your time. This could then lead to you scheduling your work and competing priorities more effectively.

Time Logs and Time Diaries

A time log involves keeping a record of how you spend your time, which may be as often as every 5 or 10 min if that is appropriate. This might be useful if you wish to know exactly how you are using your time on an activity that seems to be taking longer than you think it should and can help you to pinpoint the source of the problem and therefore provide potential solutions. However, keeping a log is time-consuming itself, so it is really worthwhile using this sparingly and only if a particular activity is causing you problems.

If you want to know more about how you generally use your time, then another option is to complete a time diary. This records how you have spent your time day-by-day and should take only a few minutes to fill in at the end of each day. You might find it easier to fill in your diary more frequently, say at the end of the morning and at the end of the afternoon, or at any other convenient break between blocks of work. In this digital era, many computers and smartphones will also have tools available to assist with time management. This includes settings reminders for tasks or dictating notes.

Scheduling Your Work

See Chapter 6, a section on setting health promotion and public health priorities.

Health promoters and public health practitioners can find that they must do far more than their time permits and that they are faced daily with too many requests and demands. This means that, first and foremost, they must be very clear about their priorities, and making this explicit will be helpful. Second, they must be assertive about saying 'no' to requests to take on non-priority tasks. Simply explaining that there are competing demands may be sufficient reason for declining. Third, they need to develop skills of organising time and scheduling work to ensure that priority work gets done.

Scheduling work into the time available can involve three steps.

1. The first is to identify how long you need to spend on a job. This depends on the following:
- The nature of the activity, for example, whether it is possible to reduce the time allowance without endangering people or public health outcomes. Sometimes, it may be necessary to ask for a time extension and negotiate this if it is required.
- How important the job is. If it is unimportant, it does not merit a large investment of your time. Will doing this job contribute to my main aims and objectives? If not, it is unimportant. If the job is important, it merits an appropriate large investment and focusing attention on delivering this within the deadline.

EXERCISE 8.2   Analysing and Improving Your Use of Time

1. ***Devise a recording format that suits you, or use the one provided below.***

Photocopy or print out a supply of the sheets or use a computer-generated format. Use as many sheets as necessary each day. Remember to include any work you do away from your organisation, for example, at home.

If you discover that particular activities, for example, telephone interruptions, are causing a problem, then make a detailed log of what happens each time. *Do this immediately* – do not leave it until the end of the day. Keep the diary for at least a week. If none of your weeks are typical, you will need to keep the log for several weeks.

Using codes will save you time. For example, you could use M for meetings, I for interruptions, P for phone calls, PI for phone interruptions and E for emails.

Time diary

Day _____   Date _____   Page no. _____

Activity   Time spent   Comments

_____   _____   _____

_____   _____   _____

_____   _____   _____

2. ***Use the time diary to analyse how you used your time***

Analyse your use of time by answering the following questions:

- How did you use your time compared with how you planned to use it?

- How much of your time do you spend on different activities, such as dealing with emails? Does this reflect the importance of the different activities? Important activities are those that help you to achieve your objectives.

- Which jobs did not get done? Does it matter? Did you finish all the important and urgent jobs?

- How much time do you lose through interruptions? Which interruptions are the most time-consuming?

- How much of your time is spent on other people's work?

- Most people have a time of day when they work more efficiently. Do you use this time for your most important work?

3. ***Now, plan how to improve your time management.***

Some of the changes you could make will be obvious. For example:

- You discover that jobs started early in the morning tend to get completed quickly. So you decide in the future to do your most important work at this time.

- You note that you spend about 2.6h each day reading and answering emails. You decide to experiment with techniques to cut down this time. See Exercise 8.3 that follows.

- You discover that urgent jobs are generally done, but important long-term projects tend to be neglected. You decide to make realistic plans to ensure that long-term projects are scheduled.

- What else can you do?

EXERCISE 8.3   Reducing Time Spent on Emails

For one week, try the following seven steps to try and cut down on email interruptions:

1. Unsubscribe from email newsletters that are not relevant to your work.
2. Turn off all email notifications.
3. Schedule a time each day for dealing with emails.
4. When sending emails, use the subject line to indicate all action required, for example, For Your Information (FYI; so people know it is information only); Action Required by...and Date or To Do By...and DATE; No Response Required (NRR; to avoid getting polite responses such as 'thank you' or 'looks interesting').
5. Keep the emails you send short, five sentences maximum or fewer.
6. If you do not have one, set up a logical filing system for emails.
7. Keep your inbox clean by deleting or filing all emails, so you start each day with a clean inbox.

At the end of the week, assess how much time you can save by being efficient with your emails. See Thomas (2021) for more time-saving ideas for emails and time management in general.

2. Identify how soon you need to have the job completed and be realistic in assessing this by considering how urgent it is. Urgent jobs are ones that have imminent deadlines. If an urgent job can be completed quickly, then deal with it right away. That means it will not interfere with you getting on with other competing demands or more important jobs.
3. Plan when the work will be done. This involves the following steps:

- Break the job or project down into manageable parts. If the job/project is big or complex, or parts of it are boring, try setting aside regular, small amounts of time to complete specific bits. Dividing it into manageable segments will help you to see that you are progressing. On big tasks, it is important to pace yourself.
- Estimate how long each part will take to complete. This may be difficult, but an informed guess will at least help you to be more realistic in future. Here are some suggestions that may help:
  - Use your experience from similar jobs if appropriate.
  - Consult with colleagues who have experience in doing the job.
  - Build in some contingency time if possible.
  - Keep a note of how long the tasks take so that you can make a better estimate next time of the time required.
- Schedule in your diary or organiser (for example, Google Calendar) when the work will be done. You may find that you need to reschedule daily to take account of changing priorities, so this is a highly dynamic process. The important thing is to ensure that the key tasks you need to undertake are scheduled to allow enough time for their completion.

The Eisenhower matrix, as shown in Table 8.1, is a tool than can be used to help with scheduling work. The top left is work that is both urgent and important, so it needs to be done. If the task is not important but urgent, then delegate if possible. If the task is important but not urgent, then schedule a time to do this. The bottom right is neither important nor urgent and therefore requires no attention and can therefore be removed from your 'to do list'.

An interesting example of the application of the Eisenhower matrix has been published by JPHMP direct, the companion site of the *Journal of Public Health Management and Practice* (Morrow, 2019). This describes the lived experience of public health practice in upstate New York, where necessity drives the priority setting agenda and is highly dynamic. This principle which has wider application, is that priority setting requires flexibility and being adaptable as unforeseen challenges may arise.

MANAGING PROJECT WORK

Planning, delivering and performance managing a health promotion or public health project can differ from other managerial activities. You might be required to implement a project from concept to delivery whilst also ensuring that the progress is controlled so that it delivers effectively and efficiently. The most obvious thing about a health-promoting project is that it has a particular and specific purpose that might be unique. This may be encapsulated in its name, such as 'community vaccination centre', 'COVID-19 testing clinic' or 'alcohol support service'. It is possibly most useful to think of a project as an instrument of change, which, when it is successfully completed, will have made an impact as defined in the original aims and objectives.

Another key aspect of projects is that they are usually time-limited; they have clearly identifiable start and finish times. Projects vary enormously in their scope. Small projects can last only a few days and involve activities by a single person. By contrast, large projects can involve many people and different disciplines and agencies and may last for several years.

All projects, however, have the same basic underlying structure and go through several stages, as set out in Box 8.3.

These stages are, of course, very similar to the basic planning and evaluation cycle that was described in Chapter 5, so this chapter should be read in conjunction with Chapter 5. The difference is that when you are delivering an ongoing service rather than a one-off project, the cycle repeats itself.

Because projects vary so much in terms of their scale and length of life, it is particularly important that they are planned systematically. It is also vital to understand how

TABLE 8.1	**Eisenhower Matrix: A Tool for Time Management**		
	URGENT		**NOT URGENT**
IMPORTANT	DO. Do it now.		DECIDE. Schedule a time to do it.
NOT IMPORTANT	DELEGATE. Who else can do it for you?		DELETE. Eliminate it.

Data from Team Asana. (2022). The Eisenhower matrix: how to prioritise your to-do list. https://asana.com/resources/eisenhowermatrix

BOX 8.3 The Stages of a Health Promotion Project

1. The start is the most important stage of any project and covers areas such as setting the overall aims, gaining approval and allocation of a budget. It will set the foundations for the lifetime of the project.
2. Specification involves defining the detailed objectives of the project. This includes what the outcomes will be and the targets for delivering these outcomes in terms of quantity, quality and timing.
3. Design stage is when the 'what' is translated into 'how'. It may take the form of detailed plans. Sometimes, it might be helpful to have a short document that can be reviewed as a reminder of the essence of the project, such as a 'term of reference'.
4. In the implementation stage, the plans are put into operation. It is important to note that the end of implementation is not the end of the project.
5. The evaluation, review and final completion stage will be marked by the delivery of the final report, which includes an evaluation of the findings and the details of a post-implementation review. This review should take place after the end of the implementation stage so that it is possible to include data on the long-term outcomes of the project, which is important from the perspective of sustainability.

the project contributes to the wider strategic plans of the organisation concerned.

Starting Health Promotion and Public Health Projects

There are numerous models on how to start a project, and as Fig. 8.2 suggests, this can often be divided into four elements. The model in Fig. 8.2 highlights the value of an initiation phase where constraints are identified, and potential problems can be anticipated.

A project will start with ideas often presented in the form of a proposal or written document. This can take a number of forms, such as terms of reference, scoping paper or report of a feasibility study. The key elements that are often described in this document include the following:

- Who is proposing to carry out the project, for example, an NHS organisation or a voluntary service such as a charity?
- Who is providing the funding or commissioning the project, for example, the local authority or possibly this may have central Government funding?
- The aims and outcomes of the project and how these will be measured, for example the number of individuals that have been helped.
- The scope of the project, for example, who will use or receive it, the setting in which it will be delivered

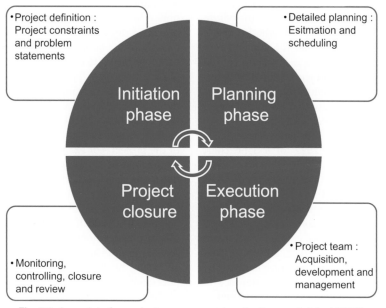

Fig. 8.2 A model of a project management cycle. Source: Adhikari (2018).

and which departments, agencies and people will be affected. It may also be important to define the limits of the project to manage expectations.

- The costs of the project in terms of staffing, travel costs, buildings, equipment and other resources.
- The project stages or milestones with timescales. It might be appropriate to grade these, and whilst a self-assessment might be limited, it does still provide some metrics on which to measure progress. For further reading on self-assessment evaluation, consult WHO (2015).
- Methods and standards: the use of any particular techniques or methods and the adoption of any recognised quality standards. This will be particularly important for the governance and accountability of the project.
- Roles and responsibilities of participants in the project, which is especially important when the project is commissioned by a partnership of a number of agencies.

Detailed Planning

For anything but the very smallest of projects, developing a detailed plan of each stage immediately before you enter it would be good practice and highly advisable. Typically, one of the last tasks in the planning of a stage will be planning the next stage. The Gantt chart, named after Henry Gantt, the man credited with its invention (see Ganttcharts.com for the history), is one tool to consider using for planning, scheduling and monitoring project tasks.

The Gantt chart is made up of a task information side on the left and a taskbar side (on the right; see Fig. 8.3 for an example). The task information side sets out the nature of each task and who is responsible for it, whether this is one or several individuals. The taskbar is a line that represents the period during which the task will be carried out. The precise content of a Gantt chart should be determined by the intended use and reflect the key milestones to be achieved. Such a chart is easy to draw and presents the plan in a visual form, which is easily understood by most people (see Hakoune, 2022 for guidance on using Gantt charts and Hirakata et al., 2022 for a Gantt chart used in COVID-19 research).

The chart can have application at every level in the health promotion or public health project planning process, from initial outline planning down to the detailed planning of individual tasks. For complex projects, any single bar on the master chart for the whole project might have to be represented by a more detailed bar for that particular task or stage. Essentially, a Gantt chart can be considered a rapid and accessible point of reference to monitor the progress of a project. It can also be used to assess what has been achieved as a retrospective tool. For

examples of the Gannt being used in practice in a variety of health-related settings, see Ohl (2017) and Hundley et al. (2019).

It follows that one major benefit of Gantt charts is that they highlight critical points, for example, where progress in X is dependent on Y already being completed. This also allows potential difficulties to be anticipated when there are contingent relationships. Planning tools such as Gantt charts are only aids to help you to achieve your purpose. Sticking to your plan will not necessarily bring success; you may have to make an adjustment because of unforeseen circumstances. However, without systematic planning you are unlikely to be able to keep your project on course at all, and many projects have to adjust. Anticipating this and being flexible is therefore important. Case study 8.1 describes the use of the Gantt chart in Fig. 8.3.

Managing Implementation

In addition to detailed plans, a project needs to have built-in control procedures. Such procedures help identify problems as soon as they arise, explore options to address them and select and implement the best solutions.

Control issues include time constraints, budgetary costs and quality. Methods for control include progress reports and progress meetings, which might include a project steering group. Large projects may need to use all these methods. Progress reports can sometimes be best presented in a standardised form, which compares progress with the project plan. Often, such considerations are agreed upon in advance of the project, for example, how often a project steering group will meet and what executive decisions can be taken or need to be referred elsewhere for approval. The use of social media can be useful to facilitate projects when there is a team of people involved with the project's development and implementation. The advantages and disadvantages of social media should be discussed before using them in a project (Stellefson et al., 2020).

Some constraints will be outside the immediate control of the project. For example, a project could be influenced by the policies of an organisation or other factors embedded in the structure and the working culture. In such cases, project managers should do what they can to reduce the impact of these issues on the project in addition to highlighting these constraints in the report. For more about quality management, see the section on working for quality later in this chapter.

Finally, health promotion and public health practitioners might be involved in more than one project, whether as the project lead or as a team member. For guidance on managing multiple projects, see Harrin (2022).

Convene local planning group – January (LA)
Appoint language translation provider – February (PG)
Receive list of refugees from Home Office – March (LA)
Assess housing, health and education needs – April (PG)
Inform Home Office of refugees to be received – May (LA)
Welcome refugees to local area – June (PG)
Repeat process with new list from Home Office – July (LA)
Assess progress and evaluate impact – ongoing (PG)

LA = Local Authority PG = Partnership groups

Case study contributed by Dr Gareth Morgan, Public Health Directorate at Hywel Dda University Health Board.

Fig. 8.3 Gannt chart for Case study 8.1.

CASE STUDY 8.1   The Syrian Vulnerable Person Resettlement Programme

The Syrian vulnerable person resettlement programme was an initiative established by the United Kingdom government. The objective was to help resettle Syrian refugees, and the programme assisted people in refugee camps from the so called MENA countries, Middle East & North Africa, such as Jordan, Lebanon, Iraq and Egypt. The programme is an example of the United Kingdom contributing to international public health programmes working with other nations. Although this was an initiative that covered the United Kingdom, the implementation and delivery of the programme was driven at a local level.

It was driven by the partnerships between the local health services, local authority and other agencies such as local and national charities. The ability of a local area to take refugees would also be dependent on multiple factors, such as the availability of housing, specialist healthcare services, translation services and capacity in schools. Community safety is also important, so local

Police officers have key roles to play. This also illustrates the broader point that public health may include multi-disciplinary and multi-agency working that also spans the 'upstream' determinants such as housing. Partnership is therefore critical.

Local partnership groups were therefore needed to ensure the successful delivery of the programme. Fig. 8.3 illustrates a possible Gantt chart for this situation. In planning a public health programme of work, such a chart gives an immediate reference point to rapidly measure progress and assess whether contingency measures need to be introduced. For example, what would happen if translation services from Arabic to English became unavailable? The Gannt chart, therefore, helps foresee potential risks and allows mitigation measures to be considered in advance. The Gannt chart presented is based on the experience of delivering the programme in a Welsh Health Board.

MANAGING CHANGE

Health promoters and public health practitioners may experience change in several ways, although these can be broadly generalised into two areas. One is being a part of an organisation that is undergoing change, perhaps a restructuring or in response to new policy. The second way is by being a change agent, by initiating and implementing changes in health promotion or public health policy or practice. This might be in response to new evidence or to a public health crisis such as COVID-19.

The first way, experiencing organisational change, is common in statutory agencies such as those in the

public sector, for example healthcare. Government policy changes affect the NHS and local authorities in particular. Understanding and surviving organisational change is outside the scope of this book (see Cameron and Green, 2015 for an overview). However, understanding how to implement and manage change successfully is a fundamental part of a health promoter's and public health practitioner's role since this competency will be required in many projects to ensure their success.

Implementing Change

You may want to introduce a change in your public health practice, such as a different way of running health promotion programmes, introducing a health-related policy at your place of work or starting off new health promotion activities. Implementing change can be very challenging, and it will help to spend some time thinking through your strategy.

Key Factors for Successful Change

The key to gaining commitment to change, and overcoming resistance to change, lies in understanding the motivation of all the people who could be affected by the change and how they feel about it. Overall, do they feel positive or negative about the proposed change? The balance between positive and negative factors can be expressed in the change equation in Box 8.4.

The basis of the equation is the simple assumption that people are rarely interested in change unless the factors or benefits supporting change outweigh the costs. As a change agent, your job is either to reduce D, the perceived costs or to increase the sum of A, B and C:

A. Dissatisfaction with the way things are. If you are dissatisfied, you may wrongly assume that others are too. If people are comfortable with the way things are, they are unlikely to support change. Consider how you could gather views on this to assess the levels of dissatisfaction.

B. A shared vision of a better future. If a vision of a better future does not exist or is unclear, people will not strive to achieve it. If there are several competing visions, energy will be dissipated in arguments. People are more likely to buy into a vision that improves their livelihood or other cherished aspects of their lives. A vision that threatens important aspects of an individual's or a group's life is almost bound to fail.

C. An acceptable, safe first step. The size of the change and the risks involved can seem overwhelming. Many of us could share a common view of what better health for all would mean. But where do we begin? The first steps are acceptable if they are small and are likely to be successful or if the risks of failure can be managed.

BOX 8.4   The Change Equation

A = the individual's or group's level of dissatisfaction with things as they are now.

B = the individual's or group's shared vision of a better future.

C = the existence of an acceptable, safe first step.

D = the costs to the individual or group.

Change is likely to be viewed positively and be implemented successfully *if*: A + B + C is greater than D.

(Gleicher, 1990).

D. The costs to the individual or group. What is important here is how people *perceive* the costs, which is subjective to them. There will always be costs, and change can be perceived as difficult or unfair. Costs can be tangible things like time, money, and resources or more intangible costs like stress or loss of status (see Case study 8.2 for an example of A–D reflected in a change in practice).

Reasons for Resistance to Change

People vary in their responses to change. Whilst one person may passively resist a change, another may actively oppose it, whereas another may embrace and facilitate change. Whether you are campaigning for a change or implementing a change in policy or practice in your work, you will need to consider that many people resist change for several reasons. In an analysis of the concept of resistance, underpinning factors included mistrust and communication barriers (DuBose and Mayo, 2020). In practice, having a strong awareness of the context will lead to appropriate strategies to overcome barriers, and further considerations include:

Self-interest. Whilst a change may be in the interest of most people, it may not be in everyone's best interest. For example, whilst many people, including some smokers, may support a no-smoking policy, others may see it as an infringement of personal liberty. Balancing these competing interests is important.

Misunderstanding. The change being proposed may be misunderstood. For example, some may think that an alcohol policy is giving an advantage to people with drinking problems by allowing different standards of work performance and behaviour compared to the rest of the workforce. Misunderstandings can occur in organisations where there is a lack of trust between the managers and the workforce.

Belief that a change is not in the interest of the people it is intended to benefit. People may believe that the costs of a change will outweigh the benefits, not only to themselves but also to others or a whole organisation.

Low tolerance for change. People may resist change because they are anxious about new demands that will be made of them. Organisational change can require people to change too much or fail to provide them with the time and support they need. This might include training or peer-support groups.

Methods for Overcoming Resistance to Change

To overcome resistance to change, it is vital to select the best approach, or a combination of approaches, for the situation and the people involved. This requires being situationally aware. Five possible options are given here:

CASE STUDY 8.2   **COVID Case Study**

The National Health Service was formed in 1948, and one of the greatest challenges in the history of the organisation was the delivery of the COVID-19 vaccination programme in response to the global pandemic.

This was a considerable challenge of change management, taking into account the logistics of vaccine supply, staff capacity and appropriate venues to deliver the programme. There was invaluable support to this from several partners, including public sector organisations, local authorities, private sector, charities, volunteers and the armed forces.

There was also a need to ensure correct messaging, balancing the need to maintain the non-medical preventative control measures such as staying at home versus the need to reassure the public of the need to attend for vaccination. As an example of a local NHS response, staff were invited to volunteer to become vaccinators to ensure sufficient human resources were available to deliver the programme.

The response was excellent and local venues were sought within the community, some of these were purposely built for the delivery of the programme. The supply, therefore, was based on three key determinants, namely the availability of the vaccine, staff available to administer it and appropriate venues. The demand was the numbers within the targeted groups, starting with the most vulnerable to the virus, such as the elderly or those with pre-existing health conditions.

The implementation matched supply and demand; for example, if the daily capacity in vaccination clinic A was 100 and the target cohort had 500 individuals, this would be a five-day operation taking into account those who failed to attend and allowing for a catch-up, so nobody in the target group was omitted.

We can apply our change equation: A = there was a high level of dissatisfaction, so called 'lockdown' fatigue, B = the vision was to protect the community from the COVID-19 virus, C = the vaccine was offered as a measure to move out of the pandemic, and D = costs include fear of adverse events and vaccine hesitancy.

In this particular case, the intention of the programme is simply to ensure enough individuals within the community are vaccinated to achieve so called 'herd immunity'. For some, $D > A + B + C$, and they have declined the opportunity to receive the vaccine. For many individuals in the United Kingdom, more than 90% of the population, $A + B + C > D$, as there has been high uptake of the vaccine.

Case study supplied by Dr Gareth Morgan, Hywel Dda University Health Board.

1. *Education and communication.* This involves consulting, informing and educating people about a change before it happens. It also involves communicating with them in a variety of ways, including one-to-one, group discussion and written documents. This approach is perhaps best indicated when resistance to change is based on inadequate or inaccurate information. The limitation is that it can be time-consuming, especially if a lot of people are involved or across many sites, such as different hospitals within the catchment area of the NHS organisation.

2. *Participation and involvement.* Resistance to change may be reduced if those initiating the change can identify those that might be most resistant. As a follow-on action, those who are resistant could be actively involved in the process of designing and implementing the change. The initiators of the change must genuinely be prepared to actively listen and learn. A token effort may provoke more resistance because people will feel let down if their contribution is not taken seriously.

   Participation and involvement are necessary when full commitment to a policy change is needed to make it work. It follows that policies work best when people feel ownership of them because they have been involved in their development. This approach is also useful when the initiators do not have full information about the implications of the change for certain groups of people or certain departments, so meaningful and constructive discussion is important. It could also be the preferred option where the initiators of change have little power because it harnesses the power of others as a force for change.

   Nevertheless, this approach does have limitations. It can be very time-consuming and demands a high degree of coordination. It can lead to a poor outcome if an attempt is made to accommodate everyone's needs. Setting realistic expectations is, therefore, crucial.

3. *Facilitation and support.* This involves helping people to identify what changes are required and providing them with support to plan options so that they might be able to manage the change themselves. This could be done, for example, by providing time for people to reflect on the situation and to identify their own objectives and how to meet them. Emotional

support to cope with the stress of change may also be required, including the delivery of mentoring schemes, where more experienced people help others with their managerial or professional development. This approach works best where anxiety and fear lie at the heart of resistance. As with participation and involvement, the limitation of this approach is that it too can be time-consuming and expensive, for example, if it is necessary to employ counsellors to support a large workforce.

4. *Negotiation and agreement*. This involves exploring potential incentives to actual or potential resisters. This might be best achieved through an intermediate, for example, through negotiating with trade unions about the effects of the change on working conditions. This could be particularly appropriate when it is obvious that some people will lose out as a consequence of the changes. It can be effective if there are specific pockets of resistance, but it could be expensive if everyone argues that they are also losing out.

5. *Political influencing*. This approach can be useful where one or a few powerful individuals are the source of resistance. Overcoming their resistance could be highly valuable as they might then champion the change. Whilst this can be relatively quick, one possible drawback is that it can lead to problems in the future if people feel that they have been manipulated.

For more details on the theory and practice of change management, see Hayes (2022).

WORKING FOR QUALITY

Working for quality involves examining the nature of the public health service and assessing how good it is when it is evaluated or judged against a number of criteria.

Criteria for Quality

What are the criteria for quality in health promotion and public health practice work? The checklist in Box 8.5 may be helpful in identifying aspects of quality. The checklist can be applied to your work overall or a particular health promotion or public health practice programme.

Improving Quality

Initiatives to improve quality are usually successful if people work together to explore ideas and generate collective solutions. This could be a group of people delegated by management to assess a particular issue or problem, such as improving the quality of patient information for COVID-19, the way in which antenatal advice is being given to prospective parents or the way a GP practice is helping patients to stop smoking.

BOX 8.5 Checklist: Criteria for Quality in Health Promotion and Public Health Practice

1. **Appropriateness**: Is it relevant and acceptable to clients – the individual, group or community concerned?

2. **Effectiveness:** Does it achieve the aims and objectives you set?

3. **Social justice:** Does it produce health improvement for all concerned, not for some people at the expense of others? In other words, is it 'fair'?

4. **Equity and access:** Is it provided to all people, whatever their racial, cultural or social background, based on equal access for equal need? (This may mean, for example, unconventional clinic times, wheelchair access, leaflets in braille and ethnic minority languages, information on audio and video cassettes, etc.).

5. **Dignity and choice:** Does it treat all groups of people with dignity and recognise the rights of people to choose for themselves how they live their lives? Is it non-judgemental, accepting that people have the right to withdraw from or reject health promotion if they so wish?

6. **Environment:** Does it ensure an environment conducive to people's health, safety and wellbeing? Does it recognise that people feel at home in different environments and may feel uncomfortable or intimidated in some settings? Is the social environment friendly and welcoming?

7. **Participant satisfaction:** Does it satisfy all those with an interest in the outcomes of the health promotion work, such as commissioners, managers, clients and other interest groups, acknowledging that the views of clients should be paramount?

8. **Involvement:** Does it involve all those with an interest, including clients, in planning, design and implementation? Does it avoid 'tokenism', with clients' views genuinely sought and incorporated in a non-patronising way?

9. **Efficiency:** Does it achieve the best possible use of the resources available and provide value for money?

Sometimes such groups are called *quality circles*. These are workgroups of up to 12 employees who do the same or similar work who meet regularly to address work-related problems. The issues to tackle are selected by the group itself, and the outcomes are presented to management. In many cases, the group is also involved in implementing the solutions. Management commitment to taking account of the outcomes and implementing recommended changes is crucial to success. Such an approach is also likely to benefit the employees, for example, boosting their professional confidence (Rohrbasser et al., 2018).

- Typically, a quality circle could start by listing issues for consideration, using techniques such as brainstorming.
- Select the issue to be addressed and focus on this specifically.
- Gather information and perceptions about the nature of the problem and analyse the causes.
- Generate a range of solutions and establish the best options or combination of options.
- Prepare a report on their findings for management decision or further discussion.

An example of a quality circle might be a colleague's commitment to improving the provision of communication support for D/deaf patients. An illustrative example of this is provided in Case study 8.3.

Developing Quality Standards

It may be helpful to improve quality by using specific standards, which are an agreed upon level of performance either mandated by the government or negotiated within available resources. Examples of standards include those produced by Public Health England (2019). These standards present a new framework for England

---

CASE STUDY 8.3 Inclusive Communication With D/deaf People

People who were born deaf may learn to communicate through sign language, such as British Sign Language. Sometimes abbreviated to BSL, this is one of the official languages of the United Kingdom and may be one of the primary communication strategies of the culturally D/deaf community. However, sometimes other methods are also used, such as lip reading.

The importance of providing communication support to a D/deaf person in a healthcare setting cannot be overstated, not least because good communication is important to understand treatment options and ensure informed consent is provided. It is also important to allow the D/deaf person to participate equally within the consultation and ask questions.

The provision of communication support to D/deaf patients can be variable in healthcare settings. One negative extreme of this is that no support is offered, which as a minimum, will make for an unsatisfactory patient experience. The opposite of this is to provide choice to D/deaf patients via an active offer and ensure the episode of care is a positive experience. In practice, there is likely to be a mix of both, and it is therefore important to work toward a positive experience as far as possible for as many patients as possible.

This provision needs to be considered a core service, underpinned by considerations of safety, dignity and patient experience. The framework could be used in two ways. Firstly, if the service was being planned, then this framework could help shape how to design, deliver and evaluate it. Secondly, if the service was already in existence, the framework could help performance manage it and identify areas for further improvement.

Appropriateness: Patients requiring communication support are offered an appropriate service according to their individual needs, such as the provision of a British Sign Language interpreter.

Effectiveness: An effective service model will be proactive and deliver on the core requirement of providing high-quality communication support to D/deaf patients.

Social justice: Do D/deaf patients feel comfortable receiving this service? Do they have an opportunity to provide feedback, improvement suggestions, or make complaints if they feel unhappy?

Equity and access: This brings into consideration issues about fairness and accessibility. Is there a fair distribution of service uptake? Are some D/deaf people still not receiving the service? If so, how do we address this?

Dignity and choice: At the core of this is to offer D/deaf patients an opportunity to work with an interpreter of their choice, as they might have a preference.

Environment: There might be ways to create a D/deaf friendly environment. For example, training reception staff to greet someone through the medium of BSL could be a small but greatly valued gesture to help patients.

Participant satisfaction: It is important to record measures that indicate satisfaction, for example, an increase in the uptake of communication support. If the uptake of the service is declining, this might reflect low satisfaction.

Involvement: D/deaf patients are involved in the ongoing improvements of the service. This might include calling a patient experience group meeting or seeking views in other ways, such as via confidential questionnaires.

Efficiency: There might be an economy of scale by having some dedicated sessions for D/deaf patients accessing healthcare. The provision of the service might then be able to help support more D/deaf patients per session.

Case study produced by Dr Gareth Morgan. For further reading, consult the Wales Audit Office (2018).

intended to raise the quality in public health services and functions. Another example of a quality standard is from Wales relating to housing, published by the Welsh Government (2019). This is important as housing can be a key determinant of health and wellbeing. As for health promotion and public health leaflets, the following criteria could be used:

- Content consistent with the values of health promotion.
- Relevant and easily understood by the people for whom the leaflets are intended. Knowing your audience is key.
- Developed with the involvement of the target audience to ensure it meets their needs and is owned by them.
- Not biased or discriminatory.
- Accurate, up-to-date information informed by facts and evidence.
- Free of inappropriate advertising or supporting a political cause.

See the section on guidelines for selecting and producing health promotion resources in Chapter 11.

A further challenge is to develop standards that are *quantifiable* in some way. This is a difficult task, but you could, for example, develop a five-point scale for assessing the quality of your leaflets so that you score them out of five for the extent to which they fulfil each quality standard. Another example could be that you decide that a quality management issue is to respond quickly to requests from your clients. You could develop this by setting a standard such as returning telephone calls within 24 hours and writing requests within three days.

Monitoring and reviewing quality standards can involve a great deal of time and effort. The benefit comes from seeing clearly identified improvements in service.

Another quality assessment technique is the use of the five whys.

The five whys are a method to assist with root cause analysis to determine i) what is causing a difficulty and ii) what are the potential solutions. Although this has limitations and may provide an oversimplistic analysis (Card, 2017), asking why repeatedly can be helpful as a reflective tool. For example, housing can be a major determinant of health and wellbeing, with cold homes leading to hospital admissions and winter deaths (NICE, 2016, Rolfe et al., 2020). See Box 8.6 for an example of the use of the five whys in practice focusing on the housing agenda.

PRACTICE POINTS

- Management skills underpin delivering effective and efficient projects, including information management, report writing, time management, project management, managing change and developing quality.

> ### BOX 8.6 Implementing the Housing Agenda
>
> The five whys were:
> 1. Why does the housing agenda have variable implementation by the NHS? Not seen as a priority
> 2. Why is housing not seen as a priority? Because of competing demands
> 3. Why are there competing demands? Because the NHS is under pressure
> 4. Why is the NHS under pressure? Because the housing agenda is not being fully realised
> 5. Why is the housing agenda not being fully realised? No good practice guide.
>
> Therefore, a good practice guide could help NHS providers with a more systematic approach to ensure patients have their housing needs addressed.

- Good information management systems involve storing the essential paperwork and/or electronic files in the simplest way possible and avoiding duplication. Retrieving information is also key.
- Good report writing involves having clarity about the report's purpose and following a coherent and logical structure. Always review your report before publication, ideally seeking views from colleagues. Try also to see the report from the perspective of your audience.
- There are many ways to ensure good time management, including using time logs, diaries and scheduling tasks appropriately. This could be done in hardcopy form or electronically.
- Project work involves detailed and systematic planning of the tasks to be delivered. A Gantt chart is a useful tool as it gives a visual reference point for the work.
- Managing change requires an effective strategy and is more likely to be successful if people have a shared vision. There may be opposing views and a need to negotiate with those resisting change by addressing their barriers.
- Working for quality is best achieved collaboratively with partners and stakeholders. These may be outside your organisation. Management support and involvement are essential for success.

References

Adhikari, S. (2018). *Project management cycle (PMC), it's phases and characteristics*. https://www.publichealthnotes.com/project-management-cycle-pmc-its-phases-and-characteristics/

Broddy, D. (2017). *Management: an introduction* (7th edition). Oxford: Pearson.

Cameron, E., & Green, M. (2015). *Making sense of change management: a complete guide to the models, tools and techniques of organisational change* (4th edition). London: Kogan Page.

Card, A. J. (2017). The problem with '5 whys'. *BMJ Quality and Safety* https://doi.org/10.1136/bmjqs-2016-005849.

DuBose, B., & Mayo, A. M. (2020). Resistance to change: a concept analysis. *Nursing Forum*, 55(4), 631–636.

Gleicher, D. (1990). Open business school/institute of health services management/NHS training authority managing health services: *Managing change* (pp. 36–37). Milton Keynes: *The Open University Book*.

Hakoune, R. (2022). *Gantt charts explained*. https://monday.com/blog/project-management/everything-you-want-to-know-about-gantt-charts/

Harrin, E. (2022). *Managing multiple projects: how project managers can balance priorities, manage expectations and increase productivity*. London: Kogan Page.

Hayes, J. (2022). *The theory and practice of change management* (6th edition). London: Bloomsbury Academic.

Hirakata, V. N., Oppermann, M. L. R., Genro, V. K., et al. (2022). Exploring the Gantt chart as a tool to highlight double report in case series published during the first wave of the COVID-19 pandemic. *Systematic Review*, 11, 155. https://doi.org/10.1186/s13643-022-02024-0.

Horine, G. (2022). *Project management: absolute beginners guide* (5th edition). New Jersey: Que Publishing.

Hundley, H. E., Hudson, M. E., Wasan, A. D., & Emerick, T. D. (2019). Chronic pain clinic efficiency analysis: optimisation through use of the Gantt diagram and visit diagnoses. *Journal of Pain Research*, 12, 1–8. https://doi.org/10.2147/JPR.S173345.

Morrow, C. (2019). *Summer at a local health department and the Eisenhower matrix*. https://jphmdirect.com/2019;08/26/eisenhower-matrix-cynthia-morrow/

NHS England. *Information governance*. https://www.england.nhs.uk/ig/about/

NICE. (2016). Preventing excess winter deaths and illness associated with cold homes. Quality standard [QS117]. https://www.nice.org.uk/guidance/qs117

Ohl, M. (2017). *Gannt chart*. https://publichealthprac.wordpress.com/2017/07/29/gannt-chart/

Public Health England (2019). *Quality in public health: a shared responsibility*. https://www.gov.uk/government/publications/quality-in-public-health-a-shared-responsibility

Reid, M. (2018). Report writing: *Pocket study skills series* (2nd edition). London: Red Globe Press.

Rohrbasser, A., Harris, J., Mickan, S., Tal, K., & Wong, G. (2018). Quality circles for quality improvement in primary health care: Their origins, spread, effectiveness and lacunae- a scoping review. *PLoS One*, 13(12), e0202616. https://doi.org/10.1371/journal.pone.0202616.

Rolfe, S., Garnham, L., Godwin, J., Anderson, I., Seaman, P., Donaldson, C. (2020). Housing as a social determinant of health and wellbeing: developing an empirically-informed realist theoretical framework. *BMC Public Health*, 20,, 1138. https://doi.org/10.1186/s12889-020-09224-0.

Stellefson, M., Paige, S. R., Chaney, B. H., & Chaney, J. D. (2020). Evolving role of social media in health promotion: updated responsibilities for health education specialists. *International Journal of Environmental Research and Public Health*, 17(4), 1153. https://doi.org/10.3390/ijerph17041153.

Team Asana. (2022). The Eisenhower matrix: how to prioritise your to-do list. https://asana.com/resources/eisenhower-matrix

Thomas, M. (2021). *7 tips to save time on emails and get back an hour a day*. https://maurathomas.com/time-saving-email-tips/

UK Government. (2018). *Data protection act*. https://www.legislation.gov.uk/ukpga/2018/12/contents/enacted

Wales Audit Office. (2018). *Speak my language: overcoming language and communication barriers in public services*. https://audit.wales/sites/default/files/speak-my-language-2018-english_6.pdf

Welsh Government. (2019). *Welsh health quality standard*. https://gov.wales/wales-housing-standard

World Health Organisation. (2015). *Self-assessment tool for the evaluation of essential public health operations in the WHO European region*. https://www.euro.who.int/_data/assets/pdf_file/0018/281700/Self-assessment-tool-evaluation-essential-public-health-operations.pdf

YouTube

Change management (overview). https://www.youtube.com/watch?v=9yysOwXbzRA

Cranfield University. Successful change management. https://www.youtube.com/watch?v=t0siBRHKbIU

How I manage my time – 10 management tips. https://www.youtube.com/watch?v=iONDebHX9qk

Martin G. Skills and competencies for public health. https://www.youtube.com/watch?v=H6mghZmVPlc

Project health: 3 ways to check on the health status of your project – project management. https://www.youtube.com/watch?v=I54uELDdnZA

Report writing. https://www.youtube.com/watch?v=FXIuHOFAxos

Working Effectively With Other People

Gareth Morgan, Angela Scriven

CHAPTER OUTLINE

SUMMARY

This chapter focuses on developing practical skills for working effectively with other people and organisations. This will assist you to plan and implement health promotion and public health programmes. The following key aspects that are discussed all relate to practice when delivering your specific portfolio of work: communicating with colleagues, coordination and teamwork, participating in meetings, effective committee work and working in local public health partnerships with other agencies. Practical exercises and case studies are included to help illustrate underpinning theories as well as help embed the skills and learning opportunities provided.

Although some health promoters and public health practitioners plan and undertake their health promotion work entirely on their own, most are likely to be working with other people. This will be drawn from the wide range of professional backgrounds that make up the multidisciplinary workforce with a remit for promoting health, including:

- Colleagues may be peers, managers or people you manage.
- Colleagues in other parts of your own organisation.
- People drawn from the community and/or from different statutory and non-statutory agencies (local, national or international) who are working with you on a health promotion activity of mutual interest and importance.
- There may also be volunteers who want to assist with a project. For example, in the United Kingdom, during the COVID-19 pandemic, many volunteers were recruited from the community to assist with the response (Gov. UK, 2022).

A key aspect of success will be how well you work with other people, and this chapter discusses the knowledge and skills needed for interprofessional communication and collaborative and partnership working. Building relationships with colleagues is a critical determinant of success. Indeed, the UK Faculty of Public Health (FPH) has published a good public health practice guide, and one of the key elements of this is communication, partnership and teamwork (FPH, 2016)

COMMUNICATING WITH COLLEAGUES

Some of the fundamental principles of effective face-to-face and written communication are dealt with in Chapter 10. Whilst these are presented primarily with client contact in mind, they are also applicable to contact between health promotion and public health colleagues. It also needs to be highlighted, however, that many meetings were undertaken online during the COVID-19 pandemic, primarily as a method to avoid transmission of the virus between participants. There is evidence that this approach to multidisciplinary working was an effective alternative (Sidpra et al., 2020) with the additional advantage of saving resources of time and travel costs. Whether this is fully sustained as the world learns to live with COVID-19 is unclear, and potentially a hybrid model combining face-to-face meetings with virtual ones may emerge.

The following factors are particularly Important to ensure effective working relationships:

- Working in a team which recognises and builds on the strengths of other team members.
- Actively listening to the people you are working with so that you understand clearly their opinions, ideas and feelings and are able to respond to their questions.

Often you will be working in a multidisciplinary team (MDT) where members will have different professional backgrounds and may work for different organisations. The Social Care Institute for Excellence (SCIE), which is a values driven improvement agency with links to the health agenda, offers a valuable commentary on MDTs and some excellent practice examples to illustrate the importance of working collaboratively to deliver effective services (SCIE, 2018).

A considerable proportion of your time may be taken up by communications with colleagues, including telephone conversations, face-to-face discussions, and written communications on paper and via email. Try Exercise 9.1 to help increase your awareness of how you communicate with colleagues and how your communication might be improved.

There are also some theoretical frameworks which can help identify personality preferences, such as the Myers-Briggs type indicator (Myers and Briggs Foundation, 2022). Myers-Briggs helps individuals understand their communication preferences and those of others. Such frameworks should be seen as neutral tools, as opposed to making assessments or judgements, that simply help understand how individuals perceive the world around them, and this can help with interpersonal relationship building. It is not about being right or wrong, but rather a tool to help understand the filters that we and others

---

EXERCISE 9.1 How You Communicate With Colleagues

Record all the types of communication with colleagues that you carry out over one working day by making a tally of all the occasions in five categories, as set out in the following table. Then add up your total for each category and your grand total for the day. You might like to compare your results with those of your colleagues. You might also like to compare this across your own working week; for example, is a Monday morning particularly busy and Friday less so? If so, what can you do to better manage your time and spread your tasks across the week? Or at least try to understand your preferred working style, for example, a busy start to the week.

	Face-to-face verbal	Telephone	Paper, letters and memos	Electronic email	'Virtual' meeting
	————	————	————	————	————
	————	————	————	————	————
	————	————	————	————	————
	————	————	————	————	————
	————	————	————	————	————
	————	————	————	————	————
	————	————	————	————	————
Totals	————	————	————	————	————

Think about whether there is anything you would like to change or improve, for example:

- If you spend too much of time on the telephone, could you improve your telephone skills? For example, pre-empting the call with an email setting out points to be discussed with attachments.
- Could you use your time more efficiently if you used less time-consuming methods of communication (for example, teleconferencing or email) instead of having meetings? This will be especially true in a situation where travel is considerable, for example, working in rural areas.
- Are there ways that you can use technology to communicate more effectively and efficiently with colleagues? One of the positive outcomes of COVID-19 is the increased use of virtual meetings.
- Do you need to selectively spend more time face-to-face to understand colleagues and establish a closer working relationship? If so, how best would this be achieved, for example, in an informal setting or a more formal environment?

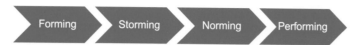

Fig. 9.1 Illustration of stages of group life. Source Adjusted from Tuckman's (1965) and Tuckman and Jensen's (1977) seminal work. Data from Tuckman, B. W. (1965). Developmental sequence in small groups. Psychological Bulletin, 65(6), 384–399 and Tuckman, B. W., & Jensen, M. A. (1977). Stages of small-group development revisited. Group and Organization Studies, 2(4), 419–427.

experience the world through. There are 16 personality profiles based on the combination of four preferences:

Favourite world: Do you prefer to focus on the outer world or on your own inner world? This is called Extroversion (I) or Introversion (I).

Information: Do you prefer to focus on the basic information you take in, or do you prefer to interpret and add meaning? This is called Sensing (S) or Intuition (N).

Decisions: When making decisions, do you prefer to first look at logic and consistency or first look at the people and special circumstances? This is called Thinking (T) or Feeling (F).

Structure: In dealing with the outside world, do you prefer to get things decided, or do you prefer to stay open to new information and options? This is called Judging (J) or Perceiving (P).

COORDINATION AND TEAMWORK

As highlighted previously, health promotion often involves multiagency and multidisciplinary working; therefore, effective coordination and teamwork are required. Teamwork is particularly important and appears to be a key determinant in safe, high-quality outcomes (Rosen et al., 2018).

Poor coordination of interventions and projects can result in losses in the efficiency and effectiveness of programmes, and it is especially difficult when big organisations like the National Health Service (NHS) and local authorities are working together. There are several ways of coordinating, and it is important to use the one best suited to the situation. Fig. 9.1 below offers a framework on which to progress coordination, and the text below uses an example of ways housing and health professionals can coordinate their work. Exercise 9.2 also offers an opportunity to reflect on this framework from the perspective of your own professional situation.

Appointing a Coordinator

As suggested by the term coordinator, this is a person who can keep an overview of the project. The ideal qualities of the coordinator are that they are committed, enthusiastic and able to understand the breadth of the project. So, in the case of housing and health, this might be someone with experience in providing supported accommodation services for patients with alcohol problems.

EXERCISE 9.2   Improving Coordination and Teamwork

In the health promotion or public health work you do that involves working with other people, can you think of any ways you could improve coordination and teamwork?

- What steps could you take to enhance the reputation of your health promotion work? Consider your strengths and how you showcase these.
- With whom could you build a better relationship to improve coordination or teamwork? Are there colleagues with a particular influence?
- What have you got to offer if you are bargaining? Think creatively about this and consider what resources are available. How could you maximise this?
- Can you think of any health promotion activities that you undertake routinely together with other people which could be more efficient with a set procedure?
- Are there any ways by which you could develop stronger links with other staff at your level in different departments or agencies to facilitate joint working in health promotion? Equally important, are there other colleagues that need to be involved?
- Have you any opportunities for joint objective setting or joint planning that could help to coordinate health promotion in your situation? How would this be helpful?
- Can you think of anything else? Have you missed anything? Discuss this with colleagues who are also involved in health promotion and public health.

Using Your Reputation

Building a reputation can be achieved in different ways. For example, you may have a reputation for having professional expertise, for example in delivering housing services to vulnerable people, such as the homeless community. Or your reputation may be one of being able to work well with colleagues or perhaps deliver projects on time and within budget.

Establishing Good Relationships

Continuing with the example of housing and health, this field of professional practice might involve a range of partners. This could include healthcare services, local authority departments, housing organisations and support services from the charity sector, such as alcohol treatment providers. Building good relationships can be achieved through an inclusive approach.

Bargaining

In practice, there may need to be trade-offs, such as exchanges of resources without the transaction of any finance. For example, an alcohol treatment charity may provide services for free if a housing agency provides free access to a meeting room along with refreshments.

Out-Ranking

Inevitably a project will involve hierarchies, even if these are implicit rather than explicit. In organisations, there are often grades of staff where these hierarchies are clear, although, across organisational boundaries, this is more difficult. There may be a need on some occasions to use the rank structure, although in practice, 'soft powers' such as influence are important.

Discussion and Negotiation

It is always worth being open to new ideas and negotiating novel solutions. In the case of housing and health, fuel poverty brings with it a major risk of living in a cold home, which can worsen health conditions. Is it possible to discuss solutions to this and negotiate a way forward? For example, could work be done with local advice services to explore how to support individuals who might be most at risk?

Another potentially helpful framework is the Belbin team roles. This offers a perspective on how teams function in respect of the key role.

The nine Belbin team roles are:

Resource Investigator, Team Worker and Coordinator (the social roles);

Plant, Monitor-Evaluator and Specialist (the thinking roles), and

Shaper, Implementer and Complete-Finisher (the action or task roles). For a fuller discussion on Belbin team roles, see Belbin (2022).

See Chapter 13 for further consideration of Belbin.

Policies, Procedures and Protocols

Making and implementing policies is discussed in Chapter 16.

Policies are important in coordinating health promotion and public health work. Using *set procedures* are ways of coordinating routine tasks. *Protocols* are agreed written procedures that everyone follows, ensuring that everyone carries out a particular task in the same way.

For example, tackling COVID-19 required many protocols, such as the wearing of face masks. On the former, there were face mask wearing protocols in GP surgeries and other health centres during the COVID-19 pandemic for the protection of both patients and staff. The protocol ensures that whoever is dealing with a patient (the doctor, practice nurse, district nurse or health visitor) offers the same level of protection with face masks or makes a reasonable adjustment if this was not possible, for example, if a patient needs to lip read. For a further review on face mask wearing during the COVID-19 pandemic, see Martinelli et al., 2021.

The UK government published national protocols for COVID-19 vaccines across the different products available and for different members of the community, such as children. This ensured governance and consistency in the way the vaccine programme was implemented (NHS England, 2022).

Joint Planning

In this approach, the parties involved not only agree on objectives but also meet regularly to develop and implement a joint plan. This may reduce the demands placed on one individual as a coordinator and also prevent the problem of one agency or department being perceived as controlling the agenda. Although it can be difficult to get everyone together, notwithstanding the possibility of virtual meetings, as described previously, there can be significant advantages to doing so. For example, the huge potential of public health practitioners working on the health agenda jointly with spatial planners and professionals with an interest in the built environment (Ige-Elegbede et al., 2021).

Joint Working Through Creating Teams

An autonomous team is given the authority, training, money, staff, premises and equipment to carry out the health promotion programme. There is no need for a coordinator because the whole team is working together from the same base and usually with a shared vision. Joint working of this kind is usually not suitable for short-term programmes but can be excellent for long term projects such as those involving community development. The NHS England document 'Building Collaborative Teams' is an interesting resource that provides a workshop guide to bring teams together to deliver joined-up services (NHS England, 2014).

Creation of Lateral Relations

This type of coordination depends on strengthening relationships between individuals in broadly equivalent jobs in different departments or agencies. Sometimes this may be appropriate and can result in setting up project teams, which are dissolved once the particular project is completed. It could also be done by forming interdepartmental or multidisciplinary teams or partnerships, which are given more authority for making decisions without having to refer them up the different hierarchies. In practice, this can lead to conflict with the existing vertical lines of command and often works best where there are good links between the various managers.

Characteristics of Successful Teams

There are different sorts of teams. The teams being considered here are associations of people with a common public health work purpose, for example, a primary healthcare team. Successful teams have the characteristics set out in Box 9.1. If you experience a team that does

---

BOX 9.1 Characteristics of Successful Teams

A Small Number of Meaningful Objectives
A set of compelling objectives that your team members share responsibility and accountability for achieving helps to create a sense of shared purpose, trust and collective achievement.

Clear Roles and Responsibilities Among Team Members
Team members need to be clear about what activities need to be undertaken and who is responsible for completing them so that nothing slips through the gaps. This is especially important when teams are forming, but roles and responsibilities may shift as your team matures and you get to know each other's strengths. These roles and responsibilities should be revisited regularly to ensure that expectations about how things would work are indeed how they are working.

Reflect on How the Team Is Working Together
All teams benefit from taking time out to reflect on how they are working together and how they might improve. You might want to do this in the form of team time-outs, away days or regular huddles, covering both technical aspects of work and how people are feeling. This time will be wasted, however, if people do not feel able to contribute freely, regardless of their role or position in the management hierarchy. So it's important to think about how you will create a safe environment for your colleagues to speak up.

Baird et al. (2020).

---

not seem to be working well, it can be helpful for the team to consider this list together to identify the cause of the difficulties (for more information on how to lead successful integrated team working, see Smith et al., 2020).

EFFECTIVE COMMITTEE WORK

A committee is a group of people appointed for a specific purpose accountable to a larger group or organisation. Examples are the management committee of a voluntary organisation or the health committee of a local authority. There are many common routines and procedures that help facilitate committees, and it is useful to be familiar with them in your situation. By doing this, you are more likely to be able to engage constructively with the committee and therefore have an influence on their work priorities.

Although details often vary from committee to committee, the underpinning principles are usually similar. For example, some committees start their life with recommendations from a steering group, which include proposals for the interim committee rules and associated timelines for the delivery of outputs. These are then reviewed and approved at the first committee meeting. After review and modification, if required, a set of rules will be agreed upon for the committee.

Committees need to be 'fit for purpose'; namely, their form fits their function. For example, the UK Health and Social Care Committee (HSCC) is a House of Commons cross-political group that holds the Department of Health and Social Care to account. This Committee examines policy, spending and administration on behalf of the electorate, and inquiries include Coronavirus: Lessons Learnt (House of Commons [HSCC], 2022). Fig. 9.1 below summarises some of the considerations of effective committee work, and Case study 9.1 illustrates their application.

Officers

The officers service the needs of the committee and carry out its instructions. Committees have key officers, usually the chair, the secretary, and the treasurer, but larger committees may have additional appointments, for example, a minutes secretary. Often several officers will be working on a committee, especially if the workload is high or the work needs to be delivered quickly.

Chair

Although much of the work of the chair may be done between meetings, constructing the agenda, it is at the meetings when the chair is most visible. The chair has overall responsibility for ensuring that the committee successfully completes their tasks or to introduce contingency

CASE STUDY 9.1   Example of COVID-19 Mass Vaccination Committee

A small team within the Public Health Department of the NHS formed an informal working committee that was tasked with helping to organise the mass vaccination programme in their area. The Head of the Department called, convened and chaired a daily team meeting to ensure work was delivered by officers as well as identify challenges and offer staff support. One of the officers also doubled up as secretary by taking brief contemporaneous notes by way of record and audit trail. There was no formal treasurer, although there were resource discussions, for example with payroll regarding the remuneration of staff for overtime.

The work needed to be agile, and standing agenda items for the meeting were rotas for the vaccination clinic, recruiting new staff to deliver the programme and barriers to delivery, such as vaccine supply. The main determinants of the effectiveness of the work with regard to behaviour were a supportive Head of Department, clarity of purpose, collective responsibility between the members of the team and mutual peer-to-peer support. Providing at least one-third of the committee were present, it was considered quorate.

Dr Gareth Morgan, Hywel Dda University Health Board, NHS Wales.

BOX 9.2   Sample Agenda for Alcohol Treatment Service Committee

It will often include standard items such as 'apologies for absence', 'minutes of the previous meeting', 'matters arising from the previous meeting' and 'any other business'. The important point is that the agenda acts as an advance organiser for everyone attending the meeting so that they are able to prepare. The committee members need to receive the agenda and associated papers in good time before the meeting, usually a week in advance at least.

Alcohol Treatment Service Committee: Agenda
- Introduction and welcome
- Apologies for absence
- Minutes of the previous meeting
  - For accuracy
  - For matters arising
- Report on alcohol treatment service
  - Activity report (Service manager)
  - Financial status (Treasurer)
  - Staffing issues (Personnel officer)
  - Future demands (For discussion)
- Any other business
- Date, time and venue of the next meeting

action if required. Effective chairs speak clearly and concisely, involve other members of the committee in discussions and delegates to ensure the active involvement of all members. The chair also has the responsibility of succession planning, for example, preparing the next chair and providing opportunities for the vice chair to develop their skills.

Secretary

The secretary has general responsibilities for all the non-financial papers and reports. The secretary will often work in collaboration with the other officers and ensure that the committee's work is coordinated and nothing is forgotten or any actions omitted. Good organisation, coordination and computing skills are needed. There are several software programmes (such as SharePoint or BoardEffect; see websites in the reference section at the end of the chapter) that can help with this work.

The secretary is responsible for compiling the agenda for the committee meetings in conjunction with the chair. This is the list of things to be done or agreed upon during the meeting. A sample agenda is shown in Box 9.2. The secretary is also responsible for the final version of the

minutes and for agreeing on these with the chair, even if a minutes secretary takes the notes at the meetings. Minutes are accurate records of the meeting and should always identify precisely who has responsibility for what action, by what date and when a report back will be made to the committee.

Treasurer

A treasurer is crucially important if the committee is responsible for any financial matters. Treasurers will provide reports on the financial position quickly and precisely at any time by recording and summarising every transaction. It is important committee members are able to see and understand the current situation; for example, spending may need to be slowed if the budget is being used too quickly. At the end of the financial year, all financial transactions are summarised in an annual statement, a clear one-page summary.

Quorum

It is unlikely that all committee members will be able to attend all meetings. The rules usually state the minimum number of members who must be present for the meeting to be considered representative of members' views and to have the authority to make decisions. This is called a quorum and is usually one-third or one-half of the total voting membership. Each committee will set their own rules, and sometimes a discussion can only really proceed if certain members are present to bring the required expertise to the committee.

Committee Behaviour

Committees can be either informal or formal, although certain behaviours are important. For example, having only one person speaking at a time without interruption allows a fair hearing for everyone. The chair should not allow an individual or particular viewpoint to dominate the meeting.

To avoid subdiscussion, members may address the meeting through the chair, although sometimes, it may seem more natural and helpful to address another committee member directly. Ultimately, the chair sets the tone that encourages all members to participate whilst keeping the meeting under control.

Sometimes, committees evolve and go through stages of group development. Tuckman's seminal work on team and group development (see Tuckman, 1965 and Tuckman and Jensen, 1977) has suggested the following: an initial 'forming' stage, where the committee first comes together, and there might be initial 'storming'. That might be where the committee starts exploring differences of perspective, and the chair will again have a key role to help work through any disagreements. 'Norming' relates to the stage where the committee is beginning to establish a work pattern before progressing to 'performing', where the delivery of the functions starts to reach optimum levels. Fig. 9.1 offers a representation of this, although, in practice, the stages may not happen always in the sequence; for example, a committee may go through several cycles of the stages of storming and norming before moving on to performing. (See Chapter 13 for further discussion on Tuckman.)

Understanding Conflict

Group conflict is inevitable at times because of differences in needs, objectives or values. The results of conflict may be positive or negative depending on how it is handled. Handled well, conflict can be a creative source of new ideas and can help a group to change and develop. It can also strengthen the ability of group members to work together. Conflict is badly handled when it is either ignored so that negative feelings develop or approached on a win/lose basis rather than a compromise or a win/win position. Undertake Exercise 9.3 to assess your conflict resolution style. This is based on the Thomas Kilman

---

EXERCISE 9.3   Your Conflict Resolution Style

Review Table 9.1 with other members of the groups you work in. Identify situations in your own practice where these different approaches to conflict resolution were used. Discuss what worked and what did not and determine why they may or may not have worked. Explore what could have been done differently to improve the outcome and what lessons can be learned. Reflect on this and assess what is your preferred conflict resolution style. What do you think is the most effective conflict resolution style? Finally, what do you need to do to achieve a better conflict resolution style?

TABLE 9.1   Approaches to Conflict Resolution

Style	Characteristic behaviour
Avoidance	Side-stepping the conflict
Accommodating	Trying to satisfy the other person's concerns at the expense of your own
Competing	Trying to satisfy your concerns at the expense of others
Compromising	Trying to find an acceptable settlement that only partially satisfies group members
Collaborating	Trying to find a win/win solution which satisfies group members

---

model (see Mishra, 2021, for an overview). For a wider exploration of conflict management in health settings, see Piryani (2019).

Conflict Resolution In The COVID-19 Pandemic

Both public health teams and the NHS needed to balance multiple and competing demands during the COVID pandemic. With reference to Case study 9.1 regarding the mass vaccination committee, the Head of Department needed to steer a narrow path between managing high expectations from the public and realistic programme delivery within constrained resources. This would require dynamic negotiation to achieve 'win/win' outcomes. For example, negotiating staff availability to deliver the vaccine programme would need agreement from line managers who faced multiple pressures.

A balance would therefore be agreed upon to free staff for defined intervals from their substantive roles whilst not compromising other non-COVID healthcare services that also needed to be maintained as part of a routine healthcare provision.

WORKING IN PARTNERSHIP WITH OTHER ORGANISATIONS

See Chapter 3 for details on the range of public health agencies and organisations.

Health promotion programmes and projects often require people from different organisations to work together; it is an established way of working in health promotion. Health promotion partnerships may be formally structured with partners or members at different levels, from chief executives to field workers. There may be a written constitution, and terms of reference or arrangements may be informal. They may be long term or set up for a time-limited period to work on a specific project (see Faculty of Public Health, 2022, for detailed guidance on partnership working in health promotion).

- The main reasons for setting up local partnerships are to harness a range of complementary skills and resources to work towards common public health goals,
- To avoid duplication and fragmentation of effort, and
- To avoid gaps in public health services or programmes.

For an excellent example of partnership working, see Estacio et al. (2017). In this example, there was a community-based health promotion project which focused on health literacy. Health literacy is the achievement of a level of knowledge, personal skills, and confidence to take action to improve personal and community health by changing personal lifestyles and living conditions (WHO, 2022). Health literacy is vital in helping individuals make informed health decisions.

A partnership approach to improving health literacy is an example of an important programme of work being undertaken by a range of stakeholders with a commitment to improving the situation locally.

Recent UK government health reforms have created the opportunity for new styles of partnerships (GOV.UK, 2022). Public health work often involves health services and local authorities pooling their budgets for joint initiatives and forming partnerships for planning, commissioning and delivering services. These new-style partnerships are genuine joint enterprises with local authorities and others. However, whilst there is a long history of partnership working to deliver health improvements, there is little evidence to date that partnership working has led to demonstrable improvements in what really matters – health outcomes. More recent analysis, however, does suggest the pooling of budgets does stimulate additional

integration activity, although the impact on health outcomes in the longer term still remains unclear (Stokes et al., 2019).

The public health reforms in the UK have created an environment that facilitates joint health and wellbeing strategies. In practice, establishing a local partnership with processes and planning mechanisms might also be driven by an unforeseen event, such as an outbreak of infectious

---

CASE STUDY 9.2 Outbreak Control Team (OCT) for Mycobacterium Tuberculosis (M.TB)

Purpose of the OCT

The primary purpose was to bring together key organisations to implement evidence-based strategies to control an outbreak of TB in a village in West Wales. The secondary purpose was to performance manage the control measures and implement further actions if required.

Responsibilities of the OCT

To collate epidemiological data on the outbreak in terms of the classic triple indicators of TIME, PERSON and PLACE.

To commission specialist services to provide both the expertise and the capacity to effectively control the outbreak.

Manage an effective communication campaign to raise awareness of the outbreak and ensure media messages were accurate.

Oversee the implementation of the control measures and ensure an appropriate data driven response to the outbreak.

Manage the programme budget and ensure that resources were used with good stewardship to achieve value for money.

Core Membership of the OCT Included

- Public Health Wales – Chair
- Carmarthenshire County Council
- Hywel Dda University Health Board

Wider Partnership Group Included

Primary care practices and GPs

A specialist 'find and treat' TB service for the X-ray screening

Oxford Immunotec to take and test blood samples

Local community councillors

Community organisations

disease such as COVID-19. Case study 9.2 is an example of the focus and wide-ranging professional and community partnerships that may be required in a real example from Wales of an outbreak of a bacterial disease of the lungs, tuberculosis.

In general, public health partnerships can take different forms and vary in terms of how closely members work together. It is useful to think of three main ways of working, spanning a range of degrees of involvement between partners: networking – cooperating – joint working.

Networking

In practice, networking means building relationships with other people from different agencies, resulting in the exchanging of information and ideas on activities and plans. This is useful for coordinating activities, learning from each other, avoiding duplication, and sharing knowledge of mutual interest. Members meet and talk, but they do not actually work together. Networking has the lowest degree of involvement between organisations and is often informal, yet it can be most important by allowing the rapid exchange of information. This might be true for a health risk; for example, services providing support to patients who misuse substances might become aware of adverse effects among those they are supporting. Networking can be digital, for example, WhatsApp, allowing rapid messages to be disseminated between practitioners. This could be a valuable health protection approach, for example, if there is sharing of injecting equipment which can predispose to risk of infection, for example, blood-borne viruses such as hepatitis which can causes liver disease.

Cooperating

Cooperating means that member agencies help each other in ways that are compatible with their own goals. They meet, talk and agree to participate in each other's work when this is helpful for their own work plans. For example, in an accident prevention partnership, people who work in the accident and emergency (A&E) department of a hospital may cooperate with a local alcohol advisory service (a voluntary organisation) to ensure that patients brought in with a drinking problem know that they can go to the alcohol agency for help. This cooperation helps the alcohol agency to reach potential clients and helps the A&E department fulfil its role of helping patients with longer term health needs. This way of working in partnership means a moderate degree of involvement between partners. Such an approach can provide a good return on investment as the cooperation can lead to positive outcomes.

Joint Working

Joint working means coming together to agree on a mutually acceptable plan and working together to carry it out. This necessitates a high degree of involvement between partners. For example, the police, the probation service, road safety officers from the local authority and a local alcohol advisory service may all work together to plan, implement and evaluate a joint programme of work to reduce drink-driving levels. This will be more formal than simply networking and would involve structured agenda items, and the discussions would be informed by data, for example, trends in road traffic accidents related to alcohol.

Partnerships can operate in one, two or all these ways. Sometimes joint working is thought to be the most effective, but networking and cooperating can be useful when it is not always feasible or worthwhile to aim for full joint or integrated working. Case study 9.3 sets of the non-statutory partnerships (which include cooperation and joint working) between a national body, Public Health Wales and commercial and local authority partners.

Factors for Successful Public Health Partnership Working

- Public health partnerships are formed for many reasons, and the successful ones are usually the result of investing a considerable number of resources, skills, and time to enable members to work well together.
- Key factors for success are that all partners need to be working towards a shared vision of what the partnership should achieve with an agenda and goals to which all partners concur.
- There must be an agreed approach. All partners need to feel a sense of ownership with no one partner dominating the agenda.
- Commitment from the highest level of member organisations is vital to ensure that belonging to the partnership fits in with the organisation's strategic aims and that there will be management support for input of time and other resources. This might be the Chief Executive of an organisation, or sometimes this may have a ministerial mandate from a high-ranking political official or their civil servant department.
- There must be a commitment of sufficient time and resources and realistic expectations. Such commitment needs to be meaningful as partnership working is time-consuming, so it may take months or years to develop a shared understanding and joint plans or achieve outcomes from joint health promotion activities.

CASE STUDY 9.3   Non-Statutory Partnerships Between a National Body, and Commercial and Local Authority Partners

During the spring of 2019, plans were made by the local NHS provider, Hywel Dda University Health Board, to implement measures to control an outbreak of TB in a village. A multidisciplinary and multiagency group was convened and chaired by a Consultant in Communicable Disease in Public Health Wales.

The primary control measure was to screen the village community with two tests. The first was a blood test which could show if there was an exposure to TB. The second was an X-ray which would detect active disease. A positive exposure blood test is known as latent TB that could become active in the future. Therefore, the interventions available to control this were treatment with antibiotics for positive cases and vaccination for negative cases.

Factors for Successful Working

- Good leadership and clarity of purpose regarding the delivery of the work programme.
- Transparency of discussion and an action log with clear accountabilities for delivery.
- Individuals feeling psychologically safe to raise concerns or challenge a decision taken.
- Clear communication and mutual respect between members of the outbreak team.
- Ability to innovate or introduce a contingency plan should the situation require this.

- Robust and rigorous evaluation of the programme by analysis of the data being collected.
- Introduction of additional measures should the evaluation suggest that this is required.
- Reflective practice of the group to ensure that lessons are learned and people supported.
- Listening to 'soft intelligence' that may be received from partners in the community.
- Being proactive and ensuring that advanced planning is factored into the discussions.

With the TB outbreak control programme, the team was highly cohesive, and the chair of the group ensured all members had an opportunity to engage. Questions and debate were encouraged, leading to decisions being taken by consensus building. Members were also empowered to think creatively, and one of the screening centres established was at a local sports stadium to accommodate a large uptake from the community.

During the summer months of 2019, the first phase of community screening was undertaken. The data analysis suggested there would be further cases in the community, so an additional screening was established during the autumn of 2019. This was highly effective by targeting specific individuals within the community. The work continues to monitor the community for further cases. For further details, see NHS Wales (2021).

Adapted from NHS Wales 2021 https://hduhb.nhs.wales/news/press-releases/independent-review-announced-into-response-to-llwynhendy-tb-outbreak/

- There must, however, be demonstrable achievements; otherwise, the partnership will be regarded as ineffective. This may lead to reputational damage, especially if there has been a significant use of resources.
- Someone acceptable to all partners should take responsibility for running the partnership (for example, setting up, chairing and servicing meetings) and coordinating action. A full-time coordinator can be employed.
- Mutual respect between partners is essential, and all partners need to feel that others welcome and value their input.
- Effective working relationships need to be characterised by openness and trust. Partners need to recognise and resolve potential areas of conflict.
- There must be an agreed upon framework for reviewing the partnership, changing the way of working if necessary and even bringing it to an end if it has outlived its usefulness or is proving unproductive.

- Awareness and understanding of partner organisations should be promoted through joint training programmes and incentives to work across organisational boundaries – ask.

See also earlier sections in this chapter on coordination and teamwork.

Potential Difficulties With Public Health Partnership Working

Partnerships, by their very nature, require different organisations or departments to work together. Collaboration between might seem straightforward in theory, although the practice can be difficult. There may be competing demands, and there may need to be compromise in what can be delivered and when.

These challenges can be intensified by a lack of top-level commitment or failure to provide adequate resources. Such resources might include staff time, capital, including equipment or premises or an adequate budget to run the public health intervention. Other factors that can impact partnership working include:

- Organisational change, which can compromise long term commitment and planning.
- Competition rather than collaboration between member agencies for funding.
- Lack of resources, which can include financial and staff capacity.
- Failure to secure a top-level commitment from members of the partnership.
- Domination by an individual or of a certain viewpoint.
- An imbalance of input from different agencies, which can lead to resentment and issues about ownership of joint activities and who takes the credit for success.
- Professional jealousy or rivalry and unwillingness to share expertise and information.
- Differences between agencies and individuals in terms of different goals and values, different organisational cultures and ways of working, and different levels of expertise and experience.

Not all partnerships are successful. Many fade out or are wound up. Partnership working is not an end in itself, it is a means to an end. Sometimes, goals might be better achieved by an organisation working alone.

For further reading on public health partnerships and how the organisational changes happening to the UK public health and health systems as this 8th edition of the book is being written might impact on partnership working, see Adebowale and Jamieson (2021).

PRACTICE POINTS

- It is important for you to reflect upon how you communicate with colleagues, including the methods you use, the time spent doing this and the quality of your professional relationships.
- How well you and other health promoters and public health practitioners work together is a key determinant of successfully implemented health promotion and public health programmes.
- Public health interventions often involve partnerships with different professionals and disciplines working together, and there is a range of ways in which you can encourage good teamwork and coordination.
- For effective meetings and committee work, you require knowledge of and competencies in the roles and responsibilities of committee members.
- Public health partnerships between two or more organisations work at varying levels of involvement, from networking at a local or national level to full joint working and from local partnerships to a strategic partnership.

References

Adebowale, V., & Jamieson, J. (2021). *Place is key to successful public health partnerships*. NHS Confederation. https://www.nhsconfed.org/articles/place-key-successful-public-health-partnerships.

Baird, B., Chauhan, K., Boyle, T., Heller, T., Price, C. (2020). *How to build effective teams in general practice*. https://www.kingsfund.org.uk/publications/effective-teams-general-practice

Belbin, M. R. (2022). *Team roles at work*. Abingdon: Routledge.

Estacio, E. V., Oliver, M., Downing, B., Kurth, J., & Protheroe, J. (2017). Effective partnership in community-based health promotion: lessons from the health literacy partnership. *International Journal of Environmental Research and Public Health*, *14*(12), 1550. https://doi.org/10.3390/ijerph14121550.

Faculty of Public Health. (2016). *Good practice public health framework*. https://www.fph.org.uk/media/1304/good-public-health-practice-framework_-2016_final.pdf

GOV.UK. (2022). *Volunteer opportunities, rights and expenses*. https://www.gov.uk/volunteering

GOV.UK. (2022). *Policy paper: build back better: our plan for health and social care*. https://www.gov.uk/government/publications/build-back-better-our-plan-for-health-and-social-care

Faculty of Public Health. (2022). *Partnerships: principles and practice of health promotion: health promotion and inter-sectoral working*. https://www.healthknowledge.org.uk/public-health-textbook/disease-causation-diagnostic/2h-principles-health-promotion/partnerships

House of Commons [HSCC], (2022). *Coronavirus: lessons learnt to date*. House of Commons. https://committees.parliament.uk/publications/7496/documents/78687/default/.

Ige-Elegbede, J., Pilkington, P., Bird, E. L., Gray, S., et al. (2021). Exploring the views of planners and public health practitioners on integrating health evidence into spatial planning in England: a mixed-methods study. *Journal of Public Health*, *43*(3), 664–672. https://doi.org/10.1093/pubmed/fdaa055.

Mishra, A. (2021). *Thomas Kilmann conflict model*. Management Weekly. https://managementweekly.org/thomas-kilmann-conflict-resolution-model/.

Myers and Briggs Foundation. (2022). The Myers-Briggs type indicator. https://eu.themyersbriggs.com/en/tools/MBTI?gclid=Cj0KCQiAveebBhD_ARIsAFaAvrFESIDCKgvO-6V_HH1iQhd4Gp1gKgPh2SJ9dA0v_jBhN_z7lQgotz8aAggdEALw_wcB

NHS England. (2014). Integrated Care and Support Pioneers Programme. Building Collaborative Teams. A workshop guide for service managers and facilitators. https://www.england.nhs.uk/improvement-hub/wp-content/uploads/sites/44/2019/01/Building-Collaborative-Teams-workshop-guide-2014-1.pdf

NHS England. (2022). Building collaborative teams. https://www.england.nhs.uk/improvement-hub/wp-content/uploads/sites/44/2019/01/Building-Collaborative-Teams-workshop-guide-2014-1.pdf

NHS Wales. (2021). *Independent review announced into response to Llwynhendy TB outbreak.* https://hduhb.nhs.wales/news/press-releases/independent-review-announced-into-response-to-llwynhendy-tb-outbreak/. Accessed 30 September 2021.

Martinelli, L., Kopilaš, V., Vidmar, M., Heavin, C., Machado, H., Todorović, Z., Buzas, N., Pot, M., Prainsack, B., & Gajović, S. (2021). Face masks during the COVID-19 pandemic: a simple protection tool with many meanings. *Frontiers in Public Health, 8*, 606635. https://doi.org/10.3389/fpubh.2020.606635.

Piryani, R. M., & Piryani, S. (2019). Conflict management in healthcare. *Journal of the Nepal Health Research Council, 16*(41), 481–482.

Rosen, M. A., DiazGranados, D., Dietz, A. S., Benishek, L. E., Thompson, D., Pronovost, P. J., & Weaver, S. J. (2018). Teamwork in healthcare: key discoveries enabling safer, high-quality care. *The American Psychologist, 73*(4), 433–450. https://doi.org/10.1037/amp0000298.

Social Care Institute for Excellence (SCIE) (2018). *Multidisciplinary teams: what are MDTs and why are they important to integration.* scie.org.uk/integrated-care/research-practice/activities/multidisciplinary-teams

Sidpra, J., Chhabda, S., Gaier, C., Alwis, A., Kumar, N., & Mankad, K. (2020). Virtual multidisciplinary team meetings in the age of COVID-19: an effective and pragmatic alternative. *Quantitative Imaging in Medicine and Surgery, 10*(6), 1204–1207. https://doi.org/10.21037/qims-20-638.

Smith, T., Fowler Davis, S., Nancarrow, S., Ariss, S., & Enderby, P. (2020). Towards a theoretical framework for integrated team leadership (IgTL). *Journal of Interprofessional Care, 34*(6), 726–736. https://doi.org/10.1080/13561820.2019.1676209.

Stokes, J., Lau, Y. S., Kristensen, S. R., & Sutton, M. (2019). Does pooling health & social care budgets reduce hospital use and lower costs? *Social Science and Medicine, 232*, 382–388. https://doi.org/10.1016/j.socscimed.2019.05.038.

Tuckman, B. W. (1965). Developmental sequence in small groups. *Psychological Bulletin, 65*(6), 384–399. https://psycnet.apa.org/doi.org/10.1037/h0022100.

Tuckman, B. W., & Jensen, M. A. (1977). Stages of small-group development revisited. *Group and Organization Studies, 2*(4), 419–427. https://doi.org/10.1177/105960117700200404.

UK Government. *National protocols for COVID-19 vaccines.* https://www.england.nhs.uk/coronavirus/covid-19-vaccination-programme/legal-mechanisms/national-protocols-for-covid-19-vaccines/

WHO. (2022). *Improving health literacy.* https://www.who.int/activities/improving-health-literacy

YouTube

Matrix teams in healthcare. https://www.youtube.com/watch?v=6xbWL6AkHrE

Websites

BoardEffect. *For board effect committee management software.* http://www.boardeffect.com/g-committee-software

Mindtools. *For toolkits on leadership, communication and management skills.* https://www.mindtools.com/CommSkll/RunningMeetings.htm

NHS England. *Partnership pages.* https://www.england.nhs.uk/ourwork/part-rel/

Sharepoint. *For software for teamwork coordination.* https://products.office.com/en-us/sharepoint/collaboration

The Myers and Briggs Foundation. www.myersbriggs.org

The Nine Belbin Team Role. www.belbin.com/about/belbin-team-roles

Facebook

Mindtools. *For ideas and information on being more effective in management and leadership.* https://www.facebook.com/mindtools

Blogs

Public Health Matter. *Partnership working in the North.* https://publichealthmatters.blog.gov.uk/2015/02/09/partnership-working-in-the-north-2/

YouTube

For information and issues linked to Health and Wellbeing Boards. https://www.youtube.com/watch?v=l4xDOB9lxQA

Twitter

One You at Twitter. https://twitter.com/OneYouPHE

Competencies in Health Promotion and Public Health Practice

PART CONTENTS

PART SUMMARY

Part 3 aims to provide you with guidance on how to assess, develop and improve your competencies in health promotion and public health practice.

Competencies are the combinations of knowledge, attitudes and skills needed to plan, implement and evaluate health promotion and public health practice activities in a range of settings. You will also need to develop other competencies, such as communicating and educating, marketing and publicising, facilitating and networking and influencing policy and practice. Some chapters of Part 3 will be more important to some professions or disciplines than others. So you may wish to start by studying the chapters most relevant to you rather than going through them in sequence. Cross-referencing is provided to help you to identify which sections of other chapters may also be relevant to your particular needs.

In Chapter 10, the fundamentals of communication are addressed, including establishing relationships and the links with promoting self-esteem and assertiveness. Four basic communication skills are identified, and guidance is provided on how to improve them. Communication and language barriers, nonverbal communication and written communication, are discussed.

In Chapter 11, some principles governing the choice of communication tools in health promotion are covered. The advantages and limitations of a variety of teaching and learning resources are considered, and guidance is provided on how to produce and use displays, written materials and statistical information. The use of mass media in health promotion is explored, including practical help about working with the local press, radio and television. There is a section included on the use of information technology in health promotion.

In Chapter 12, the principles of adult learning are outlined. How you can enable people to learn and evaluate the learning outcome is described, along with guidelines on giving talks and patient health education.

Chapter 13 covers the health promotion competencies required to work effectively with groups, covering how to lead groups and how to understand group behaviour.

Chapter 14 concentrates on how to enable people to change their behaviour towards healthier living, including information on models of the process of changing health-related behaviour. Strategies that can be used, such as working with a client's own motivation and counselling to help people to make decisions, are discussed alongside the principles that help with using these approaches.

In Chapter 15, the focus is community-based work in health promotion, including community participation, community development and community health projects.

Chapter 16 is about how local and national policies, programmes, plans and strategies are made and how they can be influenced. The methods that health promoters and public health practitioners can use to challenge health-damaging policies and develop, implement and evaluate public health policies are outlined, including sections on the principles and the planning of campaigns.

10

Fundamentals of Communication in Public Health

James Woodall

SUMMARY

This chapter starts with an exploration of client/professional relationships and a discussion of the links between self-esteem, self-confidence, and communication, accompanied by a case study on relationship skills. Discussion on four basic communication skills (listening, helping people to talk, asking questions, and getting feedback) is followed by a consideration of communication and language barriers and nonverbal communication (NVC). The chapter ends with a section on written and wider forms of communication and on health literacy. Exercises are provided on overcoming communication barriers and on each basic communication skill.

See also Chapter 12, which focuses on educating for health.

Health communication is the practice of communicating promotional health information, such as in public health campaigns, health education, and between health professionals and patients. The purpose of disseminating health information is to influence personal health choices by improving health literacy.

Health communication may seek to:
- Increase audience knowledge and awareness of a health issue.
- Influence behaviours and attitudes towards a health issue.
- Demonstrate healthy practices.
- Demonstrate the benefits of behaviour changes to public health outcomes.
- Advocate a position on a health issue or policy.
- Increase demand or support for public health services.
- Argue against misconceptions about health (Cross et al., 2017; Hubley et al., 2020).

Effective communication in a range of contexts is core to success in health promotion and public health practice. Communication in all its forms should be clear, unambiguous, and without distortion of the message. This chapter covers some of the fundamentals of relationships with clients, communication skills, and barriers to effective health communication. For more detailed coverage of spoken, written, and electronic health communication, see Cross et al. (2017) and O'Neil (2019).

EXPLORING RELATIONSHIPS WITH CLIENTS

Health promoters and public health practitioners should ask themselves some fundamental questions. For example, what is your basic attitude towards the people to whom your health promotion is directed? Do you accept them on their own terms, or do you judge them by your own standards? Do you aim to enable people to be independent, make their own decisions, take control of their health and solve their own health problems? Or are you actually encouraging dependency, solving their problems for them and thereby decreasing their own ability and confidence to take responsibility for their health? It may be useful to work through the following questions, thinking about how you relate to your clients.

Accepting or Judging?

Accepting people is demonstrated by:

- Recognising that clients' knowledge and beliefs emerge from their life experiences, whereas your own have been modified and extended by professional education and experience.
- Understanding your own knowledge, beliefs, values, and standards.
- Understanding your clients' knowledge, beliefs, values, and standards from their point of view.
- Recognising that you and your clients may differ in your knowledge, beliefs, values, and standards.
- Recognising that these differences do not suggest that you, the professional health promoter, are a person of greater worth than your clients.

Judging people is demonstrated by:

- Equating people's intrinsic worth with their knowledge, beliefs, values, standards, and behaviour. For example, saying that someone who drinks beyond safe limits is foolish both judges and condemns that person and takes no account of personal circumstances, life experience, and cultural background. Saying that drinking beyond safe levels may damage health does not judge the person in the same way.
- Ranking knowledge and behaviour. For example, 'I am the expert, so I know better than you' is judgemental; 'I know a considerable amount about this particular health issue' is a statement of fact. 'My standards are higher than yours' is judgemental; 'My standards are different from yours' is not.

Autonomy or Dependency?

There are a number of ways in which you can help clients to take more control over their health.

Autonomy can be enabled by:

- Encouraging people to think things through and make their own health decisions, resisting the urge to dominate the decision-making process.
- Respecting any unusual ideas they may have.

Autonomy can be hindered if:

- You impose your own solution on your clients' health problems.
- You tell them what to do because they are taking too long to think it through for themselves.
- You tell them that their ideas are not good and will not work without giving an adequate explanation or an opportunity to try them out.

An aim which is compatible with health promotion principles and ethical practice is to work towards as much autonomy as possible – this is a key value in health promotion practice. By doing this, you are helping people to increase control over their own health. Obviously, there are times when working towards autonomy may not be feasible. For example, it is more demanding of resources, and clients may be dependent on a health promoter or public health practitioner because they are ill, uninformed or likely to put themselves or other people in danger.

A Partnership or a One-way Process?

Do you think of yourself as working in partnership with people in pursuit of public health aims, or do you see health promotion as your sole responsibility with yourself as the expert?

A partnership means:

- There is an atmosphere of trust and openness between yourself and your clients so that they are not intimidated.
- You ask people for their views and opinions, which you accept and respect even if you disagree with them.
- You tell people when you learn something from them.
- You use informal, participative methods when you are involved in health promotion, drawing on the experience, and knowledge that clients bring with them.
- You encourage clients to share their knowledge and experience with each other. People do this all the time, of course (for example, knowledge and experience are discussed between participants in an alcohol awareness programme and parents in a baby clinic), but do you actively foster and encourage this?

A one-way process means:

- You do not encourage clients to ask questions and discuss health needs.
- You imply that you do not expect to learn anything from your clients (and if you do learn, you do not say so).
- You do not find out people's health knowledge and experience.
- You do not encourage people to learn from each other.
- You use formal health promotion and public health approaches rather than participative methods.

Clients' Feelings – Positive or Negative?

A change in people's health knowledge, attitudes, and actions will be helped if they feel good about themselves. It will rarely be helped if they are full of self-doubt, anxiety or guilt.

Clients will feel better about themselves if:

- You praise their progress, achievements, strengths, and efforts, however small the consequences of unhealthy behaviour, such as smoking, are discussed without implying that the behaviour is morally bad.
- Time is spent exploring how to overcome difficulties, such as practical strategies to help a client stop smoking. This will help to minimise feelings of helplessness.

Clients will feel bad about themselves if:

- You ignore their strengths and concentrate on their weaknesses.
- You ignore or belittle their efforts.
- You attempt to motivate them by raising guilt and anxiety (such as 'if you do not stop smoking, you will damage your baby').

To sum up, the health promotion and public health aim of enabling people to take control over and improve their health are best achieved by unconditional positive regard and working in non-judgemental partnerships. This should seek to build on people's existing knowledge and experience, move them towards autonomy, empower them to take responsibility for their health and help them to feel positive about themselves. See McKinnon's (2021) edited collection covering a full range of health communication approaches and strategies.

SELF-ESTEEM, SELF-CONFIDENCE AND COMMUNICATION

The ability to communicate is closely linked to how people feel about themselves. People with low self-esteem tend to be over-critical of themselves and underestimate their abilities. This lack of self-confidence is reflected in their ability to communicate. For example, they may lack assertiveness and thus may either fail to speak up for themselves or react with inappropriate anger and even violence (Mind, 2019).

Assertiveness means saying what you think and asking for what you want openly, clearly, and honestly. It does not mean being aggressive or bullying, but it is in contrast with hiding what you really feel, saying what you do not really mean or trying to manipulate people into doing what you want.

- Assertiveness helps people to create win–win situations (situations where everyone involved feels that they have achieved a reasonable outcome) through

direct and open communication and through avoiding aggressive behaviour (which can result in win–lose situations, where one party feels that they have won and the other party feels they have lost) or manipulation lose–lose situations, where, for example, one party in a negotiation walks out). It builds the self-esteem of all concerned. Successful negotiation is a good example of how assertiveness can work. In a successful negotiation, both parties are more likely to come away with the following thoughts: this is an agreement which, while not ideal, is good enough for both of us to support.

- Both of us made some compromises and sacrifices.
- We will be able to have successful negotiations with each other in future.

Many clients with low self-esteem will need to learn how to feel better about themselves before they can communicate effectively with health promoters and public health practitioners. People with low self-esteem require key life skills to take control of their health (see Mind (2019) for communication ideas on how to improve self-esteem).

LISTENING

As a health promoter and public health practitioner, you need to develop skills of effective listening so that you can enable people to talk and identify their health needs.

Active listening and effective interpersonal communication are very important in health promotion (Woodall and Cross, 2021). Listening is not the same as merely hearing words. It involves a conscious effort to listen to words, to the way they are said, to be aware of the feelings shown and of attempts to hide feelings. It means taking note of the NVC and the spoken words. The listener needs to concentrate on giving the speaker's full attention, being on the same level physically as the speaker and adopting a nonthreatening posture. Fig. 10.1 demonstrates that

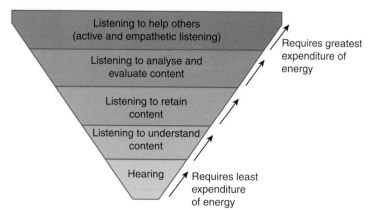

Fig. 10.1 Spectrum showing the transition from hearing to listening. (Source: Rowan, 2013 citing Gamble and Gamble, 2005).

listening and hearing are not the same thing. Most people are born with the ability to hear but not with the ability to be good listeners. Hearing occurs automatically and requires no conscious effort. If the physiological elements in your ears and your brain work, then the impulses will be received. However, what you do with the impulses after you receive them belongs to the realm of listening.

Listening effectively is a deliberate process and requires that we expend energy. The greater the amount of energy we put into listening, the more effective we will be at understanding and helping others identify and meet their health needs.

Active listening requires energy and involves searching for an understanding of the underlying meaning behind the words used by the client. There are various levels of listening which require different skills and energy.

When hearing, it is easy to allow attention to wander. Some of the things you may find yourself doing instead of listening are planning what to say next, thinking about a similar experience, interrupting, agreeing or disagreeing, judging, blaming or criticising, interpreting what the speaker says, thinking about the next job to be done or just plain daydreaming.

The task of listening to help others is to encourage people to talk about their situation unhurriedly and without interruption, enabling them to express their feelings, views, and opinions and to explore their knowledge, values, and attitudes. This reinforces the speakers' responsibility for themselves and is essential for helping them towards greater responsibility for their own health choices. See Gamble and Gamble (2013) and Hubley et al. (2020) for more information and ideas on effective listening. To practise listening skills, work on Exercise 10.1.

ENABLING PEOPLE TO TALK

The main task of the listener is to encourage and enable someone to talk. There are several useful techniques, as follows.

See Chapter 14, a section on strategies for decision-making, which discusses counselling skills.

Giving an Invitation to Talk

To get someone started, it may be helpful to give out a specific invitation to talk. Examples are:

'You do not seem to be your usual self today. Is something on your mind?'

'Can we talk some more about that matter you raised briefly at yesterday's meeting?'

'You look worried – are you?'

EXERCISE 10.1   Learning to Listen

Work in groups of three to six people. Appoint someone as a timekeeper.
1. Person A speaks for 2 min, without interruption, on a health subject of her choice to do with work or other interests (for example, sensible drinking guidelines, keeping fit and active). Everyone else in the group listens without interrupting or taking notes.
2. Person B repeats as much as they can remember without anyone else interrupting. Person B may not:
   • Add anything extra to what A said.
   • Give interpretations (for example, 'It is obvious from what they said that …').
   • Give comments (for example, 'They are just like me …').
3. Person A and the rest of the group identifies what was inaccurate, forgotten or added.
4. Repeat, with a different topic, until everyone has had a turn at being A and B.
5. Discuss the following questions:
   • What helped me to listen?
   • What helped me to remember?
   • What hindered my listening?
   • What hindered my remembering?
   • What did I learn about myself as a listener?

Giving Attention

This means listening closely to what is being said and being fully aware of all the channels of communication, including nonverbal behaviour. It requires effort and concentration to listen hard and give full, undivided attention.

Encouraging

This means making the occasional intervention to encourage someone to continue talking. It tells the speaker that you really are listening and want to hear more. Such interventions include noises or paralanguage like 'mm mm,' words such as 'yes …' and short phrases such as 'I see …,' 'And then …?' or 'Go on …'.

Another useful intervention is the repetition of a key word that the speaker has just used. For example, if the speaker says, 'I am worried by my weight gain,' you could repeat the word 'weight …?'

Paraphrasing

This means responding to the speaker using your own words to state the essence of what the speaker has been saying. Use key words and phrases, for example, 'So you are not sure whether to have the baby vaccinated or not?' or 'So you are feeling unhappy because you are overweight and being unhappy triggers overeating?'

Reflecting Feelings

This involves mirroring back to the speaker, in verbal statements, the feeling he is communicating. To do this, it helps to listen for words about feelings and to observe body language. Examples are 'You seem pleased' or 'You are obviously upset about this.'

Reflecting Meanings

This means joining feelings and content in one succinct response to get a reflection of meaning:

'You feel ... because ...'
'You are ... because ...'
'You are ... about ...'
For example:
'You feel pleased about your weight loss progress.'
'You are depressed because your children have grown up and left home.'
'You are angry about all the traffic pollution on the streets of your neighbourhood.'

Summing Up

This is a brief restatement of the main content and feelings which have been expressed throughout a conversation. Check back with the speaker to ensure that the statement is accurate. For example, say 'It seems to me that the main things you have been saying are ... Does that cover it?'

Exercise 10.2 gives you the opportunity to practise skills in enabling people to talk.

ASKING QUESTIONS AND GETTING FEEDBACK

Skilful questioning will help people to give clear, full, and honest replies. It is useful to distinguish different types of questions.

Types of Questions

Closed questions are questions that require short, factual answers, often only one word. Examples are:

'What is your name?'
'Is this address correct?'
'Are you able to see me again next Tuesday?'

Closed questions are appropriate when brief, factual information is required. They are not appropriate when the aim is to encourage talking at more length. So 'Did you get on OK with your healthy eating plan last week?,' which could be answered by 'yes' or 'no', is not the best way to encourage people to express their experiences of trying to

---

EXERCISE 10.2 Helping People to Talk

Work in pairs. Each person chooses a topic they feel strongly about (which might be a personal experience or topic of general concern such as sex education, traffic jams, cuts in the health service or increase in childhood obesity). Stay with the same topic for all three stages of the exercise. (The whole exercise takes about 45 min).

Stage 1. Giving attention

One person speaks for 2 min, and the other listens, giving only nonverbal feedback. Then swap roles. After both of you have had your turn, spend 10 min discussing these questions:

When you were listening:
- What did you find difficult about listening?
- Did your mind wander?
- Did you maintain eye contact?
- What did you notice about the speaker's NVC?

When you were speaking:
- What did the listener do which helped you to talk?
- Did the listener do anything that made it difficult for you to talk?

Stage 2. Encouraging

One person speaks for 2 min. The other listens and gives encouraging interventions (such as 'mm mm'), words ('yes ...') and nondirective comments ('I see ...') or repeats key words. Swap roles. Then spend 5 min discussing these questions:

When you were listening:
- What sort of interventions did you make?
- How did you feel about making them?

When you were speaking:
- What interventions did you notice?
- Did you find them helpful?

Stage 3. Paraphrasing, reflecting back and summing up

One person speaks for 5 min, and the other listens. The listener makes encouraging interventions as in stage two but *also* paraphrases, reflects feelings and reflects meaning when they feel it is appropriate. At the end, they make a brief statement summing up the main content and feelings of the speaker, checking with the speaker that their summing up is accurate. Exchange roles. Then spend 10 min discussing these questions:

When you were listening:
- What sort of interventions did you make?
- How did you feel about making them?

When you were speaking:
- What interventions did you notice?
- Did you find them helpful?

change what they eat. A better question would be, 'How did you get on with your healthy eating plan last week?' This is an open question.

Open questions give an opportunity for full answers. Examples are:

'How did you get on at the meeting yesterday?'

'What situations do you feel trigger overeating?'

'What do you think about trying to take a short brisk walk every day?'

Note that words like 'how,' 'what,' 'feel' and 'think' are useful for encouraging a full response.

Biased questions indicate the answer the questioner wants to hear or expects to hear. In other words, biased questions are likely to bias the response by leading the person who answers in a particular direction. Examples are:

'You are feeling better today, aren't you?' (This is biased because it would be easier to answer 'yes' than 'no').

'You have been doing what we discussed last time, haven't you?'

'Surely you aren't going to do that, are you?'

Multiple questions contain more than one question. Multiple questions are likely to confuse because the listener will not know which question to answer and probably will not remember all of them. Examples are:

'Is this a serious problem for you – when did it start?'

'Does your store have a policy on promoting healthy foods – do you stock low-alcohol drinks, and did you promote displays of low-fat products during the special campaign last September?'

'What are you going to do to get the Council to take all this rubbish away, and are you going to get more bottle banks and newspaper recycling bins?'

'Are you sure you know what to do, or would you like me to explain it again?'

Exercise 10.3 is an opportunity to practise asking appropriate questions.

Getting Feedback

After people have been given some information or have been taught a skill, it is very important to check to make sure that they really have understood what was said and remembered it or mastered the skill. This is especially important when there is any doubt about how much has been understood, perhaps because, for example, someone is in a state of anxiety or has a limited command of English. There are two key points to note about getting feedback.

1. It is your responsibility to ensure that the communication has been received and understood. It is not the fault of the listener if they tried but did not understand.

> **EXERCISE 10.3   Asking Questions**
>
> Work in groups of about ten people.
>
> Decide on a topic on which it is easy to think of health-related questions, such as exercise levels, diet or my family.
> - Person A volunteers to answer questions.
> - Person B observes the length of A's response to questions.
> - Person C observes A's nonverbal behaviour (body language).
> - Everyone else has the task of asking questions.
>
> First, everyone in turn asks a *closed* question on the topic.
>
> Second, everyone in turn asks an *open* question on the topic.
>
> Third, everyone asks *biased* questions on the topic.
>
> After these three rounds of questions:
> - Person A says how they felt about having to answer the three different kinds of questions (e.g. clear? muddled? irritated? angry? confused?).
> - Person B says what they observed about the length of A's responses to the three kinds of questions.
> - Person C says what they observed about A's nonverbal behaviour when answering the three different kinds of questions.
>
> Discuss the application of what you found out to your health promotion and public health work.

It can be helpful to ask a question in a way which shows that it is your responsibility as a health promoter and public health practitioner to be understood. For example, say 'May I check to make sure I have covered everything – could you just recap what you understand so far?' Avoid questions such as 'Let us see if you have learnt it yet; could you show me?' or 'I do not think you have totally understood; tell me what you think the main points are.'

2. Ask open questions. Closed questions such as 'Do you understand?' are not an adequate way of getting feedback. People may answer 'yes' because they are embarrassed or intimidated. Or they might just want to draw the conversation to a quick conclusion. Ask open questions, such as 'Could you please tell me what you are going to do …'

COMMUNICATION BARRIERS

As health promoters and public health practitioners, you may encounter numerous difficulties in communicating. Recognising that communication barriers exist is the necessary first stage before work can begin on tackling the problems. There are no easy solutions, but increased awareness and skill can go a long way towards improvement.

Common communication barriers may be categorised into the following six types.

1. Social and Cultural Gaps

A number of factors can cause gaps, including:
- Different ethnic or social groups, which may be apparent in dress, language or accent.
- Different cultural or religious beliefs, for example, about hygiene, nutrition or contraception.
- Different values, reflected in a different emphasis on the importance of health issues.
- Different gender or sexual orientations reflected in different approaches, interests or values.

2. Limited Receptiveness

You might want to communicate, but the reverse is not always true: people might not want to be communicated with. They may be unreceptive for many reasons, including:
- Learning difficulty or confusion.
- Illness, tiredness or pain.
- Emotional distress.
- Being too busy, distracted or preoccupied.
- Not valuing themselves or not believing that their health is important.

3. Negative Attitudes to the Health Promoter and Public Health Practitioner

Some people may be resistant to you even before you have met them. This may be caused by the following:
- Previous negative experiences.
- Lack of trust in anyone seen as an authority figure.
- Lack of credibility of the health promoter.
- Perceiving you as a threat, coming to criticise or pass judgement.
- Thinking that they already have the knowledge and skills.
- Believing that advice will be given that they cannot comply with because of financial or social constraints or being asked to change a lifestyle or behaviour that they enjoy.
- Not wishing to confront issues such as personal health problems or the need to change policies and practices at an organisational level.

4. Limited Understanding and Memory

There may be difficulties because people:
- Understand and/or speak little or no English.
- Have limited education or learning difficulties and may be unable to read and write.

- Are being confronted with technical words, jargon or medical terminology that they do not understand.
- Have poor or failing memories and cannot remember what was discussed previously.

5. Insufficient Emphasis by the Health Promoter

Communication may fail because you do not give it sufficient time and attention. The reasons may be:
- Communication was given a low priority in basic training, so it is given low priority in practice.
- Lack of confidence, skills and knowledge, which may be the result of inadequate training.
- Being too busy with other things and unable to find the time.
- Managers not being supportive about time spent on health promotion.
- Reluctance to demystify and share professionally acquired health knowledge.

6. Contradictory Messages

Communication barriers are often created when people receive different messages from different people. For example:
- Different health professionals give different advice.
- Family, friends or neighbours contradict health promoters and public health messages or evidence.
- The media can contradict professional viewpoints.
- Health advice changes as evidence is updated.

To identify communication barriers in your public health work, undertake Exercise 10.4.

EXERCISE 10.4 Identifying Communication Barriers

This exercise can be done alone, but it is best carried out in pairs or small groups so that ideas can be shared.

Consider the six types of communication barriers discussed.

1. How many of them can you identify in your own health promotion and public health practice experience?
2. What other communication barriers can you add to this list?
3. What communication barriers cause you the most problems?
4. What suggestions can you make for helping to break down communication barriers? (Share examples from your own experience and make additional suggestions).

OVERCOMING LANGUAGE BARRIERS

Language is only one facet of the gulf that may exist between people of diverse backgrounds. The root of communication problems may be racism. This is a huge topic, largely outside the scope of this book, but critical commentaries have argued that health promotion as a discipline needs to take a more active stance against racism and its impact on the health of society (Ndumbe-Eyoh, 2020).

However, when we focus solely on the question of language barriers, learning a few essential words and phrases in the other person's language may help. Help with learning the language may be available from multicultural education centres run by local education authorities.

When faced with a language barrier, there are some useful guidelines which you can follow to help someone with limited English to understand what is being said. See Box 10.1 and Exercise 10.5.

NONVERBAL COMMUNICATION

Nonverbal communication (NVC) includes the ways people communicate other than by the spoken word. It is

EXERCISE 10.5   Overcoming Language Barriers

The following five extracts come from the district nurse's side of a conversation with a patient whose English is very limited.
1. 'Hello – Oh, we are looking brighter today!'
2. 'Have you been visited by the doctor today yet? Did he give you a new prescription?'
3. 'I'll see about your insulin after I have seen how your leg's getting on.'
4. 'The doctor says you should take one of these tablets three times a day … I do not think you understand – I'll say that again … We want you to take one of these tablets three times a day … Oh dear … (louder) … DOCTOR SAYS YOU TAKE TABLET THREE TIMES A DAY.'
5. 'I'll leave this list of foods for you. There are ticks and crosses on it to show you what you can eat and what you should not eat. Do you understand? Your son can read English, can't he?'

Using the guidelines in points 1 through 8 in Box 10.1:
- Identify what is unhelpful about the way the district nurse speaks to the patient.
- Suggest better alternatives.

BOX 10.1   Guidelines for Health Promotion and Public Health Communication With Individuals or Small Groups Who Speak Little English

If you are engaging in health promotion and public health with individuals or small groups whose spoken English is limited, you should attempt to find out whether a translator could be present. If you use a translator, allocate more time for the session. Give information concisely and in stages; this will allow time for the translator to explain to the clients and to translate back information from the clients. Using children or relatives to translate information to clients can be less reliable than using trained translators.

If you do not have a translator, the following points may be helpful:
1. Speak clearly and slowly, and resist raising your voice in an effort to be understood.
2. Repeat a sentence if you have not been understood using the same words. If you use different words, you are likely to cause more confusion by introducing even more words which are not understood.
3. Keep it simple. Use simple words and sentences. Use active forms of verbs rather than passive forms, so say, 'The nurse will see you' rather than 'You will be seen by the nurse.' Do not try to cover too much information, and stick to one topic at a time.
4. Say things in a logical sequence: the sequence in which they are going to happen. So say, 'Eat first, then take the tablet' rather than 'Take the tablet after you eat'. If the listener does not pick up the word 'after' correctly, they will take the tablet first because that is the order in which he heard the instruction.
5. Be careful of idioms, such as 'spending a penny,' which may be totally incomprehensible.
6. Do not attempt to speak pidgin English. It does not help people to learn correct English and sounds patronising.
7. Use pictures, mime and simple written instructions, which may be read by relatives or friends who understand written English. Be careful of symbols on written material; ticks and crosses, for example, might not convey what you intend.
8. Check to ensure that you have been understood, but avoid asking closed questions that require a one word answer, such as 'Do you understand?' A reply of 'yes' is no guarantee that your client really has understood.

See the section on asking questions and getting feedback earlier in this chapter.

sometimes called body language. The main categories of NVC are as follows:

Bodily Contact

Bodily contact is people touching each other, how much they touch, and which parts of the body are in contact. Shaking hands, holding hands or putting an arm around someone's shoulders, for example, all convey a meaning from one person to another. However, many of these social courtesies, which include physical contact, have been re-evaluated as a result of COVID-19. Some health promoters, such as nurses, obviously touch patients frequently in the course of their work, whereas others, such as environmental health officers, do not. Touching people is governed by rules dictated by cultural expectations and taboos and by expectations of professional distance, which may be barriers to the positive use of touch. For example, a handshake can say 'I am glad to see you – welcome' and touching a distressed person can say 'I am here for you'.

Proximity

Proximity is how close people are to each other. Different messages are conveyed to a patient confined to bed by someone who talks to him from 6 feet away at the foot of the bed and by someone who comes closer and sits on the bed or a chair. However, people vary in the amount of personal space they need and may feel uncomfortable when others come too close.

Orientation

How individuals position themselves in relation to other people and objects is known as orientation. A useful example is to consider the messages conveyed by the arrangement of a room where a small group of people are meeting. Chairs in rows facing one separate chair (perhaps with a table in front of it) imply that one person will dominate and control the meeting, whereas chairs placed in a circle without a table to act as a barrier imply that everyone is encouraged to join in and that no one individual is expected to dominate.

Level

This refers to differences in height between people. Generally, communication is more comfortable if people are on the same level, so it feels better to bend down or sit down to talk to a child or a person in a wheelchair, for example. Talking to someone on a different level can leave one or both parties feeling disadvantaged. Sometimes this is done deliberately; for instance, not offering a chair to someone entering an office conveys a message that the visitor is not welcome to stay.

Posture

Posture is how people stand, sit or lie. For example, are they upright or slouched, arms crossed or not? Posture can convey a message of tension and anxiety, for example, by being hunched up with arms crossed or one of welcome by being upright with arms outstretched.

Physical Appearance

All kinds of messages may be conveyed by physical appearance, such as a person's social standing, personality, tidy habits or concern with fashion. Physical appearance can be very important to health promoters because of the messages it conveys. A uniform may convey an impression of professional competence but may also convey an unwelcome image of authority. Casual dress in a formal committee may convey the impression (perhaps a false one) that the committee's work is not being taken seriously.

Facial Expression

Facial expression can obviously indicate feelings such as sadness, happiness, anger, surprise, or puzzlement.

Hand Movements and Head Movements

Movements of the hands and head can be very revealing. Nods and shakes of the head obviously convey agreement and disagreement without the need for words. It is important to note that movements of the head and hands do not convey the same meaning in all cultures. Clenched fists, fidgeting hands (and sometimes tapping feet) reveal stress and tension, whereas still, open hands usually denote a relaxed frame of mind. Mental discomfort, such as confusion or worry, is often shown by putting the hands to the head and playing with the hair, stroking a beard or rubbing the forehead.

Direction of Gaze and Eye Contact

Direct eye contact is significant. As a general rule, a speaker looks away from the listener for most of the time when talking (because they are concentrating on what they are saying) and looks directly at the listener when they want a response. The general rule is that the listener will look the speaker straight in the eye while they are paying attention to what they say but will look elsewhere if their attention has wandered. This is particularly important if you work with people on a one-to-one basis; a person who is talking to you will infer that you are not listening if you are looking anywhere other than at them. It is critical when counselling someone in distress; the counsellor needs to be giving the client full attention, and if the client looks up and sees the counsellor gazing elsewhere, the implication is that

> **EXERCISE 10.6   Nonverbal Communication in Your Health Promotion and Public Health Practice Work**
>
> Work through the following questions and exercises with a partner.
>
> 1. When do you touch people in your health promotion and public health role, if at all?
>
>   What rules govern when it is acceptable/unacceptable to touch them?
>
>   Would people you work with be helped if you touched them more?
>
> 2. Carry on a conversation with your partner, first standing too close for comfort, then standing too far away.
>
>   What does it feel like? What is the most comfortable distance?
>
>   What implications does this have for your work?
>
> 3. When you talk to an individual in the course of your work, where do you sit or stand in relation to that person? For example, is furniture a barrier between you?
>
>   If you talk to people in groups, how do you seat them?
>
>   Do you think communication could be improved by making changes? If so, what changes?
>
> 4. Have a conversation with your partner, with one of you sitting and the other standing. Both describe your feelings.
>
>   Do you ever communicate with people who are on a physically different level from you?
>
>   What are the implications for your health promotion effectiveness?
>
> 5. Practise tense and relaxed postures, then welcoming and rejecting postures.
>
>   Which do you normally adopt with people?
>
> 6. Identify a few people you have studied or worked with whom you know fairly well. Think back to your first impressions of these people.
>
> Do you think that your first impressions were right?
>
> What were the important features of their appearance which led to your first impressions?
>
> What is the importance of physical appearance in your health promotion work?
>
> If you wear a uniform or a white coat, how do you think it affects your relationships with the individuals and groups you work with?
>
> 7. Look around at other people in the room.
>
>   What can you infer from their facial expressions or hand and head movements?
>
>   What is the importance of noticing facial expressions or hand and head movements in your job?
>
> 8. Hold a conversation with your partner while first staring into each other's eyes all the time and then without looking at each other at all.
>
>   Describe your feelings.
>
>   Watch two people talking.
>
>   Do they look directly at each other, or do they frequently look away?
>
>   Do they look more at each other when speaking or listening?
>
>   How important is eye contact in your job?
>
> 9. Say 'I do not know' in as many ways as possible, trying to convey a different feeling each time, such as despair, confusion and irritation.
>
>   How important is it for you to pick up on nonverbal aspects of speech in your health promotion work?
>
>   To consolidate your understanding of NVC, read Burgoon et al. (2021) and watch the TED talk under the YouTube references at the end of this chapter.

they are not listening. Eye contact is a critical mechanism in establishing lots of positive rapport (Jongerius et al., 2020).

Nonverbal Aspects of Speech

Consider how many ways a word like 'no' can be said. The way in which it is said can convey meanings such as anger, doubt or surprise. Tone and timing are two nonverbal aspects of speech which convey messages to the listener.

Raised awareness of NVC can help you to improve communication between you and the people you work with. For example, a person who says 'Yes, I understand' in a doubtful tone of voice with a puzzled frown clearly requires further explanation. Words alone are only part of a message and can be misleading. See Burgoon et al.

(2021) for more information and insights into NVC, and undertake Exercise 10.6 to explore NVC in your work.

OTHER FORMS OF COMMUNICATION

Writing is a craft, as well as an art that all health promoters and public health practitioners need to develop. The 12-point guidelines in Box 10.2 may help with written communication, and Box 10.3 offers guidelines for all forms of public health communication, including the use of social media.

Public health communication and campaigns apply integrated strategies to deliver messages designed, directly or indirectly, to influence health behaviours of target audiences. The communication of messages comes

BOX 10.2   Guidelines on Professional Writing

1. The point of writing is clear communication. On the whole, the more simply and briefly you write, the more effective your writing is likely to be.
2. Think about what kind of document you are writing. For example, is it a paper for a formal committee, a memo to your manager or an email to a client? This will help you to know what style to write in: formal in a set layout for a committee, brief and to the point for a manager, or business-like but friendly to a client.
3. Think about who is reading what you write and what sort of communication they will welcome: how long should it be, how detailed, how formal or chatty, first-person or third-person?
4. Use clear, simple language, and avoid long or obscure words if you can find shorter or more familiar ones.
5. Avoid technical terms if you can. If you must use them, explain them in the text or a footnote the first time you use them.
6. Keep sentences short.
7. Break the text up into paragraphs. A paragraph should usually deal with one point and its immediate development. A new point needs a new paragraph. In formal papers and reports, use numbering, headings and subheadings to break up the text and guide the reader through.
8. Use active rather than passive verbs where possible, as this is stronger and simpler. For example, write 'the health promoter advised the client on healthy eating' rather than 'the client was advised on healthy eating by the health promoter.'
9. Make sparing use of adjectives and adverbs to make your writing more striking. For example, 'the client was really very upset, cried and sobbed a lot and said they would never, ever come back to the smoking cessation programme again' (25 words) could be better expressed as 'the client was distressed and said they would never return to the smoking cessation programme' (15 words).
10. Use language accurately.
11. Use a spell and grammar checker on a word processor or ask someone to proofread.
12. If you have the time, finish a piece of writing and then put it aside for a few days. This gives your subconscious mind a chance to think about it, and you can take a fresh look and edit it. Check for clarity, simplicity and coherent structure.

through various channels that can be categorised as: mass media (such as television, radio, and billboards), small media (for example, brochures and posters), social media (Facebook, Twitter, blogs), and the interpersonal communication (one-on-one or group education) previously covered. Box 10.3 offers guidelines for effective communication across all forms of public health communication, including mass media, small media, and social media.

Health Literacy and Health Communications

One of the aims of effective communication in health promotion and public health is to improve health literacy, both in individual clients and with target groups and whole populations. Health literacy is the personal knowledge and competencies needed for individuals and communities to access, understand, appraise, and use information and services to make decisions about their health (Nutbeam and Muscat, 2021). Functional health literacy is low in the United Kingdom (UK). Health information in current circulation is written at too complex a level for 43% of working age adults (16 to 65 years); this figure rises to 61% if the health information includes numeracy (Health Literacy UK, 2022). We do not know how many people are additionally burdened by low interactive and critical health literacy skills, but the numbers are likely to be even higher.

The important point to note here is that health literacy has been shown to have an effect on health and illness. For example, a systematic review showed that there is a relationship between health literacy and adolescents' health behaviours (Fleary et al., 2018). Health literacy is a social determinant of health and follows a social gradient (Nutbeam and Lloyd, 2021). Where health literacy differs from these other social factors is that it is potentially open to positive change through health promotion and public health interventions. Improving health literacy, therefore, should be a goal for health promoters and public health practitioners.

At the present time, scholars have noted the importance of health communication during COVID-19 and the importance of critical health literacy (Abel and McQueen, 2020). Indeed, the continuous, rolling news channels, politician briefings, and endless commentary on digital platforms creates information overload. This causes confusion at best and, at worst, panic and anxiety for many (Abel and McQueen, 2020). There are several examples where untrustworthy sources have caught the public imagination and have provided illegitimate concerns, especially during the COVID-19 pandemic (Woodall, 2020). One essential role for health promoters is to promote public understanding and awareness of 'fake news' and moreover provide accurate and timely

BOX 10.3   A Guide to Effective Public Health Communications Across Contexts

Attributes of effective health communication

- **Accuracy:** The content is valid and without errors of fact, interpretation or judgement.
- **Availability:** The content (whether targeted message or other information) is delivered or placed where the audience can access it. Placement varies according to audience, message complexity and purpose, ranging from interpersonal and social networks to billboards and mass transit signs to prime-time TV or radio, to public kiosks (print or electronic), to the internet.
- **Balance:** Where appropriate, the content presents the benefits and risks of potential actions or recognises different and valid perspectives on the issue.
- **Consistency:** The content remains internally consistent over time and also is consistent with information from other sources (the latter is a problem when other widely available content is not accurate or reliable).
- **Cultural competence:** The design, implementation, and evaluation process that accounts for special issues for select population groups (for example, ethnic, racial and linguistic) and educational levels and disabilities.
- **Evidence base:** Relevant scientific evidence that has undergone comprehensive review and rigorous analysis to formulate practice guidelines, performance measures, review criteria and technology assessments for telehealth applications.
- **Reach:** The content gets to or is available to the largest possible number of people in the target population.
- **Reliability:** The source of the content is credible, and the content itself is kept up to date.
- **Repetition:** The delivery of/access to the content is continued or repeated over time, both to reinforce the impact with a given audience and to reach new generations.
- **Timeliness:** The content is provided or available when the audience is most receptive to, or in need of, the specific information.
- **Understandability:** The reading or language level and format (including multimedia) are appropriate for the specific audience.

Source: Healthy People (2010); Archive (2016)

information in culturally specific ways (Woodall, 2020). For further, in-depth reading on health literacy, see Cross et al. (2017), who offers a critical perspective on health literacy and health communication.

PRACTICE POINTS

- The quality of your relationships with your clients is at the heart of your health promotion and public health role. It is important to review and consider how your attitudes and values are reflected in your professional communication.
- Good communication and the development of health literacy are fundamental to health promotion and public health goals.
- Words, whether verbal or written, are only a small part of public health interaction, and it is important to consider all aspects of communication.
- Written and multimedia communication are core competencies in health promotion and public health practice and need to be reviewed and developed.

References

Abel, T., & McQueen, D. (2020). Critical health literacy and the COVID-19 crisis. *Health Promotion International*, 35(6), 1612–1613. https://doi.org/10.1093/heapro/daaa040.

Burgoon, J. K., Manusov, V., & Guerrero, L. K. (2021). *Nonverbal communication*. London: Routledge.

Cross, R., Davis, S., & O'Neil, I. (2017). *Health communication: theoretical and critical perspectives*. Cambridge: Polity.

Fleary, S. A., Joseph, P., & Pappagianopoulos, J. E. (2018). Adolescent health literacy and health behaviors: a systematic review. *Journal of Adolescence*, *62*, 116–127. https://doi.org/10.1016/j.adolescence.2017.11.010.

Gamble, S. K., & Gamble, M. W. (2013). *Interpersonal communication: building connections together*. London: Sage.

Gamble, T. K., & Gamble, M. W. (2005). *Contacts: interpersonal communication in theory, practice, and context*. Cambridge: Pearson.

Health Literacy UK. (2022). *What is health literacy*, why is it important? https://www.healthliteracy.org.uk/why-is-health-literacy-important#:~:text=We%20know%20that%20levels%20of,the%20health%20information%20includes%20numeracy

Healthy People. (2010). *Archive 2016 health communication*. http://www.healthypeople.gov/2010/document/html/volume1/11healthcom.htm

Hubley, J., Copeman, J., & Woodall, J. (2020). Practical health promotion: *3rd edition*. Cambridge: Polity Press.

Jongerius, C., Hessels, R. S., Romijn, J. A., Smets, E., & Hillen, M. A. (2020). The measurement of eye contact in human interactions: a scoping review. *Journal of Nonverbal Behavior*, 44(3), 363–389. https://doi.org/10.1007/s10919-020-00333-3.

McKinnon, M. (2021). *Health promotion. A practical guide to effective communication*. Cambridge: Cambridge University Press.

Mind. (2019). *Self-esteem*. http://www.mind.org.uk/information-support/types-of-mental-health-problems/self-esteem/#.V5X0uVVTGUk

Ndumbe-Eyoh, S. (2020). What would it take for health promotion to take structural racism seriously? *Global Health Promotion, 27*(4), 3–5. https://doi.org/10.1177/1757975920972259.

Nutbeam, D., & Lloyd, J. E. (2021). Understanding and responding to health literacy as a social determinant of health. *Annual Review of Public Health, 42*, 159–173. https://doi.org/10.1146/annurev-publhealth-090419-102529.

Nutbeam, D., & Muscat, D. M. (2021). Health promotion glossary 2021. *Health Promotion International, 36*, 1578–1598. https://doi.org/10.1093/heapro/daaa157.

O'Neil, I. (2019). *Digital health promotion: a critical introduction*. Cambridge: Polity.

Rowan, C. (2013). *Listening to need*. The Achievement Centre. http://www.tac-focus.com/article/listening-needs#.V5dKTVVTGUk

Woodall, J. (2020). COVID-19 and the role of health promoters and educators. *Emerald Open Research, 2*, 28. https://doi.org/10.35241/emeraldopenres.13608.2.

Woodall, J., & Cross, R. (2021). *Essentials of health promotion*. London: Sage.

Websites

Centre for Disease Control and Prevention. Gateway to health communication & social marketing practice with examples of communication campaigns. http://www.cdc.gov/healthcommunication/campaigns/

For health literacy, see http://www.healthliteracy.org.uk/

YouTube

TED talk. By body language expert Mark Bowden at TEDxToronto – The importance of being inauthentic 2013. https://www.youtube.com/watch?v=rk_SMBIW1mg

TED talk. Reading body language | Janine Driver published on 1 Oct 2019. https://www.youtube.com/watch?v=lvxJoUuG018&t=33s

Twitter

Health Literacy UK. https://twitter.com/LiteracyHealth?ref_src=twsrc%5Etfw

Health Literacy Europe. https://twitter.com/HL_Europe_net

11

Using Communication Tools in Health Promotion and Public Health Practice

James Woodall

SUMMARY

The first part of this chapter offers some principles governing the choice of communication tools and a summary of the uses, advantages, and limitations of the main types of health promotion communication resources. There are guidelines for making the most of display materials, for producing written materials (including guidance on inclusive and culturally sensitive forms of writing) and for presenting statistical information. This is followed by a section on mass media, including identifying the key characteristics of mass media, the variety of ways in which the mass media and social media are channels for health promotion and public health, what they can be expected to achieve and how they can be used effectively. Guidelines are given for working with radio, television and the local press. There is a case study on the use of mass media advertising and exercises on writing plain English, preparing and presenting material on television and radio, writing a press release, and writing a letter to the editor. The chapter ends with a section on using social media to promote health.

The range of communication tools outlined in Table 11.1 are used extensively by health promoters

and public health practitioners in their health-promoting activities but may not always be employed with maximum effectiveness. How communication tools are selected and used is as crucial as the quality of the resources themselves.

SELECTING PUBLIC HEALTH RESOURCES

There are a range of different types of communication tools available, with a constant turnover as items become out of date. You could find yourself with the task of selecting a leaflet, poster or display items from a range of possibilities. Or you may find that there is very little available, and you have to decide whether the one item you have found is suitable.

The following guidelines are designed to help you select any kind of material, such as leaflets, audio-visual or social media, and you can also use them as a checklist when producing your own.

Is It Appropriate for Achieving Your Aims?

Think about the item in the context in which you intend to use it. For example, if you are working with a group of young people on the harms of gambling, a leaflet on raising awareness in this regard may be ineffective. Materials which trigger discussion (perhaps a YouTube video) or setting up a peer support group via WhatsApp might be better.

Is It the Most Appropriate Kind of Resource?

Will something else be cheaper and just as effective, such as a tweet or social media post instead of leaflets, which can be expensive to print? Could you use the real thing, such as a young person who has successfully stopped gambling talking about their experiences instead, or actual food, instead of pictures or models, in a nutrition talk with a weight management group?

TABLE 11.1   HEALTH PROMOTION RESOURCES

Type of Resource	Uses and Advantages	Limitations
Leaflets and handouts	Clients can use it at their own pace and discuss it with other people. The educator and client can work through this together. It can be easy and cheap to produce basic written information. Can reinforce points in a talk and add further detailed information. It can be produced in different languages	Commercially produced leaflets can be expensive and may contain advertising. Mass-produced leaflets are not tailored to everyone's needs. Not durable, easily lost. Mass distribution can be wasteful
Posters and display charts	Can raise awareness of issues. Can convey information and direct people to other sources (addresses, telephone numbers, 'pick up a leaflet'). Simple posters and information displays can be cheap to produce	High-quality posters and display materials are expensive to make or buy. They are difficult to maintain. Need to ensure any writing is big enough to be read at a distance most people will see it. Displays need to change frequently to attract attention
Flipcharts, whiteboards	Good for brainstorming and involving groups in producing ideas which can be stuck up around the room for discussion. Useful for recording notes to be written up later. Can be prepared in advance. Useful where no whiteboard is available. Cheap	The educator needs to turn back to the audience to write on the board. Flip-chart paper is easily torn and dog eared
PowerPoint presentation	Useful in large rooms or lecture theatres with a big screen. Complex information (such as graphs) can be seen clearly	Needs equipment, and screen, and blackout
Podcasts/ downloaded audio files	Good for certain skills development, e.g. relaxation and exercise routines. Equipment is cheap and easy to use and transport	Lack of visual material requires extra concentration to hold the attention
Health websites	Websites have the potential to reach a worldwide audience and are useful for raising awareness of health issues, conveying information, and delivering self-help materials	There is an enormous amount of health information that can be accessed on the internet, and no control over the quality
Facebook	Reaches a mass audience, can be accessed easily from websites, leaflets can carry the URL, health information posts can be updated daily and shared amongst large audiences for very little financial cost	The quality has to be evaluated, and judgements have to be made about its suitability as a resource
YouTube	Reaches a mass audience. It can contain visual public health campaign material and a wide variety of health information that spreads the dissemination of a campaign	If you direct your clients to YouTube, they will also have access to other YouTube videos which may not be health-enhancing
Micro Blogs and Twitter	Dynamic and concise flow of information. Web logs (blogs) and numerous microblogging platforms, such as Twitter, allow users to publish messages (such as tweets). Tweets can be supplemented with hyperlinks to other online media, such as videos (for example, those on YouTube) or websites. Tweets can also include 'hashtags', a form of information indexing that allows people to search for tweets that are related to a particular discussion or topic	It is difficult to control the quality of a range of people accessing microblogging platforms. It might increase the inequality of access for those people who are not proficient in the social media

Is It Consistent With Your Values and Approach?

If your approach is to work in a non-judgemental partnership with your clients, the materials you use should reflect your values. You need to avoid material that is patronising, authoritarian, scaremongering or victim-blaming. Resources should not attribute or imply blame to individuals experiencing ill health when that ill health is rooted in their socioeconomic circumstances, for example, low income or poor housing caused by the cost of living crisis. See the section on exploring relationships with clients in Chapter 10.

Recent studies have shown various ways in which public health messaging related to facemask wearing during the COVID-19 pandemic (see Fig. 11.1). Oxman et al. (2022), for instance, has shown how messaging can vary from persuasion and information giving to coercion and manipulation. The latter approach is less consistent with the values of health promotion.

Is It Relevant for Your Clients?

Does it take account of the values, culture, health concerns, age, ethnic group, sex and socioeconomic circumstances of your clients? Does it reflect local practice and health services available?

Obvious examples of irrelevance are social media posts or YouTube clips portraying the lifestyles of affluent families, which are unhelpful if you are working with people who have limited financial resources or are struggling with increased energy bills and accommodation costs. Materials designed for one ethnic group may not be appropriate for another, not just because of language but because some aspects (such as sexual behaviour or attitudes to bereavement) are seen differently in different cultures.

Is It Racist, Sexist or Ageist?

All resources should be non-racist, non-sexist, and non-ageist. Racist materials stereotype people, attributing certain roles or character attributes based on ethnic group alone. Implicit in this are the assumptions that one ethnic group is superior to another and represents the desired norm (see Luquis and Pérez, 2021 for an overview of culturally appropriate and sensitive health promotion approaches). Sexist materials stereotype gender roles, behaviours or character attributes. Resources should also not make assumptions about sexual orientation. Guidance on non-sexist writing is provided later in this chapter. Resources should reflect the fact that we live in a multiracial society where the roles of men and women have changed and continue to do so. Strong, positive messages and images should be provided of people of all ages, ethnic groups, and both sexes.

Will It Be Understood?

Is it written in plain English, which people will readily understand? Are there any incorrect assumptions about the level of literacy or existing knowledge? Does it need

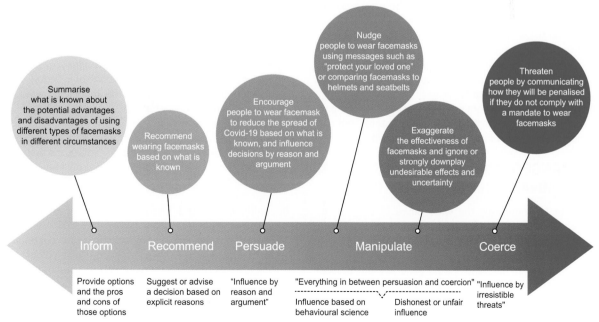

Fig. 11.1 How values and approach can influence messaging: an example of facemask wearing. (Oxman et al., 2022).

to be produced in other languages to make it accessible to people from minority ethnic groups? Do the materials need to be produced in other formats so that they are accessible to people with disabilities, such as in large type or Braille, or for audio-visual media, for example, with sign language or subtitles inserted on the screen?

Is the Information Reliable?

Is the information in the materials accurate, up to date, unbiased, and complete? Or does it contain one-sided information on controversial issues and out of date or incomplete messages? There is a big challenge for health promoters currently in relation to challenging 'fake news' and those with unsubstantiated views that may impact on individual and community health and well-being. Using reliable, evidence-based sources can overcome this.

Does It Contain Advertising?

Commercial companies, such as drug companies, baby food manufacturers or makers of safety equipment, who produce material will produce leaflets and posters that will carry the name of the company or its products or include advertisements. Using these resources can imply that you (or your employer) are endorsing the product. It may also damage your image as a credible source of unbiased health information and lead people to doubt the value of the information.

For these reasons, resources containing company names, products and advertising should be avoided whenever possible. However, the item may be just what you want, and there may be no alternative. In which case:

- The product or service advertised must be ethically acceptable as healthy and environmentally friendly. This excludes tobacco, alcohol and confectionery advertising, for example.
- The advertising content must be low key. The company name on the front or back cover is acceptable, but constant references to name-brand products are not.

THE RANGE OF PUBLIC HEALTH RESOURCES: USES, ADVANTAGES AND LIMITATIONS

Table 11.1 summarises the wide range of communication resources available for promoting health and the key points about their uses, advantages, and limitations. It is also important to note:

- Resources are aids and should generally not be seen as substitutes for the health promoter or public health practitioner. Leaflets should be used in conjunction with face-to-face discussion. Audio-visual aids, including YouTube and social media, are best presented with

an introduction and, when appropriate, a follow-up discussion and evaluation.
- It takes time and competencies to become familiar with developing and using all the health promotion and public health communication resources available.

See the section on public health teaching and learning in Chapter 12.

PRODUCING HEALTH PROMOTION AND PUBLIC HEALTH RESOURCES

Some resources, particularly posters, leaflets, and audio-visual and web-based materials, come ready made, but you might want to work with a community group to help them to produce materials that target their particular need or produce some yourself.

See Chapter 10, a section on written communication, and Chapter 12, a section on improving patient communication.

This chapter does not offer a comprehensive guide on how to produce materials, but approaching the task in a systematic way using the planning and evaluation flowchart in Chapter 5 may be helpful. If you are producing a resource such as a public health leaflet, you will need to consider who will write the draft, who will edit it, whether and how to pilot the draft, what it will cost and whether you need the services of a desktop publisher, designer, illustrator, translator or printer.

Making the Most of Display Materials: Posters, Charts, Display Boards, and Stands

Be brief and to the point. Keep the public health goal firmly in mind. Do not include material that is irrelevant; it will only distract from the main message.

Emphasis on the key point(s). Use the size of lettering, style or colour to achieve this. Place the important messages just above the centre of a display, which is the point of maximum visual impact.

Use language the audience understands. Explain any unfamiliar technical terms. If possible, express the message in both pictures and words. Test it out on a few people to ensure that you have no unexpected ambiguities in your message.

Be bold. Words and pictures should be as large as possible.

Make the most of colour. Colour can create continuity; for example, a repetition of background colour can link a series of posters. Colour can be used to identify parts of a diagram or highlight important information. Choose colours with care because responses to colour are emotional (for example, green is soothing) and because colours may be associated with certain messages, images, and places (such as red for danger, purple for funerals, and white for clinical cleanliness).

Improve the display site. If all you have is a blank wall or a wall covered with distracting wallpaper, fix a rectangle of coloured card to the wall as a background display board. If a display board has a rough or marked surface, give it a coat of paint or a covering of coloured paper, hessian or felt.

Use the display site to the best advantage. Busy corridors can only be useful sites for posters with immediate appeal and few words. More information can be conveyed in a waiting area, and it may be possible to supplement displays with leaflets to take away. Ensure that writing on displays is at eye level and large enough to read without people having to move from the queue or their chair.

Be aware of lighting. Daylight is unreliable; spotlights directed onto a display are ideal.

Making the Most of Written Materials: Instruction Sheets and Cards, Leaflets, and Booklets

Pilot materials on a sample of consumers. Do not assume that you know what they like, want or need. *Ask them.*

Use colour, layout, and print size to improve clarity. Larger print may be helpful for those people with a visual impairment.

Use plain English. Use everyday words; avoid jargon and explain any technical or medical words. Aim for short sentences of 15 to 20 words. Use active rather than passive verbs; for example, say, 'Increase your fruit and vegetable consumption …' rather than 'Your fruit and vegetable consumption should be increased …'. Undertake Exercise 11.1 to practise plain English.

Do a readability test on your written materials. Many word-processing packages are able to give readability statistics, as well as the average sentence length and the percentage of passive sentences used. They give a rough measure of readability for adult readers based on the principle that the combination of long sentences and long words is harder to comprehend. But note that many other factors that affect readability are not taken into account, such as how the text is laid out, the use of illustrations and the size of the print.

Non-Sexist Writing

The importance of material being non-racist and non-sexist has already been discussed, but using language in a non-sexist way presents particular challenges. One is the use of 'man' as a generic term for a person. For example, people talk about manning an exhibition stand when it is just as likely to be staffed by a woman or by people who do not identify as either a man or woman. Many job titles

---

> ### EXERCISE 11.1   Writing Plain English
>
> Write plain English versions of the following. The first two are very similar to the instructions found on the packages of medication bought over the counter in chemist shops. The last two are very similar to passages in health promotion and public health leaflets.
>
> 1. *Wheezoff* paediatric syrup is specially formulated for children. It is indicated for the relief of cough and its congestive symptoms and for the treatment of hay fever and other allergic conditions affecting the upper respiratory tract. Contraindications, warnings, etc. Hypersensitivity to any of the active constituents. If symptoms persist, consult your doctor.
> 2. *Notwinge* cream – Directions for use. Apply a sufficient quantity of balm to the part affected. Massage lightly until penetration is complete.
> 3. The baby lies curled up in what is called the foetal position. It lies in a bag of water, and the membranes which make up this fluid-filled balloon are enclosed in the womb.
> 4. Vitamin B1, also called thiamine, is required for the functioning of the nervous system, digestion and metabolism. Insufficient vitamin B1 can cause anorexia and fatigue.

end with 'man' and date from the time when only men performed these duties, for example, postman.

Another problem is the generic use of the male pronoun. For example, 'Each doctor presented a case from his own practice' assumes that all the doctors are men. Although it may seem clumsy to say 'he' or 'she', it can sometimes usefully emphasise that both sexes are involved. An alternative which has been used in this book is to turn the singular into a plural and use the words 'they' or 'their', changing 'A health promoter and public health practitioner must be a fluent communicator. He must also be a good listener.' to 'Health promoters and public health practitioners must be fluent communicators. They must also be good listeners.'

It may be possible to rephrase a passage to eliminate the pronouns altogether. So, instead of 'Information given to a social work agency is confidential in the same way as communications between a doctor and his patients', say '… in the same way as communications between doctors and patients'.

Another way is to use 'you' instead of 'he', 'she' or a noun that implies male or female. For example, in a leaflet on parenting, you could change 'A mother often finds difficulty in persuading her two-year-old to eat' to 'You may find difficulty in persuading your two-year-old to eat' or

'Parents may find difficulty …' This avoids the implication that only mothers (not fathers) have a parenting role.

Or avoid 'he' by finding another noun. Thus, in 'You may find it difficult to persuade your two-year-old to eat. He may prefer throwing his food around' instead, you could say '… A child at this age may prefer throwing food around instead.'

It is also important to avoid sexism when speaking and writing. So, for instance, a health promoter or public health practitioner who refers to the women who attend a smoking cessation programme as 'the ladies' could affront the women in the group. It is far better to refer to the women who attend as 'patients' or 'clients'.

For further discussion of language barriers, see the section on overcoming language barriers in Chapter 10.

PRESENTING STATISTICAL INFORMATION

Numbers may be meaningless to lay people unless they are carefully presented in a visual way, such as in Fig. 11.2. Graphs are one way of presenting statistical information, and these have been commonplace in health communication techniques. A wide range of other computer software programmes facilitates the production of information in ways that are visually appealing and easy to understand. Infographics have become increasingly popular ways of communicating complex information and serve as an effective educational strategy for synthesising, analysing and sharing key messages with a targeted audience (see Barlow et al., 2021).

Consider Figs 11.2 and 11.3 and analyse how effective these figures would be as a resource for use by health promoters in advocating for more funding and resource for upstream ways of tackling health inequalities that focus on the social determinants of health – such as geography and gender. Discuss:

1. How and where they might be used.
2. How you might modify them for use.
3. How you might combine them with other resources.
4. Whether there are any ethical issues with using figures such as these.
5. Overall, how effective do you think they are as a resource to persuade.

USING THE MASS MEDIA TO PROMOTE HEALTH

The mass media are channels of communication to large numbers of people and include television, radio, the internet (see the section on social media in the following section), magazines and newspapers, books, displays and exhibitions. Leaflets and posters are also mass media when they are used on a stand-alone basis, as opposed to being used as a learning aid in face-to-face communication with an individual or a group. However, usually, when people talk about the media, they are referring to television, radio, newspapers and magazines.

Health promoters and public health practitioners are most likely to become involved with mass media when undertaking public health programmes or campaigns with the public or when a public health issue becomes a news item, such as during the COVID-19 pandemic. Probably most involvement will be with local newspapers and local radio or television. However, it is useful to put this into

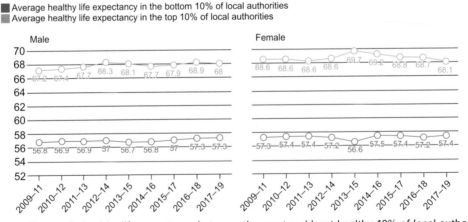

Fig. 11.2 The gap in healthy life expectancy between the most and least healthy 10% of local authorities has remained over the past decade. (Source: Health Foundation (2022) (https://www.health.org.uk/news-and-comment/charts-and-infographics/healthy-life-expectancy-target-the-scale-of-the-challenge)).

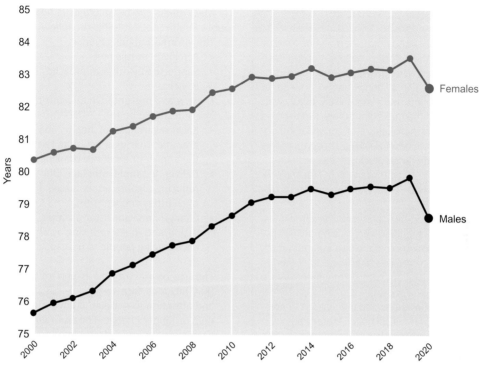

Fig. 11.3 **Life expectancy at birth in England, 2000–2020.** (Source: Kings Fund 2021 ONS and OHID (https://www.kingsfund.org.uk/publications/whats-happening-life-expectancy-england)).

a wider context and to appreciate the range of ways in which health issues and messages are portrayed via mass media.

Mass Media as Tools for Health Promotion and Public Health

Health messages and information are sent through the mass media in a number of different ways:

- Planned health promotion interventions and campaigns which harness the benefits of television advertising, cinema, radio, print and online advertising. For example, Western Australia's *LiveLighter* healthy weight and lifestyle campaign focussed on decreasing the consumption of sugar-sweetened beverages using these approaches (Morley et al., 2019). Moreover, in the United Kingdom, the *Change4life* campaign (a campaign that aims to prevent people from becoming overweight by encouraging them to eat a healthy diet and take more exercise) utilised posters, leaflets, displays and exhibitions as well as mass media approaches such as TV and radio (NHS, 2016).

- Health promotion by transnational companies – such as Coca-Cola and McDonalds – can have mass appeal and indeed laudable goals, but health promoters should be acutely aware of the challenges that such mass media approaches bring (Anaf et al., 2020).
- Books, television, newspapers, and magazine articles about contemporary health issues (e.g. COVID-19). The problem here is that the media may distort the evidence with attention-grabbing headlines, which can give out unhealthy messages, see Box 11.1.

Further ways health is addressed in the media are:

- Discussions of health issues as a by-product of news items ('Rock star dies from drug overdose') or entertainment programmes, notably soap operas/serial dramas where a character has a health problem, such as being abused as a child or suffering from cancer.
- Health (or anti-health) messages conveyed covertly or incidentally, such as well-known personalities or fictional characters refusing cigarettes or, conversely, smoking. The portrayal of alcohol on television, for example, can convey a norm of heavy drinking and

---

> ## BOX 11.1   COVID-19, The Media and Conspiracy Theories: A Challenge for Health Promoters
>
> During the COVID-19 pandemic, there were several examples where untrustworthy sources caught the public imagination and have provided illegitimate concerns (Shimizu, 2020), and evidence shows how some (right-wing) media outlets were more likely to run with COVID-19 conspiracy theories than others (Romer and Hall Jamieson, 2020). The plethora of conspiracy theories and misinformation, often published in some media outlets, covered a wide range of issues. This included:
>
> - The origins of COVID-19 and links with 5 G technology.
> - Insinuation that COVID-19 was being used as a bioweapon.
> - COVID-19 is a 'big plot' by pharmaceutical companies.
> - Anti-vaccination perspectives and vaccine hesitancy.
>
> There were, and continue to be, challenges for health promoters to communicate effectively and to challenge media reports when working with communities. While the power of the media is undisputed, often misinformation can perpetuate challenges and inequalities in communities where levels of critical health literacy are low.

associates consumption of alcohol with benefits rather than costs.

- There is increasing evidence about the role of mass media approaches in sports advertising on television and at live events and how this can negatively (Dixon et al., 2019) and positively (Scully et al., 2020) influence behavioural decisions in relation to lifestyle choices.

Using Mass Media to Promote Health

The fact that the message is sent via a medium, such as television, makes it difficult to obtain immediate feedback and modify the message to respond to the needs and characteristics of the audience. There can be some two-way communication through radio and television phone-ins or through online chat facilities, but mostly it is one way, which has implications. For example, it is not possible for the sender to repeat, clarify or amplify the message. In general, it is best to use mass media to convey simple rather than complex messages.

There is research focusing on the efficacy of mass media for public health interventions and communications, and studies have shown that they can be both effective and cost-effective (Worthington et al., 2020). It is important for you to know what success you can realistically expect when you use mass media in your health promotion and public health work. The research evidence tells us how

mass media can be used effectively and what it cannot be expected to achieve, as follows.

Mass media *can* be an effective health promotion and public health tool if it fulfils the following criteria:

1. The information portrayed is:
   - Perceived as relevant.
   - Supported by other approaches such as one-to-one advice.
   - New and presented in an appropriate context.
2. The aim should be to:
   - Raise awareness of health and health issues (for example, to trigger action to raise awareness about the impact of excessive drinking).
   - Deliver a simple message (for example, to make reducing alcohol intake easier by providing details of charities and websites).
   - Change behaviour (for example, to reinforce motivation and make reducing alcohol intake easier by encouraging people to perhaps download a support app).
3. The use of mass media is part of an overall strategy that includes face-to-face discussion, personal help, and attention to social and environmental factors that help or hinder change. For example, mass media campaigns are just one strand in a long-term programme to influence people's knowledge and behaviour in relation to climate change (Junsheng et al., 2019).

A systematic review showed that mass media campaigns could improve knowledge in relation to alcohol consumption, and there were some signs that attitudinal change could occur, but there was little evidence that a mass media approach could impact alcohol consumption, i.e. create behavioural changes (Young et al., 2018). Therefore, it is useful to consider what mass media *cannot* be expected to do. This includes:

1. Conveying complex information.
2. Teaching skills.
3. Severely shift people's attitudes or beliefs.
4. Changing behaviour unless it is a simple action, easy to do, and people are already motivated to change.

Creating Opportunities

You may be motivated to use the mass media, but you may have misgivings and feel the need for further training. For example, you may feel apprehensive about interviews with reporters from the local news media because of concerns about being misquoted or that the media might sensationalise the issue or that you will not perform effectively.

What can be done to overcome these concerns? Many NHS organisations, local authorities, and non-government organisations have guidelines for dealing with the media (for example, Mind, 2022), and some professional bodies offer advice to their members in terms of media involvement. Contact local journalists to establish a mutually beneficial relationship. You can give exposure to health topics, and they want items for their reading, listening or viewing public. Get to know how they work and their special areas of interest. Also, remember that it is in both your interests to have good skills in communicating via the mass media, so ask for help with training needs. Short courses on using the media may also be available.

Keep a record of what you find out about local media and update it regularly. Include information on names and special interests of journalists and the copy dates (deadline for submitting written information) for each of the media in your area. The daily newspapers should be able to respond immediately to a press release; radio often needs a few days to prepare coverage; television may need longer advance notice to allow time for booking a film crew.

Working With Radio and Television

Using radio or television effectively requires research, preparation, and skill. The following checklists are prepared to help you get your health promotion story to the right person and have the best chance of getting coverage. You need to monitor your local radio and television to see which programmes might be interested in your kind of news.

Basic Information

- What hours do they broadcast?
- What region do they cover?
- Who are the listeners/viewers? Does the profile alter according to the time of day?

The Programmes

- What is covered in the news items?
- How many minutes of current affairs and local interest items are broadcast?
- Are interviews used, or is it straight reporting?
- What are the different kinds of programmes, and what is the proportion of time they occupy (news, current affairs, weekly events, phone-ins, music)?
- Which programmes use guests or experts?
- Is there any local programme that regularly covers health issues?
- Is there a round-up of events in the week ahead? What is the deadline for information?
- How much detail do they give? What sorts of events are covered?

Interviews

- Which programmes use interviews?
- How many minutes?
- What is the tone (bland, chatty, aggressive)?
- How long is the average answer before the next question? Time it!
- Are they on location or in the studio?
- Are they recorded or live?
- Who are the presenters or interviewers on the programmes who might be interested in health? What is their style?

Finding Out About a Specific Programme

- What programme is it? What sort of approach does the programme have? How long is it? When is it transmitted? What kind of audience does it have?
- Why is your topic of interest *now*? Is there some local or national controversy or news item that sparked off interest? If so, do you know all about it?
- How are you going to be presented: an information spot, an interview or a discussion panel?
- If you are going to be interviewed, who will do it? Will it be in the studio, on location or a telephone or online interview?
- If you are going to take part in a discussion, who else will be taking part?
- Will it be broadcast live or recorded first?
- How much time are you likely to have on the programme?
- When and where is the broadcast or recording to take place?

Preparing the Message

- Do your homework. You may know a lot or a little about the subject, but in either case, you need to identify exactly what it is you want to get across and to have this very clearly in your mind *before* you go on air.
- Be positive. Emphasise the good news, *not* a series of don'ts. Tell people what they *can* do and emphasise the benefits.
- You should have two or three key points to put across, and *no more*. You can expand on these and describe them in different ways but do not overload your audience with too much detail or too many points. They will not remember the additional information and may even forget the key points.
- Use anecdotes and analogies to illustrate what you mean; simple messages do not have to be bald and boring. Tell stories (short ones) and use real-life experiences. Put complex points over with everyday analogies.

- Avoid technical terms (unless these are essential, in which case use them and explain them) and jargon, but do not be patronising. It helps pitch the level right if you imagine that you are talking to an intelligent 14- to 15-year-old whom you have never met.

Presenting Your Message

- If you are nervous, regard it as positive; it means that you will be keyed up to do your best. Remember that the interviewer is there to help you tell your story and to put you at ease.
- Perform with liveliness and conviction. Be alert and (if you are on television) look alert at all times. Always assume that the camera is on you even when you are not talking. Make sure you look convincing and involved.
- Speak with your normal voice; if you have a regional accent, this will make you more interesting to listen to. Speak clearly and distinctly, and (especially on radio) vary the pitch and speed.
- Make sure you say what you want to say. You do not have to follow the line of the interviewer's questions if, for a good reason, you do not wish to. Provided you stick to the broad framework of agreed subjects, you have every right to steer the interview or discussion in such a way that you get over what you want to say. Regard the questions as springboards from which to make your points. For example, if you do not like a question, you can say:

  'I can't really answer that question without explaining first that …'

  'The real problem behind all this is …'

  'We don't know the answer to that at the moment, but what we do know is …'
- When the interview is over, remain still, quiet, and alert until you are *told* it is over.
- On television, wear what makes you feel comfortable and confident. Avoid wearing blue or bright red, predominant stripes, small patterns or flashing jewellery. As the camera will be on your face for most of the time, pay special attention to what you wear in the neckline area.

  Practise your media skills by undertaking Exercise 11.2.

Working With the Local Press

Local community newspapers are an excellent medium for promoting health, and journalists will be interested in newsworthy health issues. These newspapers still attract a great deal of interest with some sections of the local population. This is a checklist of what to look for when researching a newspaper.

EXERCISE 11.2   Being Effective on Television and Radio

1. **Prepare your message.**

   Select a health promotion topic that you are familiar with, such as healthy eating, sensible drinking, breast-feeding, keeping fit or avoiding home accidents.

   Identify *three* key points you would want to put across in a 5 min radio or television interview. Be clear in your mind:
   - What the three key points are.
   - How you will explain them in an interesting way and what illustrations, analogies or anecdotes you could use.
   - How you will develop your point further if you have time.

2. **Practise your presentation.**

   Get a colleague to act as your interviewer and record your interview on an audio or a videotape. Ask a third person to be an observer. Play the tape back and assess your performance:
   - Did you sound/look lively, alert, and convincing?
   - Was your voice clearly understandable? What did it sound like for speed and pitch?
   - Did you get your key points across? Did you do so in an interesting way?
   - Were you able to deal with difficult questions?

Basic Information

- Is it published daily or weekly?
- What are the copy deadlines?
- What locality does it cover?
- How many readers, and who are they?

The Copy

- What is the style (bright, sober, campaigning)?
- What is the average length of articles (often different for news, business, and features)?
- What percentage of articles have photos?
- How many photographs per page?
- How are photographs used generally?
- How are quotes used?

The Subjects

- What sorts of stories are used (local, controversial, educational) and how are they treated?
- What is the ratio of coverage for news, features, business, diary, and advertisements?
- How long and how full is the section publicising events ahead?

- Are there special sections or supplements on health, education or women? How long and on what day?
- Are there regular columnists? What are their special interests?

The Language

- What is the average length of sentences?
- What is the average length of paragraphs?
- What kind of language is used (multisyllabic, slang, turgid, lively, short and simple)?

Your Special Interests

- Anything in the papers that may be of special use to you or your organisation?

Gradually build up expertise with a fact sheet on each newspaper. This will be indispensable for targeting your press releases.

How to Write a Press Release

To write a press or news release, you need to consider the following:

Headline. Create a catchy headline that is short and simple, using less than ten words. It should convey the key point made in the opening paragraph in a light-hearted manner that catches imagination and attention but does not mislead or sensationalise.

Collate and organise your facts. A simple rule is to find answers to questions pertaining to the five Ws: who, what, when, where, why, and then how. Identify your story's angle. A good story angle must have the following attributes. It must be the most important fact in your story; it must be timely; it must be unique, newsworthy or contrary to trends. The story angle must be presented in the first paragraph. Make your points in order of importance. Use short sentences, brief paragraphs and easy language with no abbreviations or jargon. Put the most important message down into a quote. Journalists use quotes from the newsmakers to add an authoritative voice to their reports. If the press release contains quotes that are important and relevant, they have more chance of being replicated in full in the published article.

Keep to one page if possible. If longer, type 'More follows …' at the bottom right-hand corner. Do not carry over paragraphs or sentences to the next page. Type 'ends' after the last line of the release. End the press release with brief background information on your organisation and who to contact for further information.

Be specific. Focus on people rather than making generalised statements or quoting dry statistics. For example, say 'Last week, three Bloggsville children were admitted to the Royal Infirmary after accidentally swallowing weed killer. This brings the number of children accidentally poisoned this year to over 100. Sister Florence Nightingale, in charge of the Accident and Emergency Department, said: "It is heartbreaking to see the needless distress this causes" …'

Timing is vital. Your press release may not be used if a) it comes out on a day when there is news overload, such as on the day of the election of a new prime minister or b) the news is not topical or current. Alert newspapers a few days in advance so that they can send reporters to cover an interesting event. For example, contact on a Friday or Monday is usually best for a weekly paper published on the following Friday. If you want to launch a story at a particular time, use the embargo system. This means writing, for example, 'Not for use until Wednesday September 2nd 2022' or 'Embargoed 6 p.m. September 2nd 2022' across the top of the press release. If it is for immediate release, then state FOR IMMEDIATE RELEASE.

Presentation. Use A4 paper, headed with a logo if possible. Colour catches the eye, so a coloured heading or coloured paper will make your release stand out. Journalists work at speed, so make their task easier by:

- using only one side of the page, placing the text centrally on the page
- using a layout with double spacing
- leaving at least a 1 inch (2 to 3 cm) margin on either side
- putting a release date or embargo date at the top
- giving names and telephone numbers of people in your organisation for further information (including an after-hours telephone number)
- sending it to a named journalist if possible
- not underlining any words (because this gives printers instructions to use italics; use **bold** for emphasis instead).

Communication. Send a copy of the press release to everyone who will be affected, including your organisation's communication or press officer, and to everyone mentioned or otherwise involved in the story.

This section is based on ideas from *Pressbox: press release writing* (http://www.pressbox.co.uk). There are many websites with excellent ideas for writing press releases for the media. See also the example of a press release on Box 11.2.

Writing Letters to the Editor

Another way of using the local paper as a medium for health promotion is by writing letters to the editor. This can keep an issue in the public eye for some time and

BOX 11.2   Press Release

Press Release 1 January 2023 – Prisoners supporting each other proves successful, study shows

As the prison population in England and Wales reaches almost 90,000, a research study led by Kofftown University has assessed whether health programmes run by prisoners themselves work to improve health in prison.

The study has been looking at the use of peer-based health programmes in prison: programmes that see prisoners, rather than trained staff, providing health education, support or advice to their fellow prisoners. A prominent example in England and Wales is a Samaritan run scheme which trains prisoners to act as listeners to support fellow inmates.

The research team found that such programmes can be an effective way of reducing risky behaviours. Peer helpers offer a valuable source of support within prisons, particularly for prisoners with mental health needs. A key finding was that becoming a peer worker was associated with gaining self-confidence and improvements in personal wellbeing, but more research is needed on the impact on the prison population.

There are many examples of peer schemes already in operation in prisons in England and Wales. This study has also highlighted some of the factors that can help them run smoothly in what is, by all accounts, a challenging environment.

For further information, please contact:

Jo Goodheart, Media Contact Kofftown University, People's Lane, Kofftown KT1 2YZ

Telephone 1234 246 802 (day) or 1234 135 790 (evenings)

EXERCISE 11.3   Writing for the Local Press

1. Write a press release about a public health issue you are currently concerned about or working on, such as healthy school meals, binge drinking, drug taking by young people in local clubs, lack of play facilities for young children or poor public transport.
2. Write a letter to the editor supporting a current public health campaign or drawing attention to a specific need for health promotion.

USING THE INTERNET AND SOCIAL MEDIA TO PROMOTE HEALTH

The internet has revolutionised the way health promoters, public health practitioners and the general public gain access to health information. Because of the massive growth of web-based health information, the global nature of the internet and the absence of real protection from harm for citizens who use the internet for health purposes, quality is regarded as a problem (Daraz et al., 2019).

The internet can be used by public health practitioners and health promoters to:

- Support evidence-informed practice.
- Disseminate resources and information to other professionals.
- Provide information and support to the public.

See the section on evidence-based health promotion in Chapter 7.

Social Media

Woodall and Cross (2021) offer a useful overview of social media, describing the term as generally referring to internet-based tools that allow individuals and communities to gather and communicate; to share information, ideas, personal messages, images, and other content, and in some cases, to collaborate with other users in real-time. Social media are also referred to as social networking. Social media sites provide a variety of features that serve different purposes for the individual user. They may include blogs, social networks, video- and photo-sharing sites, wikis or a myriad of other media, which can be grouped by purpose, serving functions such as:

- Social networking (Facebook, Twitter, Instagram).
- Professional networking (LinkedIn).
- Media sharing (YouTube, Flickr).
- Content production (blogs (Tumblr, Blogger) and micro-blogs (Twitter)).
- Knowledge/information aggregation (Wikipedia).

provides good opportunities for public debate on controversial issues. Letters to the editor should be to the point, short (some newspapers restrict length) and be on one topic only.

Practise writing a press release and a letter to the editor by undertaking Exercise 11.3.

For quality criteria for consumer health information, see the Discern webpage in the reference section at the end of this chapter. These criteria can be used for judging online materials in addition to printed materials but will not judge the scientific accuracy. It is designed for healthcare contexts but can also be applied to public health information.

Participation in social media by the general public has increased sharply. The use of social media is prevalent across all ages and professions and is pervasive around the world (Ventola, 2014). Because of this global increase in people accessing social media, there are many public health benefits but also risks. Health promoters and public health practitioners can use social media to engage people in an interactive way on public health issues and facilitate individual's and group's access to information about health and wellbeing, including news about services. An example of its potential is shown by the World Health Organisation, who use social media to share news and information about their work and engage with other social media users. As well as their social media accounts, they maintain a Twitter account that deals with a range of public health subjects. See the WHO Twitter account in the reference list at the end of this chapter.

Assessing the Quality of Health Information on the Internet

The potential health risks of social media are well documented (O'Neil, 2019; Ventola, 2014). Guidelines issued by public health organisations and professional bodies provide sound and useful principles that health promoters and public health practitioners should follow to avoid pitfalls. It is important that health promoters and public health practitioners evaluate the quality of any website or social media, such as blogs or Twitter or Facebook pages they use and/or advise their clients to use before trusting the information it provides. The following guidelines offer some insights into what you should be evaluating (adjusted from Georgetown University Library, 2016):

Author

- Is the name of the author/creator on the page?
- Are their credentials listed (occupation, years of experience, position or education)?
- Is the author qualified to write on the given topic? Why?
- Is there contact information, such as an email address, somewhere on the page?
- Is there a link to a homepage, and if so, is it for an individual or an organisation?
- If the author is with an organisation, does it appear to support or sponsor the page?
- What does the domain name/URL reveal about the source of the information, if anything?

Purpose

Knowing the motive behind the page's creation can help you judge its content:
- Who is the intended audience?
  - Specialist audience or experts?
  - General public?

- If not stated, what do you think is the purpose of the site? Is the purpose to:
  - Inform or teach?
  - Explain or enlighten?
  - Persuade?
  - Sell a product?

Objectivity

- Is the information covered fact, opinion or propaganda?
- Is the author's point-of-view objective and impartial?
- Is the language free of emotion-rousing words and bias?
- Is the author affiliated with an organisation?
- Does the author's affiliation with an institution or organisation appear to bias the information?
- Does the content of the page have the official approval of the institution, organisation or company?

Accuracy

- Are the sources for factual information clearly listed so that the information can be verified?
- Is it clear who has the ultimate responsibility for the accuracy of the content of the material?
- Can you verify any of the information in independent sources or from your own knowledge?
- Has the information been reviewed or refereed?
- Is the information free of grammatical, spelling or typographical errors?

Reliability and Credibility

- Why should anyone believe information from this site?
- Does the information appear to be valid and well-researched, or is it unsupported by evidence?
- Are quotes and other strong assertions backed by sources that you could check through other means?
- What institution (public health agency, government, charity such as Mind) supports this information?

Currency

- If the timeliness of the information is important, is it kept up to date?
- Is there an indication of when the site was last updated?

Links

- Are links related to the topic and useful to the purpose of the site?
- Are links still current?

Undertake Exercise 11.4 and read Case study 11.1 to consider the benefits and risks of using social media to promote health.

Chapter 13 has more information on establishing social media groups.

EXERCISE 11.4   Does Social Media Pose a Threat to Public Health?

Read the following interview with a retiring Director of Public Health. Do you agree that social media is a threat to public health? List the ways social media could be both a threat and offer opportunities to promote public health. Do the benefits outweigh the threats?

Social media could pose one of the biggest threats to public health in the future, a leading doctor has warned.

Tom Scanlon, the outgoing Director of Public Health for Brighton and Hove, issued the warning as he prepares to leave the position after 15 years. He said emerging evidence shows that, in some areas of mental health, the use of Facebook, websites, and Twitter can have a detrimental effect. Although social media can be used as a force for good, Dr Scanlon said the existence of websites that promote anorexia and other eating disorders are harmful. He said cyberbullying and the increased access to images of super-skinny celebrities could all also have a negative impact. He said, 'The public health science on social media is in its infancy. We have managed to mine some social media use locally for our annual report, and my view is that in certain areas of mental wellbeing: eating disorders, self-harm,

anxiety, and depression, there is emerging evidence that the use of social media can have a detrimental effect. This has previously been suggested in some cases of suicides, although I haven't seen any local instances of this, and we know there can be a copycat effect. My feeling is that some of the imagery/texts/memes posted on social media becomes aspirational, particularly to certain vulnerable young people and that this select group behaviour, probably hidden from external influences like parents/teachers, feeds the problem rather than provide any positive support or solutions. This is something we are just on the cusp of, and we don't really know how it will develop. It is a real challenge.'

Dan Raisbeck, the co-founder of the internet bullying charity the Cybersmile Foundation, said the organisation recognised the risks associated with social media and the promotion of some websites. He said: 'Safeguarding is something that each user needs to learn about, how security and profile settings can be applied and the use of filtering tools or monitoring home internet use, especially if young people are involved. Learning about the risks and finding out how you can keep yourself and your family safer online is a very important part of dealing with the problem.'

Source: The Argus (2016)

CASE STUDY 11.1   The Mums2be Smokefree Facebook Support Group

Case study produced by Tracey Hellyar, N.N.E.B, Smoking in Pregnancy Coordinator, Solutions 4 Health LTD

Background

Women who smoke during pregnancy often experience feelings of embarrassment, guilt, and fear. Attending a group is often deemed uncomfortable because of the feeling of being judged. In Somerset, as a result of the rural nature of the landscape, a group was not viable. Web-based support groups offer a number of advantages, including convenience and increased access to care for individuals who would not attend groups residing in remote areas or for those suffering from social anxiety. Additionally, fewer resources are required, thus reducing costs.

Aim

Each client who engages with the Mums2Be Smokefree programme has the opportunity to receive peer support. By using an online platform, support is available continually for

24 h a day, seven days a week. An advantage to remaining in the group post-delivery is that each woman has continued support, potentially reducing the chance of relapse.

Setup and Administration

To protect the clients' anonymity, the group was set up as a secret Facebook group. This meant that the group could not be searched for, that nothing in the group is shown on the clients' timeline, and no one could see that the client was in the group except for other group members.

To join the group, the client is sent a friend request by the administrator and once accepted, they are added to the group. The friend acceptance is then removed.

There are two administrators in the group and three practitioner moderators. The group also has four users who are nominated champions who post regularly.

Clients may stay in the group for as long as they wish as there is no time frame, as it is important for the support to continue post-delivery.

CASE STUDY 11.1   The Mums2be Smokefree Facebook Support Group—Cont'd

How Is the Success Evaluated?

An online survey was carried out 11 months after the initial group was set up. The survey was anonymous, and a link was posted within the group for members to complete. The group at the time had 73 client members. There was a 31.5% response rate.

95.85% strongly agreed or agreed that participation in the group provided support and encouragement.

100% strongly agreed or agreed that participation in the group helped them to realise that any problems they encountered were not unique.

87.5% strongly agreed or agreed that participation in the group enabled them to confront difficult problems.

96% strongly agreed or agreed that participation in the group supported them to quit.

75% strongly agreed or agreed that participation within the group helped to avoid relapse.

96% would recommend the group to friends.

96% felt safe within the group.

Mums2Be Smokefree is an intensive smoking in pregnancy programme, offering one-on-one support and free nicotine replacement therapy with a named practitioner throughout the clients' pregnancy and up to six months post-delivery within the clients' home. The online support group is an extension of this service enabling the client to gain further support around the clock from their peers and maintain support post-delivery to prevent relapse.

See Chapter 13 for guidelines on setting up a Facebook page.

PRACTICE POINTS

- Communication tools for health promoters and public health practitioners are wide-ranging and need to be selected carefully and used effectively with an assessment made of the advantages, uses and limitations of each kind of resource.
- Consider factors such as location, colour, language and style when creating displays.
- Written materials should be non-sexist, non-racist, in plain English and accessible to everyone, for example, ethnic minority languages, large type or alternative formats such as audiotape instead of written materials.
- Present statistical information with appropriate use of graphics to ensure clarity.
- The mass media can be used to raise awareness of health issues and deliver simple messages.
- Work effectively with local media by researching potential opportunities and carefully preparing TV presentations and press releases.
- Social media offers a potentially effective way of promoting health but needs to be used with caution.

References

Anaf, J., Baum, F., Fisher, M., & Friel, S. (2020). Civil society action against transnational corporations: implications for health promotion. *Health Promotion International*, *35*(4), f877–887. https://doi.org/10.1093/heapro/daz088.

Barlow, B., Webb, A., & Barlow, A. (2021). Maximizing the visual translation of medical information: a narrative review of the role of infographics in clinical pharmacy practice, education, and research. *Journal of the American College of Clinical Pharmacy*, *4*(2), 257–266. https://doi.org/10.1002/jac5.1386.

Daraz, L., Morrow, A. S., Ponce, O. J., Beuschel, B., Farah, M. H., Katabi, A., Alsawas, M., Majzoub, A. M., Benkhadra, R., Seisa, M. O., & Ding, J. F. (2019). Can patients trust online health information? A meta-narrative systematic review addressing the quality of health information on the internet. *Journal of General Internal Medicine*, *34*(9), 1884–1891. https://doi.org/10.1007/s11606-019-05109-0.

Dixon, H., Lee, A., & Scully, M. (2019). Sports sponsorship as a cause of obesity. *Current obesity Reports*, *8*(4), 480–494. https://doi.org/10.1007/s13679-019-00363-z.

Georgetown University Library. (2016). *Evaluating internet resources*. http://www.library.georgetown.edu/tutorials/research-guides/evaluating-internet-content

Junsheng, H., Akhtar, R., Masud, M. M., Rana, M. S., & Banna, H. (2019). The role of mass media in communicating climate science: an empirical evidence. *Journal of Cleaner Production*, *238*, 1–10. https://doi.org/10.1016/j.jclepro.2019.117934.

Luquis, R. R., & Pérez, M. A. (2021). *Cultural competence in health education and health promotion*. New Jersey: John Wiley & Sons.

Mind. (2022). *How to report on mental health*. http://www.mind.org.uk/news-campaigns/minds-media-office/how-to-report-on-mental-health/

Morley, B., Niven, P., Dixon, H., Swanson, M., Szybiak, M., Shilton, T., Pratt, I. S., Slevin, T., & Wakefield, M. (2019). Association of the livelighter mass media campaign with consumption of sugar-sweetened beverages: cohort study. *Health Promotion Journal of Australia*, *30*, 34–42. https://doi.org/10.1002/hpja.244.

NHS. (2016). *Change4life campaign pages and resources*. http://www.nhs.uk/change4life/Pages/change-for-life.aspx

O'Neil, I. (2019). *Digital health promotion*. Cambridge: Polity.

Oxman, A. D., Fretheim, A., Lewin, S., Flottorp, S., Glenton, C., Helleve, A., Vestrheim, D. F., Iversen, B. G., & Rosenbaum, S. E. (2022). Health communication in and out of public health emergencies: to persuade or to inform? *Health Research Policy and Systems, 20*(1), 1–9. https://doi.org/10.1186/s12961-022-00828-z.

Romer, D., & Jamieson, K. H. (2020). Conspiracy theories as barriers to controlling the spread of COVID-19 in the US. *Social Science & Medicine, 263*, 1–8. https://doi.org/10.1016/j.socscimed.2020.113356.

Scully, M., Wakefield, M., Pettigrew, S., Kelly, B., & Dixon, H. (2020). Parents' reactions to unhealthy food v. pro-health sponsorship options for children's sport: an experimental study. *Public Health Nutrition, 23*(4), 727–737. https://doi:10.1017/S1368980019003318.

Shimizu, K. (2020). 2019-nCoV, fake news, and racism. *The Lancet, 395*, 685–686. https://doi.org/10.1016/S0140-6736(20)30357-3.

The Argus. (2016). *Social media could pose one of the biggest threats to public health in the future, a leading doctor has warned*. http://www.theargus.co.uk/news/14388589.Social_media_poses_one_of_the_biggest_threats_to_public_health/?ref=twtrec

Ventola, C. L. (2014). Social media and health care professionals: benefits, risks, and best practices. *Pharmacy and Therapeutics, 39*(7), 491–499. 520.

Woodall, J., & Cross, R. (2021). *Essentials of health promotion*. London: Sage.

Worthington, J., Feletto, E., Lew, J. B., Broun, K., Durkin, S., Wakefield, M., Grogan, P., Harper, T., & Canfell, K. (2020). Evaluating health benefits and cost-effectiveness of a mass-media campaign for improving participation in the National Bowel Cancer screening program in Australia. *Public Health, 179*, 90–99. https://doi.org/10.1016/j.puhe.2019.10.003.

Young, B., Lewis, S., Katikireddi, S., Bauld, L., Stead, M., Angus, K., Campbell, M., Hilton, S., Thomas, J., Hinds, K., & Ashie, A. (2018). Effectiveness of mass media campaigns to reduce alcohol consumption and harm: a systematic review. *Alcohol and Alcoholism, 53*(3), 302–316. https://doi.org/10.1093/alcalc/agx094.

Websites

The Health Foundation. A site which uses charts and infographics to explore key health and healthcare trends in an accessible way. https://www.health.org.uk/news-and-comment/charts-and-infographics

The Discern. Site for quality criteria for health information. http://www.discern.org.uk/

Free Infographic Design Tools

Piktochart. Piktochart.com

Vengage. Vengage.com

Facebook

Department of Health and Social Care [DHSC] Facebook page. https://www.facebook.com/DHSCgovuk.

Health Communication Working Group supported by the American Public Health Association [APHA]. https://www.facebook.com/APHAhealthcomm

Twitter

NSW Multicultural Health Communication Service. https://twitter.com/mhcsnsw

WHO on Twitter. https://twitter.com/WHO

YouTube

The Role of Effective Communication in Health Promotion | Dr Chioma Nwakanma. https://www.youtube.com/watch?v=Bkd9o8_DtlQ

WHO on YouTube. https://www.youtube.com/c/who

12

Educating for Health

Gareth Morgan, Angela Scriven

SUMMARY

This chapter opens with a discussion on the principles of learning, and an exercise is used to explore effective public health education as well as illustrate the principles of facilitating learning. Subsequent sections move on to delivering public health talks, approaches to patient education, and teaching practical skills. Throughout the chapter, exercises are offered to practice skills of effective patient health education.

Understanding the skills and methods used in planned public health learning experiences is important in professional development and may be built into your annual review to help with career development. Such skills can be underpinned by theories that aim to empower individuals, groups or communities by providing them with tools to acquire health information to enable them to make quality health decisions. Health education is an important area of health promotion, and many professionals have a remit that offers the potential to provide public health education. Examples include:

- A health promotion specialist giving a talk on a locally identified health topic to a large community group, such as the risks of alcohol misuse.
- An environmental health officer teaching an adult education class in food safety to help avoid foodborne diseases, such as salmonella.
- University-based services facilitating a sexual health programme for students, including risks of infections and unplanned pregnancy.

- Physiotherapy teams supporting patients with musculoskeletal conditions and how best to manage chronic pain and reduce muscular stiffness.
- A pharmacist giving information to a customer about how to use a COVID-19 testing kit.
- A public health practitioner teaching a small group of colleagues about the techniques and procedures used in a smoking cessation programme.

PRINCIPLES OF LEARNING FOR HEALTH

Health promoters and public health practitioners require an appreciation of education, teaching and learning as this is likely to be relevant in many projects and public health interventions. An important element of practice is credibility because professionals will have the training and expert knowledge that is likely to be valued and respected in the delivery of their work. However, qualifications and expertise alone do not make a good public health educator.

Achieving results in the form of measurable learning achievements includes greater retention and application of health information and skills. Public health educators, therefore, need to understand some of the basic principles of learning, such as the importance of participation. The basic principles of learning as applied to health are summarised in Box 12.1. There are at least 130 learning theories, models and frameworks that address how people learn. If you want to read more on these and how they can be applied in practice, see Bates (2019) and for health education and how it differs from but links to health promotion and public health, see van Teijlingen et al. (2021).

FACILITATING HEALTH LEARNING

Exercise 12.1 will help you to identify factors that have helped and hindered your learning and to assess your own qualities and abilities.

BOX 12.1   Principles of Learning as Applied to Public Health Education

- Learning for health is most effective when the learner identifies their own learning needs and has involvement in helping to set their own goals, which gives a sense of ownership.
- The public health educator's role is to enable or facilitate learning rather than to direct it. Public health educators who adopt this approach often refer to themselves as facilitators.
- Learners are generally most ready to learn things that they can apply immediately to existing health problems or to their own situation. This also fosters a sense of ownership.
- Learners bring with them life experience, which should be seen as a key resource and to which new health learning should be related as it builds upon their previous knowledge
- Learners can help each other because of their experiences and should be encouraged to do so. This could work best if the group is mutually supportive and gives encouragement.
- Health learning is best when active (not passive), by doing and experiencing, for which learners need a safe environment where they feel accepted and able to ask questions.
- Learners should be encouraged to continuously evaluate their own learning. Public health educators should use this evaluation to fit the learning process to the learners' needs.

EXERCISE 12.1   What Helps and Hinders Health Learning?

Think of at least two occasions when you have had an opportunity to be a learner. This might be from when you were a student or perhaps if you have listened to a talk or a conference lecture, which are sometimes available on the internet.

These learning occasions may or may not have been connected with your professional role, for example, listening to a history documentary or attending a yoga class. One should be when you felt the experience was positive, whilst the other was less positive. Reflect on this and try to understand the underpinning factors that shaped your experience. In each situation, reflect on the factors that helped you to learn and those that hindered your learning. Think of these factors in four categories:

1. *Environment*. What made it good, e.g. a spacious, comfortable room? What made it less good, e.g. too noisy or too hot or too crowded?
2. *Qualities of the health educator/facilitator*. Were they engaging with a good sense of humour? Or did they come across as unfriendly?
3. *Presentation*. Was this clear and well thought out, or was it muddled and too long?
4. *Myself*. Reflect on how you learn best. Are certain times better? Do you learn best with short sessions with lots of breaks, perhaps with a walk? Or by a longer

session for a deeper exploration of the topic? Or perhaps a combination?

	Environ-ment	Educator	Presen-tation	Myself
Factors helping				
Factors hindering				

If you are working in a group, compare your chart with those of other people:

- What have you learnt about the importance of the environment? What can you change to improve this for your own preferred style?
- What qualities of a good public health educator do you think you already possess? How do you ensure you use these qualities to the best effect?
- What helpful points about presentation do you think you already use or will use in your own work? What preparation techniques do you also use?
- What points about your own qualities or presentation skills would you like to improve? How could you go about making these improvements?

Plan Your Session

However skilled and knowledgeable you are about the public health topic, it is vital to put thought and time into preparation. You need to think through what you aim to achieve, how you are going to introduce and develop your session, as well as how and when you will involve your audience. Also, think about how long the session is going to be and avoid having too much material for the time available.

Preparation is especially important when facilitating health learning is new to you, and it is well worth practising ahead of the session. This is time well spent, as even the most experienced and self-confident public health educator needs to spend some time in preparation. Active participation of the attendees is a more complex process and will require greater attention to planning for it to be effective.

Start With What Is Known

Wherever possible, it is worth trying to find out ahead of the session what the attendees already know. If this is not possible, use the start of the session to find out what people know; for example, a smoking cessation group might be worth starting with some well-known facts about the health risks of using tobacco products. For example, most people would know that smoking is a causal factor of lung cancers, although fewer might know that it is also a factor in other cancers, such as cancer of the mouth and a range of other diseases (see Pietrangelo, 2019, for an excellent diagram of the effects of smoking on the body). Very often, the audience will have mixed knowledge, and this can be delivered in practice by saying that 'Although many of you will know that smoking is a causal link in most lung cancers, perhaps fewer of you might be aware of the full range of diseases linked to smoking'.

Your aim is to add new health information and awareness, or new skills, to what is already known so you could then open up a dialogue about the other health risks of smoking. Often the attendees will have different needs and concerns. If the session has a mixed audience who might be interested in different messages, then you might need to move from the general to specific and vice-versa.

Aim for Maximum Involvement

People learn best if they are actively participating in the learning process and are not just passive listeners. For an analysis of participatory health learning in practice and for an assessment of the effectiveness of participatory approaches, see Allaham et al. (2021).

There are two key considerations in achieving maximum involvement. Firstly, where appropriate and if possible, involve your clients in deciding the aim and content of the session. You could seek their input prior to the delivery of the course, seeking suggestions for content or even asking if there are specific questions that they would like to be addressed. Doing this improves preparation and increases the chances of the session being delivered in an effective way.

If you are running a course, such as an awareness raising of the impact of a sedentary lifestyle on health and wellbeing, you might begin by explaining your aims, asking for comments and suggestions before then going on to discuss the content. This will help to increase motivation by stimulating clients to think about their own needs and to take some responsibility for their own learning. The goals and content of a one-to-one session can be established by discussion and mutual agreement at the outset. As a general rule, it is worth considering how much room for flexibility and negotiation there is in your public health education role and spending time to find out what people really want. Ask yourself, 'Is what I cover, what I want to teach or what my clients want to learn?' Matching clients' needs with the delivery of the material is likely to be a key determinant of success. A gap between what you want to teach and what is wanted has the potential for frustration, disengagement and potential reputational harm.

Secondly, aim to keep your clients involved as much as possible during sessions. This is a challenge with a large audience, but there are still methods, such as asking people to respond to a question. Suppose you were delivering a course on improving healthy behaviours, you say: 'Welcome to the session today. To start, please could you put your hand up if you made a new year resolution to take more exercise this year'. Or ask them to engage in a series of questions, for example, with healthy behaviours, ask the whole audience to stand up, then ask them to sit down if they:

- Are current smokers.
- Drink alcohol daily.
- Rarely eat fruit and vegetables.
  Or (focusing on more positive aspects of behaviour):
- Are non-smokers.
- Stay within the recommended weekly unit allowance of alcohol.
- Eat fruit and vegetables every day.

Although many will be sitting down by now, they will feel alert and involved. Another way of keeping an audience involved is to give them time to talk, and planning this into the session is important as long presentations can be information overload. There are several ways to do this, including having question-and-answer sessions or allowing short breaks to allow discussion in small groups for a few minutes. For example, in a talk to unpaid carers who look after family members, you could give your audience a couple of minutes to talk about some of the challenges involved, such as fatigue. This might even lead to supportive networks emerging from the session you are delivering by way of people facing similar challenges, both offering and seeking peer support.

It is also important to keep people involved with eye contact, making sure that you look around and scan the room rather than just focusing on the people immediately in front of you. Try to scan the room both from left to right and also front to back to connect with all attendees. Occasionally, a person may raise their hand during your session to ask a question, and you can either invite the question at the moment or ask them to pose it at a set time, depending on the running order.

Vary Your Learning Methods

It is important to consider health education from both the public health educator's point of view and also from the learner's point of view. For example, talking for 30 min demands concentrated effort and total involvement on your part, but all your audience is doing is listening, which involves only one of their senses and is highly unlikely to hold their full attention. Furthermore, this may also have disadvantages, such as a somewhat one-way communication style. Try to reflect on different ways to convey your session.

For example, if you are using a PowerPoint presentation, you could briefly pause at the end of each slide. If you are presenting on improving healthy behaviours, you might have a few slides each on alcohol, smoking, diet, and exercise. Receiving some immediate questions on these discrete sections might improve audience engagement, participation and retention of the key messages.

Variety can be brought into health teaching in many ways, including strategies that can be used with individuals, groups, large audiences, children or adults; see Table 12.1 for ideas. Part of the skill in delivering this, which will become more natural with experience, is choosing the right combination of these strategies for each session. Try different methods and reflect on the experience, as this will provide invaluable information on the most effective method of delivery that suits both your teaching style and the learner's needs.

Devise Public Health Education Activities

Activities can be helpful to assist learners in thinking through what is being said and acting on it in their own way. Whilst asking a group 'What do you think?' at the end of a health talk or after viewing a video has value, planned activities can help people to explore and apply ideas, feelings, attitudes and behaviour. It can be more effective to have several bespoke activities that are specifically tailored for a particular group of learners. As part of your professional development, it is worth seeking to develop skills of devising your own activities for your specific situation rather than relying on general learning aids. There is a range of possibilities, and examples are set out in Table 12.2. There are also ideas in some of the exercises used throughout this book.

Ensure Relevance

It is important to ensure that what you say is relevant to the needs, interests and circumstances of the clients. For example, recommendations about health-promoting activities that cost money may not be useful to an audience with no budget unless the recommendation itself will give a return on investment. A discussion on improving exercise levels may be irrelevant to a person due to

TABLE 12.1   Learning Methods Involving Clients

Client Involvement	Materials and Methods
Listen	Lectures, audiotapes and one-to-one or small group information giving
Read	Books, booklets, leaflets, handouts, posters, whiteboards, flipcharts, PowerPoint slides, websites, blogs
Look	Photographs, drawings, paintings, posters, charts, and material from media (such as advertisements)
Look and listen	Videos, PowerPoint slides, demonstrations, YouTube
Listen and talk	Question-and-answer sessions, discussions, informal conversations, debates, brainstorming
Read, listen and talk	Case studies, discussions based on study questions or handouts
Read, listen, talk and actively participate	Drama, role-play, games, simulations, quizzes, practising skills
Read and actively participate	Programmed learning, computer-assisted learning
Make and use	Models, charts, drawings
Use	Equipment
Action research	Gathering information, opinions, interviews, and surveys
Projects	Making public health education materials – videos, leaflets, etc.
Visits	To health service premises, fire stations, sewage works, playgroups, voluntary organisations
Write	Articles, letters to the press or politicians, stories, poems

For a discussion of some of these methods, see Chapters 13 and 14; for a discussion on the use of audio-visual and media aids, see Chapter 11.

having a procedure to improve their vision, as this will not meet their immediate needs. Once the person has received their treatment, for example cataract surgery, then they might be more receptive to a wider discussion on improving their lifestyle.

TABLE 12.2   Common Types of Public Health Learning Activities

Type of Activity	Example
Guidelines for discussions with specific people about a public health issue	Guidelines on 'what to do if you think your child may be experiencing cyberbullying' for discussion at a parent-teacher meeting
Analysing and discussing diary records	Ask people to keep a record of their exercise in the last week. Ask them to talk about what they are pleased about and not pleased about, ideally giving reasons for this
Sentence completion	Ask people to complete a sentence. For example in mental health awareness, such as 'I feel really anxious when …'
Using checklists	Have a list of strategies, such as increasing activity by taking the stairs rather than the lift
Identifying your own thoughts/feelings/behaviour in particular situations	Ask people to think about and discuss what they feel when offered alcohol when they are trying to reduce the amount they drink
Generate lists	Ask a group to make a list of all the ways they could support a smoker who has lung disease but resists giving up and becomes defensive when asked about their smoking
Answer sheets	A quiz with yes/no or multiple answers on 'Do you know what body mass index is and what the various measures mean?'
Drawing charts or bubble diagrams	Draw a stick-person picture of yourself in an exercise class. Draw bubble thoughts about all the things that motivate you to attend
Writing instructions	Ask unpaid carers to write down instructions for someone else on what medicines the person they care for takes in case of emergency
Practical skills development	Practise guide-walking a visually impaired person by attending a training class

You can help your clients see the relevance of your subject if you use concrete examples, such as practical problems and case studies, to explain and illustrate the points. It may be more difficult for your clients to relate to abstract statements such as quotations of statistics or population evidence, maybe from epidemiological studies. For example, saying 'one person in eight is an unpaid carer' (see Welsh Government, 2021) instead of 'X million people in this country'. Using clear language could also be helpful; for example, during the COVID-19 pandemic, the risk of becoming infected could be reduced by mask wearing and increased by mixing with lots of people. Illustrating 'reducing the risk' could be done by saying, 'Whilst wearing a mask offers no guarantee that you will avoid being infected, your chances are lower. It's like wearing a safety belt in a car; it's a safety mechanism that is intended to be helpful by offering a degree of protection'.

Identify Realistic Health Goals and Objectives

In Chapter 5, there was a discussion of the importance of clearly identifying health promotion aims and objectives. It is worth emphasising again that it is essential to be clear about what you are trying to achieve in a health education session. This might include:

- Raising awareness of a health issue, perhaps to the local community or other professional colleagues.
- Giving people more health knowledge, in which case consider what you want your clients to know, feel and/or do at the end of your session.

As previously mentioned, your clients should be involved in these decisions.

Three or four key points are all that anyone attending can be reasonably expected to assimilate from a session. Overloading information risks both diluting and rushing the key messages; for example if you are asked to give a talk on a huge theme, you will need to select what you feel to be the few points most relevant for your audience and avoid the temptation to include everything. Consider healthy ageing as a large and diverse topic where there are many factors. What are the most relevant to your audience?

Use Learning Contracts

It may be appropriate to introduce learning contracts. In summary, this is an agreement about what is expected to be learnt within a specific time interval. These can be customised to the individual and the topic to ensure they take into account the specific circumstances. Learning contracts are often used in the training of healthcare professionals and can be adjusted for use with clients in health promotion settings, see Hesketh and Laidlaw (2013).

Step 1: Assess Health Learning Needs With the Learners

First, decide on the competencies required to carry out actions, behaviour, or roles. A competency can be thought of as the ability to do something, and in practice, it is a combination of knowledge, understanding, skills, attitudes, and values.

For instance, the ability to support people who are obese may involve increasing knowledge of the health risks of obesity, nutrition information, advice concerning weight loss strategies, and the development of skills in preparing nutritious low calorie meals.

Next, assess the gap between where learners are now and where they should be with regard to each health-related competency. Learners may wish to draw on the observations of friends, family or experts to make this assessment. Each learner will then have an idea of the competencies needed and a map of their health learning needs. For example, to count calories whilst on a weight loss diet, a learner might want to develop skills in using a diet app and a greater understanding of portion control and food swapping.

Step 2: Specify the Learning Objectives of Each Learner

Translate the health learning needs identified in step 1 into objectives that describe what each learner wants to learn. All learners should state their health learning objectives in terms most meaningful to them. For example, using a smartphone or laptop, accessing websites focusing on weight loss and adopting stress management strategies to avoid emotional eating.

Step 3: Specify Learning Methods

Review the learning objectives of the learner or (if you are working with a group of learners) all the members of the learning group, perhaps through listing them on a flipchart and identifying shared objectives and areas of difference. Now think about how you could go about accomplishing these objectives. Specify the methods you would use. In the obesity example, you could specify that this needs a practical demonstration of preparing low calorie snacks followed by supervised practice with food preparation or filling in online food diaries.

Step 4: Evaluate Learning

Now describe what evidence you will need to show that these objectives have been achieved. For example, health knowledge can be tested through quizzes; understanding can be tested through problem solving; skills can be tested through demonstrations of performance; attitudes can be tested through role-play and simulation exercises; values can be tested through live debates and value-clarification exercises (see also Chapter 5, a section on planning evaluation methods).

An example of a learning contract for two different groups is provided in Box 12.2 for a young parent group on healthy eating in Boxes 12.2 and 12.3, illustrating a COVID-19 learning contract. This is derived from the NHS

BOX 12.2   Learning Contract for a Young Parent Group on Healthy Eating

Group members said they wanted to know more about how to cook cheap, interesting, healthy meals for their families as a change from the usual ready prepared foods such as frozen fish fingers, cans of beans, or frozen chips. The facilitator and group members worked out the following learning contract.

Learning Objectives	Learning Methods	Evaluation of Achievement of Objectives
Know what to eat to be healthy	Keep food diaries for two days. The facilitator to produce guidelines, and members discuss how far their food matches up with the guidelines	Be able to say what sort of food each member should aim to eat more or less of
Know where to buy healthy, cheap food	Group members share their experiences of where they buy food, as well as its price and quality	Two weeks later, members identify changes in where they buy food and whether it is of better quality and value for money
Be able to cook healthy meals that their families enjoy eating	The facilitator and group members bring recipes, choose some to try out, and cook together	Have cooked new healthy meals at home

BOX 12.3 Learning Protocol for Mass Education of the Public

As part of COVID-19 control, the public were provided with messages through a variety of sources regarding measures to break infection chains of transmission.

Learning Objectives	Learning Methods	Achievement Measure
Awareness and the implementation of measures like wearing face masks and social distancing of 2 m	Whole system information campaign through radio, television, posters and digital media, e.g. Facebook	Adhere to key messages and the potential social norm of these practices as part of the societal attempts to control COVID-19
Knowledge of key COVID infection symptoms, e.g. coughing, loss of taste or smell (anosmia), fever and need to self-isolate	Whole system information campaign as similar to the above. Also promoted in settings, e.g. work, school	Confirmed by testing numbers rising to show the participation of the public in acting on their knowledge of COVID-19
Knowledge of the key importance of vaccination in the control of COVID-19 as a way to build 'herd immunity' in the community	Whole system information campaign supplemented by health services inviting people to get vaccinated	Update of first and second vaccines. Public health impact monitored via indicators like hospital admissions

response to COVID-19 when there was a need to ensure the workforce was given the skills and learning to meet very different challenges. One such challenge was to establish a contact service for patients who tested positive for COVID-19 to undertake an exposure history. This intelligence gathering would help establish possible sources of infection and allow mitigation and control measures to be introduced. For example, supposing ten patients with COVID-19 all attended the same restaurant within the week prior to their diagnosis, action could be taken to find other cases and thus help prevent the spread of the infection. Exposure history was, therefore, an important part of the COVID-19 control, and staff needed to learn the skills.

Individuals in a group can have their own personal version of the learning contract (see Chapter 14, a section on strategies for increasing self-awareness, clarifying values and changing attitudes).

Organise Your Public Health Education Material

Whether you are talking to a group or an individual, it helps if you organise your material into a logical framework and tell your client(s) what this is, both at the beginning and during your health education session. For example, with an individual client in an alcohol support group, say:

- We are going to review your alcohol intake and the reasons why you drink every day.
- We can then try to identify the barriers to you drinking less frequently.
- We can also explore where you are in terms of your motivation to reduce your alcohol intake.
- Firstly, let us discuss your drinking behaviour and what prompts this behaviour.
- Secondly, what do you think will prevent you from stopping or reducing your alcohol consumption?
- Finally, let us see where you stand regarding your wanting to stop drinking.

The same principle applies if you are talking to a group. You do this in three stages, namely:

- To tell them what you are going to tell them.
- Tell them by delivering the material.
- Tell them what you have told them.

This helps you and the audience know where you are and where you are going. Recapping where you are at intervals is helpful: 'That concludes my session on the health benefits of exercise. So let's now explore how you can get started …' or 'Now moving onto my final two slides, which set out the local opportunities to attend an exercise class…'

Evaluation, Feedback and Assessment

Feedback is important for two reasons. Firstly, to help you assess how much your client is learning and secondly, to help improve your own performance in the future (see Chapter 5, a section on planning evaluation methods, and Chapter 10, a section on asking questions and getting feedback).

Assessing Your Own Performance

You need to ask yourself what went well, what was less good and why and how things could be improved next time. You may find it helpful to use a simple form to record your thoughts (see Box 12.4). The importance

BOX 12.4 Nutrition and Cooking Project Monitoring Form

Session no:
Date:
Time:
Facilitator:
Number of attendees:
Number in crèche:
Activity:
Positive outcomes:
Negative outcomes:
Feedback/comments from participants:
Crèche issues:
Issues needing further action:
Action plan:
Completed by:

(From Hartcliffe Health and Environment Action Group and health visitors from Hartcliffe and Withywood, Bristol. Reproduced with permission)

BOX 12.5 Evaluation Form A

Title of session:
Date:
 Please help me to get the session right for you by completing the following sentences about how you feel. Thank you.
It helps me when ....
It is difficult for me when ....
I would like more of ....
I would like less of ....

BOX 12.6 Evaluation Form B

Title of session:
Date:
 We would like your views to help us assess this session and make plans for similar sessions in the future. All your comments will be valued as well as used and treated confidentially.

	Yes	No	Partly
1. Overall, have you found this session beneficial? (please tick)			

	Yes	No	Partly
2. Did the session match up to your expectations?			

3. What did you expect to gain from the session?
Please comment:
4. Which parts of the session have you found most beneficial?
5. Which parts of the session have you found least beneficial?
6. How do you think the session could be improved?
7. Do you have any other comments you would like to make?

of doing this has been recognised by the World Health Organization, who have published instructions to organisers of events to evaluate the participants' perception by asking key questions, Did the attendees like it? Was the material presented relevant to their work? (WHO, 2019).

Getting Feedback

You could include oral feedback as part of your session. For example, at the end, ask people to do a round of sentence completion:
- 'The most valuable part of today's session was ...'
- 'The most important learning I am taking from this session is ...'
- 'The thing I found least helpful about today's session was ...'

 However, some people may find this intimidating and might not feel comfortable expressing what they feel. You may also wish to use a written evaluation as per Boxes 12.5 and 12.6, as this can also be completed anonymously.

Assessing the Health Learning Outcomes

Assessing learning outcomes is an important aspect of evaluation in health education. It is the process of measuring the extent and quality of your clients' learning, judging how successful they have been in progressing towards the goals which they set themselves. It may be carried out very informally by getting apparently casual feedback from clients about how they have applied the learning to real-life situations, or it may involve setting tests in formal situations. Here are two examples of ways in which health promoters assess how well they are doing.

 Tracy is a mental health support worker who provides a once-a-week drop-in service that offers advice to people experiencing stress. Tracy evaluates the effectiveness of the support group activities by using a self-reported stress measure, which is taken at the initial attendance and at each week for a maximum of six weeks. Tracy uses a simple system ranging from one being very calm to ten being very stressed. Not everyone is required to stay on the full course, and attendees are followed up two months after their last attendance.

Ivor provides a non-competitive and supportive exercise class to adults with learning difficulties. Ivor keeps records of their progress, for example, how many short interval runs can be done in 1 min. This is then extended to 90 s, and additional 30 s intervals are added, if appropriate, based on increasing fitness levels. Ivor is able to show his members not only the changes in their speed if they do more intervals in 1 min but also their increasing stamina if they can maintain this for a longer time.

Monitoring clients' progress by keeping records of achievements can be valuable for helping them to see what they have achieved. If your public health education is geared towards people learning to change their behaviour, it can help to keep diary-type records that reflect the nature of the provision. As long as this gives an indication of something that can be measured over time, then it will be useful.

Another method of helping to embed learning is via the use of photographic records. For example, on a course designed to help people cook and eat healthier food for their families, you could encourage people to make a pictorial record of the dishes they cooked and their family enjoying the meals. This will aid recall and also help sustain the learning from the session. It may also even have other impacts, for example, inspiring other people to make similar changes in their own life.

GUIDELINES FOR GIVING PUBLIC HEALTH TALKS

Giving a formal health education talk is often part of a health promoter's work and can be valuable for several reasons. It is important, however, to avoid this being a one-way communication process with little opportunity to assess how much people are learning or understanding.

A talk can be used to introduce a public health topic by giving a broad overview of it, which may then lead people to take further action. A talk may also be an important source of health information and awaken a critical attitude in the audience, for example, by drawing their attention to local issues such as alcohol-related assaults or providing housing support to refugees. Giving

talks is also a relatively economical way to use a health promoter's time because large numbers of people can be addressed at one time. To ensure success, the following points could be considered.

Check the Facilities

If possible, visit the place where you are going to give your talk prior to doing so. This will help you become familiar with how to get there and the layout. You can also check the seating, lighting, and audio-visual equipment, including electric power points and extension leads.

On the day of the talk, arrive early so that you can arrange chairs, open windows and check that the equipment is working. Get your audio-visual and media equipment ready for use. If you need blackout, check that you can turn the lights on and off quickly so that you do not lose rapport with the audience whilst they are left in the dark.

Make a Plan for the Session

It can be useful to make an outline plan of your whole session, indicating the sections, times and any audio-visual or media aids you are using. This is particularly useful if you are sharing a session with a colleague so that you are both clear about what you are doing. See the example in (Box 12.7) and either use this as a skeleton overall plan to guide you when you make detailed notes to speak from (see the following section), or it might be enough to enable you to speak from the plan itself.

Making and Using Notes

It is generally best to give a public health talk from notes. The more experienced you are, the fewer notes you are likely to need unless your talk is full of technical detail or likely to be taken down and quoted verbatim (for example, by the press). However, very few people can give a successful talk with no notes at all, and beginners may find it helpful to write out a talk in full before they transfer the main points to notes.

If you are writing out your talk in full to begin with, it is useful to know that a 50 min lecture consists of about 5000 words, allowing for pauses and an estimated speed of delivery of about 110 words per minute. You can then try transferring the key points as notes to cards or paper.

There may be disadvantages to giving a talk by writing it out in full and then reading it because this risks coming across as flat and stilted. Furthermore, you may find it difficult to look at your audience because you will need to keep your eyes on the notes, and if you look up, you are likely to lose your place.

BOX 12.7   Plan for Giving a Talk

Talk on 'Sense in the Sun – Preventing Skin Cancer'
Bloggshire Secondary School Parent–Teachers Meeting
21 February 2023: An hour at the end of a curriculum meeting, 8:00–8:45 p.m.
SN (school nurse) and DH (deputy head)
AIM: To give parents basic information on the risks and prevention of skin cancer

Time (pm)	Section	Content	Audio-visual aids PowerPoint (PP)	Who
8:00	Intros	Intro JAS & SNS. Why we are now concerned about skin cancer – a rising incidence?	TED YouTube lesson – Why do we have to wear sunscreen? PP graph showing a rise in skin cancer in the UK	DH
8:05	What is skin cancer?	Different types of skin cancer. How do you spot it? Who is most at risk (fair skin, sunburn, etc.)?	PP key points	SN
8:15	Prevention	Key message: Respect the sun – avoid exposure at the hottest times, use good sunscreen, and cover up with sun hats and light clothing. Be a mole-watcher	Examples of sun hats and light clothing (big, long-sleeved, cotton shirts, etc.). Examples of sunscreen creams	SN
8:25	What the school can do?	Encourage the use of cover up and sunscreen creams in outdoor physical education. Include topic in Personal, Health, Social and Economic and science teaching	Main points on PP	DH
8.30	Summary	Aim for school and parents to work together. Main points to remember: care in the sun, cover up, use sunscreen creams	PP: 3 Cs to remember: care in the sun, coverup and creams. Leaflets to take away	SN
8:35	Any questions?			SN
8:45	Concluding remarks and further information	Further reading and information: Facebook page – sun safety* NHS 2019 advise on sunscreen and sun safety. YouTube Ted Talk on the importance of sunscreen	PP	SN

*See references at the end of the chapter.

Prepare Your Introduction

- Secure the attention of your audience with your opening words. Some ways of doing this are to state a surprising fact or an unusual quote.
- Ask a question that has no easy answer.
- Use a visual image to trigger interest.
- Get the audience to do something active (some suggestions are discussed in the earlier section on aiming for maximum involvement).
- Tell a joke if you have the confidence to do it successfully.

As you deliver your introduction, it is important to establish eye contact with your audience and, if necessary, ask them whether they can see and hear you. Briefly state your aim and theme at the beginning of your talk and remember this is not the time for a complex summary of the whole talk.

For example, say, 'My talk today explores both the benefits and advantages of incorporating more physical activity into your life and ways of making small changes to ensure you are getting sufficient exercise,' which allows you to save the main details for the substantive part of the talk. By the time you have finished the introduction, you should have:

- Confirmed your aim and theme with the audience.
- Obtained both their interest and commitment.
- Ensured that they can hear and see you clearly.

If you are unsure if you have achieved this, then pause before going into the main details of the topic. For example, if people are unable to clearly see and hear you, then make reasonable adjustments where possible.

Prepare the Key Points

Identify the three or four main points you wish to make and prepare your talk around each point in turn. Illustrate and support your points with evidence from your experience or from research with examples, audio-visual materials, and other materials (see Chapter 11 on using and producing audio-visual materials, including leaflets, handouts and film/videos).

Plan a Conclusion

Some ways of concluding your talk are:

- A very brief summary of the key points, such as 'We've now covered the basics of exercising and the advantages it confers to your health.'
- A statement of what you hope the audience will do with the information you have given them, such as 'Following the session today, you might now like to consider how best you can confidently make changes to your lifestyle to include more exercise, for example joining a class.'
- A suggestion for further action: 'If anyone has any further questions, then please feel welcome to come to see me afterwards or contact me at … (provide appropriate contact details such as email or telephone number).'
- A question, such as 'Ask yourself: What small lifestyle changes can you make to include more physical activity into your life?'
- Thanking the audience for their attention and/or participation.

Ask for Questions

If possible, include a question-and-answer session in your talk. It gives you feedback and gives the audience a chance to participate. When you ask for questions, allow people time to think; do not assume that there are to be no questions just because one is not instantly forthcoming.

When a question is asked, it is often helpful to repeat it or summarise it. This gives you a little time to consider the question and ensures that everyone else in the audience has heard it. Never ignore or refuse to answer a question. If you don't know the answer, admit this and ask whether anyone else in the audience does. In any case, this helps involve the audience; you could also ask for comments on answers: 'Does anyone else have suggestions for the person who asked that question?'

Work on Your Presentation

Important points about presentation include pace and timing, which can mean consciously having to slow down your rate of speaking; the nervous beginner can speak too quickly. Other factors are looking at the audience and using notes appropriately.

Thorough preparation will help you to feel confident, but however nervous or inexperienced you may feel, do not apologise for being there. For example, if you have been asked to give a talk about your work, avoid something negative like 'I'm going to talk about the work of the COVID-19 vaccination centre, but I'm afraid I've only been working there for three months, so there's a lot I don't know yet'. Instead, present yourself positively: 'I'm going to talk about the work of the COVID-19 vaccination centre. We all have had to learn quickly to respond to the pandemic, and I'd like to share my experience of the work with you'.

The way to improve presentation is to practise. Practise giving your talk out loud or to friends or colleagues. Ask a trusted colleague to sit in when you give a talk and to give you feedback afterwards. It is also helpful to have your talk recorded so that you can assess your own strengths and weaknesses. For example, are you too slow or too fast? Or perhaps too quiet or too loud? Or perhaps a little repetitive?

Plan for Contingencies

A major fear when giving a talk is that you might lose your place or your train of thought. If this is a possibility, it is better to think beforehand about what you will do if it should happen. It is best to acknowledge that you have a problem rather than leave an embarrassing silence. You may also want to have a glass of water to drink, both in case you get a dry mouth but also to allow a few moments to think.

If something unexpected happens, just be honest. For example, say, 'Sorry, could you give me a moment to gather my thoughts'. Remember that an audience is likely to be friendly rather than hostile. So let them help by asking for time: 'Excuse me for a moment whilst I find my place' (see also the section on dealing with difficulties in Chapter 13).

Another fear is that audio-visual equipment may not work. You cannot insure against this, so it is best to have a contingency plan ready. For example, 'Unfortunately, PowerPoint is not working as planned, so I'll write the

TABLE 12.3 Summary Checklist for Giving Public Health Talks

Checklist Point	Some Key Considerations
Check the facilities	Both pre-session and on the day
Make a plan for the session	Get an outline plan with timings
Making and using notes	Helps with remembering points
Prepare your introduction	Helps get attention of the audience
Prepare key points	Three or four key points is a general guide
Plan a conclusion	Always thank the audience
Ask for questions	Allows audience participation
Work on your presentation	Think about pace and timing
Plan for contingencies	Have some backup options

stages up on the flipchart and talk through them instead', or you may wish to ensure you have a backup, such as overhead projector slides of the PowerPoint presentation. An alternative backup is to have hardcopy handouts available.

Table 12.3 provides a summary of these points, and for further advice on giving talks and public speaking, see Alexander (2020).

IMPROVING PATIENT EDUCATION

Evidence suggests that patients want health information, but some have difficulty in understanding and remembering what they have been told by their doctor, nurse, or other health worker. Obstacles that prevent understanding of and action on health information might include literacy, culture, language, age and physiological barriers. Patients who feel dissatisfied with the communications aspect of their encounters with health professionals may be reluctant to ask for more information and/or may not comply with the advice and treatment prescribed for them or may not develop the health literacy needed to fully understand and communicate with health professionals (Stewart, 2020). For a broad discussion on communication skills, see Thompson (2017).

There may be complex reasons for these apparent failures, but a common cause will be the way in which information, advice and instructions are given to patients. Often, the circumstances are less than ideal because patients are distressed or feeling unwell, and there may be little time in a busy surgery, health centre, outpatient clinic or hospital ward. This is all the more reason to ensure that the best possible use is made of the time and opportunities for patient education. See Box 12.8 for some basic principles of patient education.

All the basic communication skills discussed in Chapter 10, and the principles of helping people to learn outlined in this chapter, are important. There is also now a growing body of evidence and guidance in the field of patient education and imparting health information. For example, Morris (2022) explores ten ways to improve patient education, and for an interesting discussion on providing culturally appropriate patient education and information, see Allen et al. (2021).

Exercise 12.2 is designed to help you practise the skills of patient education and supplements the basic communication skills outlined in Chapter 10. Another useful way of learning to improve communication skills and education is via role-play, and for an interesting example of this with reference to mental health, see Bonning and Bkorkly (2019).

TEACHING PRACTICAL SKILLS FOR HEALTH

Health promoters in a number of health-related settings are often called upon to teach practical skills, such as relaxation or physiotherapy exercises, how to bathe a baby or feed them and how to give an injection or take a blood sample.

Teaching a skill is not just about giving the client information and teaching new practical skills. It is also necessary to pay attention to what clients feel. If people are afraid to do something because they are worried about looking foolish or doing it incorrectly, they are unlikely to succeed; encouragement and step-by-step progress are needed. Confidence-building is as important a part of the health educator's role as developing practical skills.

To develop clients' abilities to perform a skilled task, a three-stage approach is most effective:
- Stage 1. Demonstrate.
- Stage 2. Rehearse.
- Stage 3. Practise.

Clients will be watching and listening in stage 1, but they become actively involved in stages 2 and 3.

It may be useful to begin by using a dummy, for example, when teaching safe lifting techniques or to use a manikin in training for first aid. As skills develop, the techniques can be tried in real-life situations (lifting people, for example) and perhaps under more difficult circumstances.

BOX 12.8   Some Principles of Patient Education

- Say important things first: patients are more likely to remember what was said at the beginning of a session, so give the most important advice and instruction first whenever possible.
- Stress and repeat the key points: patients are more likely to remember what they consider important, so make sure they realise what the important points are. For example, say:
  - 'The most important thing for you to remember today is …'
  - 'The one thing it's really essential to do is …'
- Repetition of key points also helps people to remember them. Give specific, precise advice: sometimes, it is appropriate to give general guidance, but specific, precise advice is more likely to be remembered than vague guidance. For example, say:
  - 'I advise you to lose 5 pounds in the next month' rather than 'I advise you to lose weight'.
  - 'Try to take 30 min exercise every day' rather than 'Take more exercise'.
- Structure information into categories: This means telling the patient headings and then categorising your material under these headings as you present it. See 'Organise Your Public Health Education Material' discussed previously in this chapter.
- Use plain language. Avoid jargon and long words and sentences; if you need to use medical terms or jargon, make sure the patient understands what they mean. Never use a long word when a short one will do. Use short sentences. See CDC (2022) for plain language materials and resources to use in public health settings.
- Use visual aids, leaflets, handouts and written instructions (see Chapter 11 on using communication tools).
- Avoid saying too much at once; three or four key points are all you can expect someone to remember from one session. See 'Ensure Relevance' discussed previously in this chapter.
- Ensure advice is relevant and realistic to the patient's circumstances.
- Get feedback from patients to ensure that they understand (see the section on asking questions and getting feedback in Chapter 10).

EXERCISE 12.2   Skills of Patient Education

Working in groups of three, taking each role in turn.

The **first person** takes the role of the public health educator. They select the topic to be taught, drawing on their own experience, and tell the patient their medical history before role-play starts. The **second person** plays the patient. This patient should have one of the following sets of characteristics:

- Intelligent but with a very limited understanding of spoken English, no ability to read or write English and no one available to translate into their preferred language.
- Extremely worried, tense and anxious about their medical condition and prognosis, for example, a diagnosis of COVID-19 in a severely asthmatic patient.
- Has some learning difficulty and finds great difficulty in understanding and remembering instructions, although they try hard to engage and be cooperative.

The **third person** takes the role of the observer, using the observer's checklist in the following text.

Role-play the scene in which the health promoter is teaching the patient for 10 min. The observer keeps time. Then give constructive feedback as follows:

- Firstly, the health promoter assesses their own performance, saying what they felt they did well and identifying points they feel they need to work on in the future.
- Secondly, the patient describes how it felt to be the patient, identifying what the health promoter did or said that made them feel at ease, put down, anxious, reassured, more confused and so on.
- Finally, the observer gives feedback using the checklist below as a guide.
  1. Nonverbal aspects of communication (e.g. tone of voice, posture, gestures, facial expression and use of touch).
  2. Sequence and structure of key points (e.g. important things first, logical sequence, information in categories).
  3. Choice of language (e.g. appropriately simple and short, use of jargon or idioms, medical terms).
  4. Two-way communication (e.g. encourage the patient to talk and express feelings, get feedback about how much is understood, open/closed/biased/ multiple questions).
  5. Amount of information (e.g. too much or too little).
  6. Clarity of objective(s).
  7. Use of repetition.
  8. Use of emphasis to stress important points.
  9. Any assumptions made but not checked (e.g. about previous knowledge, facilities for carrying out instructions, willingness to comply).
  10. Anything else?

Individual learners need to progress at their own pace and build up confidence at each stage. For this reason, teaching practical skills needs time and patience, but it is worth the investment to get the right skills programme from the beginning. People who have lost confidence in their ability to do something are sometimes more difficult to help than a new learner.

PRACTICE POINTS

- To be successful in public health education with clients, you need to understand the principles of learning and factors that help and hinder the learning process. You may find it helpful to use informal learning contracts to provide a framework and point of reference for your activities.
- Giving talks on public health topics requires detailed planning, preparation and practice. Anticipate that this may not always run as planned.
- You can help patients to understand and remember more if you take account of some key principles of patient education.
- Use a three-stage approach of demonstration, rehearsal and practice when you are teaching practical health-related skills.

References

Alexander, M. (2020). *The public speaking bible; a survival guide for standing on stage*. Marcus Alexander Publishing.

Allaham, S., Kumar, A., Morriss, F., et al. (2021). Participatory learning and action (PLA) to improve health outcomes in high-income settings: a systematic review protocol. *BMJ Open, 12*, e050784. https://doi.org/10.1136/bmjopen-2021-050784.

Allen, C. G., Bridgeman-Bunyoli, A. M., Dominguez, T. C., et al. (2021). Providing culturally appropriate health education and information. In J. A. St John, S. L. Mayfield Johnson, & W. D. Hernandez-Gordon (Eds.), *Promoting the health of the community*. Springer Cham.

Bates, B. (2019). *Learning theories simplified: ...and how to apply them to teaching*. London: Sage.

Bonning, S. B., & Bkorkly, S. (2019). The use of clinical role play and reflection in learning therapeutic communication skills

in mental health education: an integrative review. *Advances of Medical Education and Practice, 10*, 415–425. https://doi.org/10.2147/AMEP.S202115.

CDC. (2022). Plain language materials and resources. https://www.cdc.gov/healthliteracy/developmaterials/plainlanguage.html

Hesketh, E.A., Laidlaw, J.M. (2013) Learning contracts. www.resources.nes.scot.nhs.uk/ti/LearningContracts.pdf.

Morris. G. (2022). 10 ways nurses and nurse leaders can improve patient education. Nurse Journal. https://nursejournal.org/articles/tips-to-improve-patient-education/.

NHS. (2019). Sunscreen and sun safety. https://www.nhs.uk/live-well/seasonal-health/sunscreen-and-sun-safety/

Pietrangelo, A. (2019). The effects of smoking on the body. https://www.healthline.com/health/smoking/effects-on-body.

Stewart, M. (2020). The art of science of patient education for health literacy. London, Elsevier.

Thompson, S. (2017). Communication skills. https://www.sth.nhs.uk/clientfiles/File/Communication%20Skills%20-%20Shirley%20Thompson.pdf

Van Teijlingen, K. R., Devkota, B., Douglas, F., Simkhada, P., & van Teijlingen, E. R. (2021). Understanding health education, health promotion and public health. *Journal of Health Promotion, 9*, 1–7. https://doi.org/10.3126/jhp.v9i01.40957.

Welsh Government 2021 Strategy for unpaid carers: What we will do to improve the recognition of and support of unpaid carers. https://gov.wales/strategy-unpaid-carers-html.

World Health Organization. (2019). Model of workshop evaluation form. https://www.who.int/publications/i/item/WHO-CED-PHE-EPE-19-12-04

Website

University College London. *For systematic reviews on participatory action and learning.* https://www.ucl.ac.uk/global-health/research/topics/participatory-learning-and-action

YouTube

The Ted Lesson on sun safety. Referenced in Box 12.6. https://www.youtube.com/watch?v=ZSJITdsTze0

Facebook

Facebook page on sun safety. Referenced in Box 12.6. https://www.facebook.com/search/top/?q=sun%20safety%20

Working With Groups to Promote Health

Gareth Morgan, Angela Scriven

SUMMARY

This chapter is about working with clients in groups. These can be either physical groups where face-to-face meetings occur or more virtually, such as via social media or videoconferencing. A hybrid model (combining face-to-face and videoconferencing) may also work for some groups if some members are local to the meeting and others live further away or are perhaps unable to attend.

This chapter begins by discussing the range of groups in health promotion and public health and the potential advantages and disadvantages of working in groups. Group leadership styles and responsibilities and individual group behaviour are considered, whilst the last part of the chapter focuses on the competencies needed for working successfully with people in groups. This includes the practicalities and skills of setting up a group, getting groups established, discussion skills, and dealing with difficulties. Exercises focus on identifying the benefits of joining a group, looking at your leadership style and planning a group meeting.

Health promoters and public health practitioners work with many kinds of groups in a variety of settings. Working with groups of colleagues is considered in Chapter 9, whilst in this chapter, the focus is on the public health promoter's work with groups of clients. Many of the skills discussed in Chapter 9, such as coordination, teamwork and working effectively in meetings and committees, may also apply when working with client groups (see Chapter 9).

Group work encourages members to be active participants in their own health issues and with their communities. Many of the groups with which health promoters and public health practitioners are involved will already exist. This is where members have come together for a common purpose, and health issues form part, or the whole, of the agenda. The role of the health promoter or public health practitioner may vary widely, from leading a one-off session to facilitating the development of a new group or leading a group with a defined lifespan.

Whatever the role, competencies in group work are needed. Leading therapeutic groups are excluded from the discussions in this chapter. Therapy requires in-depth professional training in a range of possible approaches, which is outside the scope of this book (see Nicholls (2019) for further details on therapeutic group activities, including what group therapy can achieve in terms of promoting health).

TYPES OF GROUPS

As shown in Fig. 13.1, groups are formed for a variety of purposes and are not simply a random collection of individuals. Members generally have a sense of shared identity, common objectives, defined membership criteria and their own ways of working. The term group work can be applied to a range of activities such as group therapy, social action or self-help. Groups in the context of health promotion and public health are usually formed for one or more of the following purposes:

For raising awareness. To increase members' interest in, and awareness of, health issues through group discussion. This may be a group already in existence, such as a club for D/deaf people, which is intended to support good mental health.

For mutual support. To support members in difficult decision making, to help each other to cope with shared health problems/disabilities or to change a health-damaging behaviour. Examples are self-help groups and fellowship groups such as Alcoholics Anonymous and Narcotics Anonymous. These fellowships can be found by searching on the internet for details of the local group.

For social action. To use collective power to campaign for social change, for example, tackling a local problem that may be impacting on health, like the lack of local and affordable recreational and sporting facilities.

For education. To impart skills, offer information and sometimes to prepare members for specific life events,

for example, a visually impaired club to help members to prepare themselves for progressive sight loss.

For group counselling. To help members find solutions through exploring a shared problem with a counsellor, for example, a support group for armed forces veterans.

Being clear about the purpose of a group is important. Confusion can result if the tasks of a group are changed, especially if this means that individual members must adopt different roles. For example, an individual will have difficulty if they attend a group to obtain support and find the purpose has changed to campaigning.

The type of task will determine the most effective size for the group; for example, educational groups may be larger than support groups. For example, for a smoking cessation group, the educational focus means that this is about providing information and possibly referring on to support groups.

Different kinds of groups may also require the health promoter or public health practitioner to take on different roles and use different skills. Leading and facilitating groups or administrating or moderating social media groups requires special skills and methods. Later in this

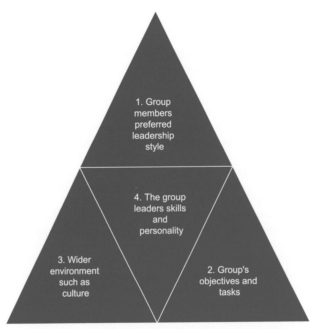

Fig. 13.1 Factors influencing group leadership style.

chapter, group leadership, and the skills you need to be effective as a group leader are discussed.

WHEN TO USE GROUP WORK

Whilst health promoters and public health practitioners may be unsure about when it is appropriate to use a group work approach to promote health, there is a growing evidence base that these types of intervention work (see, for example, research into self-management groups for diabetes and how best to target patients for the appropriate level of support Zupa, 2022).

Group work is appropriate when your plans fulfil the following criteria (see also Chapter 5, a section on deciding the best way of achieving your aims):

- You have looked critically at what other health promotion opportunities exist, and that group work is required to fill a gap.
- You have strong evidence that group work is effective for this particular client group.
- You are going to be working with a defined group of people over a period of time, which will allow the group to build up trust and be able to help each other. This might be particularly true for people with a condition that might be vulnerable to being judged for their lifestyle practices, for example blood-borne viruses such as HIV-positive or hepatitis C.
- You have access to a comfortable, private, and relaxed environment in which to run the group and which is acceptable to members, for example, a community centre. As an alternative, a virtual group could be established, providing members have the means to access this.
- You have access to support and supervision to provide you with assistance when you need it and help you develop your group work. Undertaking this alone may be too demanding and may be unsustainable, so having support is important. It is important you are proactive in seeking help and being responsible for working within your level of competence.

Even if your plans fulfil the above criteria, it is important to consider the specific context. For example, group work may be particularly helpful in some circumstances. This might include plans to work with people who are already in a close small group and possibly already used to group work, for example, a group of young people who are in a residential drug rehabilitation setting.

You will also require skills in establishing a connection with people who have a common interest and wish to develop an equal and respectful partnership with them.

This might include a group of people who have experienced domestic violence and recently moved into a group home.

You should also consider your ability to engage with the group. For example, if you want to work with a particular ethnic minority community but you do not come from that community, then you will be faced with issues of differences in culture and language. In this case, it could be helpful to run a group to look at health issues in partnership with a link worker or health advocate who can offer culturally sensitive help and skills in translation and interpretation. For example, if you wanted to work with refugees, then understanding their culture will be essential, and this will require preparation and training.

There are also times when it may not be advisable to embark on group work or to continue to run an existing group. These may include situations when you have not consulted with prospective clients to establish their needs (see Box 13.1).

BOX 13.1 Reasons When Group Work Is Not Advisable

- Members are from such a diverse range of backgrounds that they have little in common, making for a confused agenda where people feel uncomfortable.
- The cultural or psychosocial background of the group members will make it difficult for them to adapt to a group setting and thus prevent cohesive work.
- The group will meet just on a one-off basis or perhaps twice, which means that people will not have long enough to get to know and trust one another.
- The membership of a group is not stable, and people are constantly leaving or joining, which then disrupts the dynamic of the group.
- Your aim is solely to transmit information, so a one-off talk with questions and answers would be a better use of time than calling a group together.
- The purpose of the group is to encourage a change towards a healthier lifestyle, but the people are unable to make changes, e.g. lack of money, skills, and support.
- You do not have suitable accommodation for meetings, e.g. you only have available a large, tiered lecture theatre seating 100, but the group membership is six.
- You do not yet have the competencies to facilitate group work or access to the necessary training and support, so are, therefore, ill-equipped for the task.

GROUP LEADERSHIP

Two aspects of group leadership are useful to consider. One is your leadership style, and the other is your responsibility as a group leader.

Leadership Style

It is important that all group members are agreed upon who the leader is and then support the leader in this role. The leadership style needs to be compatible with the group members, especially if the group has to work together to complete complex tasks. For example, a group of highly motivated and trained professionals will work best with a leader who encourages participation and shared decision making. It is essential for leaders to be aware of which style members prefer and to develop the ability to adjust their style if the situation demands it. A key dimension of leadership style is where the leader stands on a continuum from authoritarian to participative, as shown in Fig. 13.2.

An **authoritarian style** is directive and requires the group leader to provide the expertise. If you adopt this approach, you rely heavily upon your status, credibility, and expertise to ensure acceptance of your views and leadership role. It would be unwise to adopt such as style without either the qualifications or experience to do so. To be authoritarian without such qualities risks reputational damage. The strength of this style is that members may feel secure, reassured, and protected from harm, especially if they are vulnerable. The weaknesses of this style

are that clients may become fearful, anxious, and reluctant to take independent action or to contribute to group discussions. Furthermore, it does not develop their ability to take responsibility for their own decisions and actions. In addition, clients may respond by challenging your position, leading to rebellion and a rejection of your guidance.

A **participative style** involves shifting power from the group leader so that it is shared between the leader and the group members. This means using all the skills and knowledge of the group members, as well as the leader, who is more likely to choose the title of facilitator. As a facilitator, you will need good interpersonal skills and be able to show warmth and empathy, encourage group members to express their feelings and provide support and encouragement. You will need to be tolerant of different viewpoints, showing objectivity, fairness, and impartiality. You will need skills and the ability to confront difficult issues and resolve conflict using a problem solving approach (see Chapter 9, a section on understanding conflict).

The strength of this style is that clients learn to trust their own judgements and, at the same time, appreciate other people's rights and opinions. This can foster an inclusive approach and bring advantages of shared decision making, thus leading to creative solutions and lateral thinking. The weaknesses of this style may be that strong feelings are uncovered and distress experienced by the client and yourself, which might be difficult to manage. Also, clients who are used to being told what to do may feel confused and dissatisfied because they are not receiving advice and direction. They will need

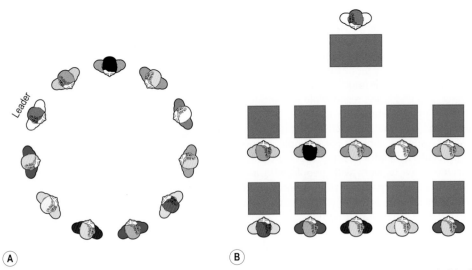

Fig. 13.2 (A) Seating in a circle – best for group work; (B) traditional seating in rows – unsuitable for group work.

to have the approach explained to them to reduce any frustration and be given suitable learning experiences to show them that it works.

Group leaders can operate somewhere between the two extremes (Busse and Regenberg, 2019), providing some authoritative leadership whilst also encouraging a degree of participation. Successful group leadership depends on a variety of factors, such as the leader's preferred style of operating and their personality. For example, if you have been used to being perceived as the expert with the authority of professional knowledge that you want to pass on, you will probably feel and look uncomfortable if you try to switch to a facilitator style without sufficient training. This may produce tension in the group and undermine the effectiveness of how it is working. Inauthenticity is, therefore, unlikely to be beneficial, and the prestigious Harvard Business School has cited that being authentic in your leadership style is associated with several benefits. These include better relationships with colleagues, higher levels of trust, greater productivity and a more positive working environment (Gavin, 2019).

Other factors should also be considered in determining the group leadership style. These are summarised in Fig. 13.1, with a more detailed exploration below.

1. The group members' preferred style of leadership in the specific circumstances of the group is a key factor. For example, if group members are low in confidence, they may need you to be more authoritarian to start with so that they feel secure. You can then gradually encourage participation and adopt a more facilitative style as members learn to trust you and each other to feel confident enough to join in.

2. The group's objectives and tasks will be highly context specific. For example, a group that has the objective of learning new skills, such as an exercise group, might require a more authoritarian leader who will tell them how to do the exercises properly. By contrast, a group of parents in a bereavement support group that aims to help them recover from the death of a child will need a facilitator to help members to express and work through their grief. The more participative style may also lead to members providing mutual support to each other.

3. The wider environment, such as the culture of the group members and of the organisations they belong to, is also important. For example, the cultural norm of some groups may be passive and see themselves as recipients of information. They may not only lack confidence about active participation in groups but may also perceive it as inappropriate and disrespectful to the facilitator. There could also be barriers to language and communication, so having appropriate translation services in place would be essential.

4. The group leaders preferred style, leadership skills, professional experience and personality.

You need to consider these factors and how they might be modified so that the group achieves its purpose. The easiest thing to modify in the short term should be your own style, but in the long term, it may also be possible to make other changes; for example, develop the group members' confidence, so they are willing to take on more responsibility and increase participation. The participative style fits best with the self-empowering client-centred approach to promoting health. However, some health promoters and public health practitioners will have been trained in an authoritarian style and will have modelled themselves on this experience. If this is true in your case, you will need to learn how to work in a participative style to become more effective in empowering your clients.

Finally, a participative style must be distinguished from a permissive style. A permissive style lets clients come to their own conclusions and aims to avoid conflict and keep everyone happy. Helping the clients to enjoy the experience is more important to the leader than achieving the goals of the group. Difficulties and conflicts are not confronted, and the clients may feel neither nurtured nor secure. This is unlikely to produce beneficial outcomes, and whilst giving group attendees options is valuable, there still needs to be some framework rather than simply a vague permissive style that is open-ended and unclear.

Leadership Responsibilities

The responsibilities of group leaders will depend on the role they take, for example whether they may be responsible for the practical organisation such as booking a venue. Whatever the role, however, a leader's responsibilities may also include the following:

- Helping members identify and clarify their interests and needs, including what they want to gain from the group in the short, medium and long term.
- Helping develop a relaxed atmosphere in which group members feel able to be open and trusting with each other as well as able to participate freely.
- Offering expertise to the group on the understanding that members are free to choose whether to accept or reject the offer that the leader is making.
- Accepting and valuing all contributions from group members providing some general principles are observed, such as respecting the view of others.

Group members also have responsibilities too. They may include:

- Participating in clarifying the aims of the group.

- Choosing whether and how much to participate.
- Identifying personal health goals and concerns.
- Deciding on challenges and risks they want to take.

The last point is related to setting appropriate boundaries and ensuring what is discussed within the group remains confidential. For example, how much are they prepared to expose their own weaknesses and vulnerability to other people in the group? This needs careful judgement and to strike a balance of sharing between what is relevant to progress the group and what is inappropriate over disclosure.

GROUP BEHAVIOUR

Health promoters and public health practitioners will be able to work with a group more effectively if they are aware of the group dynamics and the ways in which people are likely to behave when they come together in groups. There are three aspects of group behaviour that you may find particularly useful:

- The pattern of behaviour that usually develops in a group's life.
- The different roles group members may perform.
- The concept of hidden agendas.

Group Development

Groups tend to show a particular pattern of behaviour as they mature and develop. A seminal work characterised small group developmental process into four stages (Tuckman, 1965; 1977):

1. **Forming**. The group is forming. People meet each other and get to know one another, with individuals establishing their own identity and role within the group. The group's purpose and way of working are established.
2. **Storming**. Most groups go through a conflict stage when the leadership and ways in which the group is working are challenged. For example, people may question how things are being done and what the leader's role is and may get into heated discussions with each other. This can be a difficult period for both leader and members, but it is a vital stage in the group's maturing process, rather like the period of rebelling and questioning during adolescence. Successful handling of this period leads to the development of open communication, trust and shared responsibility for achieving the purposes of the group (see Chapter 9, section on understanding conflict).
3. **Norming**. At this stage, the group settles down with the norms and accepted practices of the group established.

4. **Performing**. The group is fully effective at this stage and can concentrate on its tasks (see Chapter 9 for further application of the Tuckman stages).

When the developmental process fails in some way, attempts to sabotage the group may occur. It is thus worth investing time and effort to help new groups develop successfully, such as having regular review discussions to ensure that the members are satisfied with the way the work is evolving. If this is not the case, it is important to discuss solutions and contingency plans.

Many groups have a limited life and only meet for a set number of sessions or until a particular task or aim has been achieved. At the end of a group's life, it may be helpful to have a final session, which could give group members an opportunity to express their appreciation and perhaps arrange a follow-up or reunion.

Group Members' Roles

A seminal study established the characteristics of team members, identifying that a mix of nine roles is needed for full effectiveness (Belbin, 1981). These roles may also be relevant to a group's effectiveness and are outlined in Box 13.2.

At different times, each group member may play a variety of these roles although generally, most people have personal characteristics which might result in more affinity with a particular role. If one or more of these

---

> **BOX 13.2   Roles for Working in Groups**
>
> - **The Coordinator** – clarifies goals, promotes decision making and delegates, which enables the group to work effectively.
> - **The Shaper** – is action oriented and encourages the group to get on with its tasks.
> - **The Plant** – is the creative source of ideas and proposals.
> - **The Monitor/Evaluator** – is good at analysing and criticising.
> - **The Resource Investigator** – has a good network of contacts and liaises with other people and agencies.
> - **The Company Worker** – is good at organising and administration.
> - **The Team Worker** – supports the members of the group and is a good listener.
> - **The Specialist** – provides specialist knowledge and skills.
> - **The Finisher** – contributes foresight and perseverance to ensure that the group completes its tasks.

roles is lacking, the facilitator can help to make a group more successful by consciously adopting a different role or encouraging other group members to adjust their roles.

Hidden Agendas

People will have their own individual reasons for joining a group, which may be in addition to, or instead of, the stated purpose of the group. For example, a person may attend a health group focusing on lifestyle change because they are lonely and see the group as a way of meeting people. They may not be motivated to change their lifestyle by increasing exercise or improving their diet and have only really joined as a way of alleviating their loneliness. Or a group member may seek a prominent position in a group, such as being the chair or secretary, to fulfil their need to feel valued and useful. In these examples, fulfilling these personal objectives are hidden agendas. Members will work together more effectively when there is communication about individual objectives or agendas and agreement about shared objectives. You will be more effective as a group leader if you are aware of the hidden agendas in the group and can find ways of dealing with them. There is no prescriptive way of doing this and simply being observant of the attendees. One possible theoretical framework to explore this is the Johari Window Model, which can be used to help group members better understand their relationships both with themselves and with others. As such, it's a useful technique for improving an individual's self-awareness and development in group situations. It also aids two-way communication within the group (Hampson, 2021).

SETTING UP A GROUP

Planning and preparation are essential for successful group work. The following sections take you step-by-step through the thinking and planning you need to do when setting up a group.

Why Are You Proposing to Run The Group?

- Are you reacting to a demand from clients, other professionals, a community or your own observations? How can you evidence this?
- Are you trying to develop your health promotion role and see this group as a way of progressing? What is your motive for doing this?
- Are you aiming to provide advice and support, to supply information or to help people to change health-related behaviour? Which and why?

- Are you aiming to satisfy your own needs or your client's needs? If your reasons are both, try to distinguish the respective factors.

Who Will the Members Be?

- How will members be identified? Will they be referred, for example, from their GP? Will they be encouraged to join, or will membership be entirely voluntary via self-referral?
- Have you given everyone an equal opportunity to join? This includes consideration of facilities for wheelchairs, disabled toilets, signing for those hard of hearing, hearing loops, and translation into other languages if needed. Have you made provision for people to let you know of any special needs? How can you make reasonable adjustments?
- How will you identify the potential members of your group? This could include from individuals requesting a group, from local or national registers or from people with shared characteristics. The latter includes age, sex, lifestyle, culture, job and health concerns. Or by other means?
- How will you recruit your members? Do you need to advertise? If so, how?
- How many members will you recruit? What is the ideal number, bearing in mind the purpose of the group and any constraints imposed by your location and resources available?

What Are The Group's Aims and Objectives?

- Are these within the realistic abilities of yourself and the members?
- Can all the potential membership understand them?
- Are you clear about your own objectives in setting up the group and whether these are different from the members' objectives?
- Are all members clear about their individual objectives? Have members defined the specific outcomes they hope to achieve through attending the group?

Where Will the Group Meet?

- Is the location appropriate? For example, a health centre or hospital could appear clinical and cold and remind people of illness. Neutral territory, such as a room in a community centre, may be more relaxing and inviting.
- How will you arrange the seating? If you are aiming for participative group work, seating people in a circle is best (see Fig. 13.2), with physical barriers to communication, such as tables or desks, removed.

- Are the facilities adequate for the purpose? Is there enough space for the activities you plan? Is the floor covering suitable for the purpose? Is the temperature suitable and adjustable if necessary? Are the facilities adequate for the purpose? This includes access to pushchairs, toilets, catering facilities, washing/shower rooms and crèche. Are there facilities for people with special needs, for example, wide access for wheelchairs, disabled toilets, hearing loops and language translation?
- Is access good? Is the venue accessible by local transport? Do you have transport for members who cannot manage on public transport? Can members car share? Are parking arrangements satisfactory?
- What are the security arrangements? Is the area safe? Where are the fire extinguishers, and what is the fire drill? In case of an emergency, who do you contact? Do you need insurance coverage?
- Is the location signposted, or does it have a sign on the door? For example, new mothers' group: Room 10 second floor 3-4 pm.

What Resources Do You Need?

- Do you need any special equipment, for example, audio-visual media equipment? Are you familiar with the equipment and confident you can operate it? Does the equipment have to be booked in advance? If so, are you familiar with the booking system?
- Do you need any additional resources or facilities such as Wi-Fi, leaflets, posters, books or outside speakers? If so, have you made all the necessary arrangements in advance?
- Do you need to pay for anything? If so, have you identified a source of funding? This could include a charge to the group members or a sponsor.
- Do you provide refreshments? Or ask members to provide their own? Or make a small donation to cover the cost?

When Will the Group Meet?

- Is the time you have chosen the best one for the clients, or have you chosen it to suit yourself? To encourage maximum attendance, the former is likely to be more important than the latter to have good attendance.
- Does the length of meetings suit members and consider their other commitments?
- Have you consulted potential members about timing and tried to satisfy the majority?

- Are there particular days of the week that work best for members?

How Will the Group Be Run?

- Will it be a self-help group and directed by the members or led by a public health professional?
- To what extent will the structure be flexible and the content negotiable?
- Will the group be open, meaning that anyone can join at any time, or will there be restrictions on admitting new members once the group has started?
- Will there be roles adopted by the members? For example, a nominated person who will ensure the location is open on time and another person who ensures refreshments are available.

How Will the Group Be Evaluated?

- Will this take place at the end of each meeting? Or at the end of the group? Or both? (see also Chapter 12, a section on evaluation, feedback and assessment).
- How will this be achieved? Verbally, in writing or both? How will you ask questions to obtain accurate feedback from members? One way to do this is to provide opportunities for anonymous feedback.
- How will you know that the group, individual and your own objectives have been achieved?
- Were there any unplanned outcomes of the group? Were these desirable or undesirable? What caused them?
- What have you learned? What would you do differently next time?

See Erford (2018) for more details on group work in general and for counselling specifically, and Freeman et al. (2020) for an evaluation of health promotion group work in primary health care setting.

GETTING GROUPS GOING

Some people may feel nervous about going to a group meeting for the first time, especially if they are unlikely to know other members. The initial task of the group leader is to help people to feel at ease.

Before the First Meeting

If you know in advance who is coming to a group meeting, it may be helpful and welcoming to confirm by email. A group's email list would be the most time efficient, and this can be sent to all members anonymously without revealing their contact details to each other, which can be done later if members agree.

Other methods include:

- Facebook post or messenger alert.
- Letter or telephone text that you are expecting them with the time and place.

If anyone has let you know they have special needs, contact them in advance to discuss their needs and let them know what facilities will be available. There may be a need to provide something additional; for example, if a visually impaired person attends with their assistance dog, then more space may be needed for this member.

On Arrival

It helps if clients can be greeted personally, introduced to other group members or given something to do: 'Whilst we wait for others to arrive, help yourself to refreshments on the table. There is also a welcome pack of information to read'. Ensure that anyone with special needs has appropriate facilities and assistance.

Getting to Know Each Other

Getting to know each person's name and something about them is the first step towards constructive group work because it helps them feel valued as a member of the group and is the beginning of openness and trust between members. There are many ways of going about this, some of which are as follows:

Introduction in Pairs

Ask each person to sit next to someone they have not met before. One person in each pair then interviews their partner. After a few minutes, the leader asks the partners to swap roles. Then, in turn, each member of the group introduces their partner by name and says something about them. You may like to remind people that no one has to answer any questions if they do not wish to.

The leader could also suggest appropriate questions. For example, in groups for prospective parents, the leader could suggest that partners find out if this is the first baby, where the mother goes for antenatal check-ups or where she is booked to have her baby. This can then be fed back to the whole group by way of wider introductions, for example 'I'd like to introduce Fiona, who is due to have her second baby in four months' time. Fiona enjoys meeting other prospective parents, and for any expecting their first baby, she is willing to share her experience'.

Name Games

Group members sit in a circle, and you, the leader, take an object, such as a pen, and hand it to the person on your left, saying, 'My name is A, and this is a pen'. You ask the person who now holds the pen to say, 'My name is B, and A says that this is a pen'. B then passes the pen to the person on his left, who says, 'My name is C, and B says that A says that this is a pen'. This continues until the pen gets back to the beginning. This may work best in relatively small groups, and if members forget someone's name, the rest of the group can prompt them.

Another way to do this is for the leader to make the first introduction and then ask for the person to their right to re-introduce them and then themselves. For example:

LEADER: 'Good evening. My name is Brian Jones, and I'm going to facilitate the discussion tonight. Can I move to my right and ask you to introduce yourself and then re-introduce the previous person'.

Person A: 'Good evening, my name is Peter Williams, and this is my first meeting. To my left is Brian Jones, who will facilitate the meeting'.

Person B: 'Hello everyone. My name is Alison Smith, and I have been a member of this group for six months. To my left is Peter Williams, who is new to the group'.

This helps to build a cooperative and supportive atmosphere and helps people learn each other's names. Any tensions and embarrassments are relieved by laughing, and tension is effectively broken. At subsequent group meetings, it is often helpful to do a quick round of names at the beginning, for example, 'Who would like to have a shot at naming every member of the group?' or 'I'm going to try to see if I can remember everyone's name'.

You might like to set the tone by suggesting how people are addressed, by first names or more formally. The important thing is to encourage people to use whatever feels comfortable: 'My name is Annabelle Smith, but everyone calls me Anna'.

Sharing Initial Feelings and Expectations

People may be helped to relax if they know that others also feel nervous or shy. So you could ask questions as below.

'What did you feel about coming here today? Did anyone feel nervous? Did anyone almost not come?'

Or possibly make some opening remarks, for example: 'Thank you all for coming today. Some people may be nervous, and others may almost not have come. That is all perfectly understandable, and please be assured this will be a supportive group. Sometimes the hardest step to take is the first one, and everyone is welcome.'

This can open the way for people to express their anxieties, especially if the group is there to help people who may have experienced judgement in the past, for example, individuals who drink excessive amounts of alcohol. You can also encourage them to say why they have come to the meeting and what they expect to gain from it. It might help to ask members to complete a checklist, ticking statements that are true for them about their concerns or why they came.

Such statements might include the following:

- I'm worried I won't have anything to say.
- I'm afraid I'll talk too much.
- I'm worried I'll make a fool of myself.
- I'll be too embarrassed to join in.
- I'm afraid I might get upset.
- I'm concerned I may be bored.
- I want to meet other people in the same situation.
- I enjoy talking to others.
- I enjoy a good debate.
- I want to get out of the house.
- I want to go somewhere different.
- I enjoy listening to other people.

People can then compare their list with that of one or two other people, and then it may be helpful to share what has been discovered with the whole group without attributing comments to any specific individual.

Setting Ground Rules

People joining a group will have different expectations and assumptions about how the group will run, especially if they have never attended a group before. Problems can arise if these are not brought out in the open and clarified at the beginning. For example, people may assume that what they say in a group will be treated confidentially and then be upset if they find that another member did not realise this and had discussed the issue elsewhere. Whilst confidentiality may be a reasonable expectation, this will need to be made explicit rather than assumed.

Or some members might expect the group leader to take all the responsibility for organising the group and may feel let down if they later discover that the leader expects them to do some of the work. Again, this could represent a breakdown of communication and being clear about this from the outset will help prevent such disappointment from occurring.

To prevent these difficulties, it is often helpful to establish a set of ground rules. Early in the group's life,

members need the opportunity to explore their expectations and reach an agreement about issues such as the following:

- How members are expected to behave in the group.
- Are any rules and sanctions to be set, for example, about nonattendance at group meetings or whether members can join in if they arrive late?
- What is confidential to the group?
- Can new members join at any time, or is the group closed to new membership?
- How will the leader and the members exercise control in the group?
- Who has responsibility for the practical aspects of running the group, such as bringing refreshments along or booking the room?

For example, in a self-help group, mutual rights and responsibilities will be agreed upon based on the equality of leader and clients, although in reality, the power balance may not be completely equal, and a contract could help with power sharing. In a counselling group, the power of the counsellor can be much greater than that of the clients. This brings a duty to the leader to respect the members and to promote their autonomy. There might be a need for group ground rules to be prepared (see Reid, 2020, for ideas on setting ground rules).

DISCUSSION SKILLS

A discussion may not happen just by putting a group of people together and saying, 'Let's discuss …' Discussion needs planning and preparation, and there are many ways of triggering it and providing structures that will help everyone to participate. The diagram in Fig. 13.6 below offers a useful summary.

Trigger Materials

Discussion can be triggered by providing a focus, possibly a controversial one. This can simply be a question 'What do you think about increasing the price of alcohol as a way to deter excess drinking?' It might also be a leaflet, a poster, a health promotion campaign film or an item in a newspaper or magazine:

'What do you think the organisers of this virtual exercise class are trying to convey in this advertisement?'

Choose something that people can engage with, and that is likely to stimulate discussion.

Some health promotion campaign films are specially made as trigger materials, presenting situations for people to discuss. Helpful notes for group leaders often accompany such campaign films.

Brainstorms/Think Sessions

Brainstorming is a useful way to open a topic and collect everyone's ideas. Ask an open question to which there is no single right answer, such as: 'Why do some young people misuse illicit drugs?' or, 'what do you feel you need to know before you decide on whether to stop smoking?'

Accept every suggestion without comment or criticism and write them down in a list on a flipchart or blackboard. Ask the group not to start discussing the ideas until everybody has finished. You can also make your own suggestions and write them down along with others.

In this way, all members' contributions are equally valued, and everyone has a chance to participate. Encourage shy members by asking, 'Would anyone like to add anything further?' and allowing silent pauses whilst people think. An additional strategy is to ask for contributions on post-it notes, covered later in the chapter.

Then you can set the group to work by asking them to put the ideas into categories and to identify the key features of each category. For example, people might categorise reasons for taking illicit drugs into a reinforcing category: 'It helps me to socialise' or 'It helps me to relax, to feel good', and an escape category: 'I can forget my problems' or 'It stops me from feeling stressed'.

Rounds

A round is a way of giving everyone an equal chance to participate. You invite each group member in turn around the circle to make a brief statement. You might like to start the round yourself or join in when your turn comes in the circle. For example, ask everyone to make a brief statement about one of the following:

'My first feelings when I knew I had to reduce my alcohol intake was …'

'What I think about COVID-19 vaccination is …'

'The main reason why I struggle to sustain my weight loss is…'

'The one thing that has made the most difference in my efforts to give up smoking is …'

There are four essential rules for successful rounds, which must be explained and gently enforced if necessary.

Firstly, there are no interruptions until each person has finished their statement.

Secondly, no comments on anybody's contribution until the full round is completed. This means no discussions or interpretation, not even 'I think that too' or 'I agree with that' remarks.

Thirdly, anyone can choose not to participate. Give permission, clearly and emphatically, that anyone who does

not want to make a statement can just say, 'pass'. This is very important for reinforcing the principle of voluntary participation.

Fourthly, it does not matter if two or more people in the round say the same thing. People should say what they had intended, even if someone else has said it already.

Rounds are also useful ways of beginning and ending sessions. For example:

'One thing I've started doing since last week is …'

'The main learning I've taken from today's session is …'

'One thing I'm going to try to find out by the next time we meet is …'

It is also a useful way of getting feedback. For example:

'One thing I really enjoyed during the session today was …'

'One thing that I didn't understand about today's session was …'

'One thing I wish that we could have covered is …'

Buzz Groups

Buzz groups are small groups of two to six people who discuss questions or topics for short periods, usually about 10 min. It is especially useful for large groups to be divided up in this way as it gives everyone more chance to talk. Form the groups first, then say what you would like each one to do, such as 'Make a list of the times when you want a drink of alcohol' or 'Talk about the things you find helpful when you feel anxious', and how long they have in which to do it. If you want people to share ideas with the rest of the group afterwards, it may be helpful to provide large sheets of paper and felt-tip pens so that feedback posters can be put up for everyone to see and discuss.

Safe Revelations

Sometimes people may hesitate or refuse to say what they really feel for fear of looking silly, being embarrassed or getting upset. One way of overcoming this is to give everyone a piece of paper and ask them to write down, for example, what their biggest worries are or what they really want to know. All the papers are then folded and put in a receptacle, such as a waste-paper basket or a basket. Each person, in turn, picks out one piece of paper and reads aloud what is written on it. Remind people not to reveal if they pick out their own piece of paper, and also that nobody needs to identify themselves as the author of any of the statements. The aim is to find out the concerns of the group members in the security of anonymity. Make sure that everyone listens and does not comment until all the papers have been read out. Then you can discuss what was discovered.

Post-It Notes

Often during a discussion, ideas may arise. An effective way to capture this is by writing them down – post-it notes are useful for this task. They offer a way to write down an idea and then assemble them into a structured format that can reveal themes or areas requiring further exploration. Post-it notes offer non-intrusive support to a discussion that can occur whilst others are speaking, thus avoiding the need for interruption. This can also be a useful way to ensure less confident speakers have opportunities to fully contribute.

DEALING WITH DIFFICULTIES

Acknowledge the potential difficulties of running a group and work out strategies in advance for coping should the problem arise. Ask yourself: 'What could go wrong here?' Some common problems and possible strategies for coping are as follows:

Silence

Silence can be useful as it can offer an opportunity for group members to think. Silence often does not feel as threatening to group members as it may do to the facilitator. However, you may find it helpful to run a group with a partner so that you can help each other out if either of you experience the group not contributing to the discussion. It is also important to ensure thorough preparation when you have planned activities and questions. Write down a plan and a list of questions to ask, with an additional activity ready to use if the reason for the discussion closing down is that what you have planned does not work.

Unexpected Events

Unexpected events include such things as late arrivals or finding that too few or too many people have turned up. There is no blueprint strategy to cope with the unexpected, but it will help if you acknowledge what has happened and share it with your group:

'I'm delighted that so many of you have come along, but I wasn't expecting such numbers, so we may be a bit crowded this week'.

Also share your plans for dealing with the unexpected event, such as 'I'm going to try to get a bigger room next time' or 'I'm going to start 10 minutes late'. Sharing the problem and enlisting cooperation can have the positive benefit of encouraging mutual support, whilst not sharing it openly can leave your group feeling angry or confused.

Distractions

Distractions can take many forms. This includes:
- Noises outside the room, such as road works.
- Noises inside the room, such as crying babies or coughing.
- People coming in late or leaving early or other interruptions.

Distractions can also be caused by group members themselves, for example, by someone becoming very angry or upset. Generally, there are three choices for you as group leader:
- **Ignore them**. This is seldom a good idea as it leaves people wondering whether you are going to do anything, which is in itself is a distraction. It may also undermine the confidence that members have in your leadership.
- **Acknowledge and accept them**. This is generally best with things you cannot change: 'I know the traffic is really noisy, but there's nothing we can do about it at present. So I think that just for today, we'll try to make the best of it, and I will find a different location for future meetings. I'll confirm this by email prior to our next meeting'.
- **Do something about them**. It is preferable to involve the group in the decision: 'As so many of you found it difficult to get here by 2 o'clock, shall we start at 2:15 next week?'

If someone is showing emotion, such as crying, acknowledge it: 'I can see that you're upset' and offer reassurance that it is OK to show emotion: 'There's no need to be embarrassed … we do not mind if you cry …' Offer the opportunity to talk about it: 'Would you like to tell us what is upsetting you?' or to take some time away from the group, accompanied by you or someone else: 'Shall we go outside for a few minutes?'

Do not put any pressure on people in distress. Help them to do what they want to do, whether it is cry, talk, keep silent, stay, leave or be by themselves. But do not ignore a show of emotion, as ignoring it will only cause tension and embarrassment for the person and other members.

Difficult Behaviour

How group members behave can pose difficulties for the public health leader. There are two broad categories of difficult behaviour: nonparticipation and talking too much. The latter category takes many forms, such as a person who dominates and always responds with the answers and prevents other people from contributing. Sometimes people can launch into long stories, whilst others may interrupt or talk off the point. There are also people who always disagree and others who always make jokes, which can sometimes be inappropriate. It is important to note that people often change their behaviour as they get to know others and feel more comfortable in a group. Below are some points about dealing with people who talk too much and about encouraging quiet members to engage.

- Think about why dominant people are behaving like this. Are they nervous, threatened or worried? Are they desperately in need of attention? Or under the influence of alcohol? If you can deal with the underlying cause and introduce solutions, the situation is likely to improve.
- Give people the opportunity to work in pairs or small groups, which can help quiet members join in and give others a break from the constant talker.
- Use structures in your discussion such as rounds or make a point of asking for other people's opinions: 'I'm conscious that some other people have not yet had the opportunity to contribute, so it would be good to hear from them' or 'Would someone else like to offer their thoughts?'
- Finally, it may be necessary to confront a person who talks too much but not in front of the rest of the group. For example, you could say: 'I'm delighted that you feel confident to contribute a lot, although could I ask you to be mindful of other members and perhaps keep your comments to just a couple of sentences so others can speak? Would you feel OK about doing that?'

Exercise 13.1 offers you the opportunity to apply all the previous points when planning a group meeting. Read the overview of a group intervention in Box 13.3 before starting the exercise.

VIRTUAL GROUPS

Social media, including Facebook, have become an integral part of many people's lives and offer a way that virtual groups can be formed to exchange public health-related information and support. Research has shown that some public health Facebook groups that are used for support exchanges between group members contained a) highly specialised health-related information, including information about health services use, symptom recognition, compliance, medication use, treatment protocols and medical procedures and b) tailored emotional support through comparison, empathy and encouragement. For information on the use of virtual groups to help improve cancer outcomes, both prevention and treatment, see Prochaska et al. (2017), and for details of the effectiveness

---

> **EXERCISE 13.1 Planning a Group Meeting**
>
> 1. Identify a public health issue that you have encountered or are likely to encounter where informal group work would be appropriate. For example, this could be a group of people with alcohol problems, armed forces veterans with mental health problems, an antenatal group for teenagers, a group of hospital patients recovering from a stroke, a stop smoking group or a group for weight control with both exercise and healthy eating. Assume that your group consists of about 12 people who do not know each other and that this is the first of several meetings.
>   - What do you think would be the best place and time to meet, and what are the best physical features of the meeting room?
>   - What are your aims for the first meeting?
>   - What are your objectives for your group members for the first meeting?
>   - Complete the following:
>   - At the end of the first meeting, each group member will:
>   1. ....
>   2. ....
>   3. ....
>   etc. ....
> 2. Make a plan for what you will do:
>   - As people start to arrive.
>   - To get people to become acquainted with each other.
>   - In the main part of the group meeting.
>   - To round off the meeting at the end.
>   - To evaluate whether you have achieved the objectives you set.

---

of Facebook groups to boost participation in a parenting intervention aimed at reducing adolescent substance use, see Epstein et al. (2019).

Setting Up a Social Media Group

When setting up and using a Facebook (or other social media) group, you will be the group administrator or moderator. It is important to abide by the communications protocol of your organisation. See for an example of this the Merton Council Social Media Protocol (2022) on their website referenced at the end of this chapter. It is also important to establish a set of guidelines for group conduct. See Box 13.4 for an illustration of social media guidelines.

BOX 13.3   Weight Management Group Interventions for Adults Who Are Overweight and Obese

Purpose: To offer group members the opportunity to learn behavioural techniques for losing and maintaining weight loss. The group will share their experiences and provide each other with mutual support. Being part of a group will add competition to weight loss and help to keep people motivated.

Group Membership: Criteria for joining the group will be based on a 30-plus body mass index (BMI) with the aim to engage people to lose at least 5% of their initial body weight.

Method: There will be six interactive, motivational and social/peer support group sessions, followed by long term support at three, six, nine and 12 months. At the start of the programme, group participants will be assessed on motivation, readiness and self-efficacy for weight management change. A different topic will be covered at each of the six sessions. The content will combine advice on beliefs and attitudes around food preferences, healthier eating, energy intake, food labelling, portion size and physical activity. Ten to 15 participants will be recruited for each group, and the sessions will be based on the principles of adult learning, which are designed to encourage group interaction and active learning.

Focus: Group members' personal knowledge and skills in behaviour change will be developed to enable and empower them to make small lifestyle changes to lose weight and embed those into their everyday life. Building people's self-confidence and motivation to change are key. A range of evidence-based approaches is incorporated into sessions, including patient-centred goal setting, problem solving, self-monitoring and other behavioural approaches.

Goal setting will be used in promoting changes in health behaviours, and clients will set personal goals which are crucial to success. Goal setting involves the public health practitioner and group members working together to mutually agree upon goals for dietary and lifestyle change. For many clients, being part of a group will offer social support and increased motivation to remain focused. Group members will be encouraged to discuss previous or ongoing strategies that they use to manage their weight, to plan for situations that might get in the way of change and to share their behaviour change goals with others.

The weight management groups are also designed to support and equip people with the skills they need to maintain their weight loss. This is enabled by providing support to clients beyond 12 weeks, with longer-term follow-up of at least 12 months included in the plan. This ensures that clients who achieve initial weight loss are encouraged to continue to lose weight or maintain a healthy weight. Relapse prevention techniques will be discussed, and clients will be supported to become more self-dependent by promoting self-help opportunities and incorporating peer support activities when appropriate.

Evaluation: Several outcomes are expected from the group-based weight management programmes. The specific aim is for clients to achieve a modest weight loss of 5% to 10% of initial body weight with improved dietary intake, improved physical activity levels, improved mental health and wellbeing and weight maintenance.

Group weight losses will be reported using a range of outcome measures so that the effectiveness of the different services can be compared. The measurements recorded will be height, weight, waist circumference and BMI.

BOX 13.4   Adjusted From NHS England (2022)

Please note these guidelines are for Twitter use but are equally applicable to Facebook.

Example of Guidelines for Facebook and Twitter Groups

Do
- Stay on-topic. Do not post messages that are not related.
- Be reasonably concise and not constitute spamming of the site.
- Post in English – unfortunately, we do not currently have the resource to moderate comments in other languages.
- Respect other people. Comments should not be malicious or offensive in nature.

Do not
- Incite hatred based on race, religion, gender, nationality, sexuality or any other personal characteristic.

BOX 13.4 Adjusted From NHS England (2022)—Cont'd	
• Reveal personal details, such as private addresses, phone numbers, email addresses or other online contact details. • Impersonate or falsely claim to represent a person or organisation. • Be party political.	• Include swearing, hate speech or obscenity. • Break the law – this includes libel, condoning illegal activity, and breaking copyright. • Advertise commercial products and services – you can mention relevant products and services if they support your comment.

There are two important issues to consider when setting up a Facebook page. Firstly, the mission statement should create a sense of belonging. Secondly, you will need to protect the group's privacy. The privacy setting of the Facebook page is crucial. There are three privacy settings: public, closed and secret. A closed or secret group might work best, but this would depend on the aim and mission of the group. See Facebook Help pages under the web references at the end of this chapter for more information on setting up a group. A set of guidelines, as in Box 13.4 will enable the efficient administration of the virtual group.

PRACTICE POINTS

- In health promotion and public health, groups in a number of forms, including social media, are useful for raising awareness of health issues, mutual support, social action, education and group counselling.
- Group work covers a wide range of activities and has a number of potential benefits for individual group members.
- Group work is not always the most appropriate health promotion or public health practice method to use; you need to be sure that it is right for your particular clients and public health issue.
- You need to develop skills of group leadership and facilitation, appreciate the range of leadership styles and understand the roles and responsibilities of both leaders and members and the way in which groups develop over time.
- Thorough planning and preparation are essential for successful group work, which includes having a clear rationale and aims and paying attention to recruitment, venue, facilities, resources, timing and evaluation.
- If you facilitate groups, you will find it helpful to develop a range of competencies and strategies for getting groups established, encouraging discussion and dealing with difficulties.

References

Belbin, R. M. (1981). *Management teams*. London: Heinemann.

Busse, R., & Regenberg, S. (2019). Revisiting the "authoritarian versus participative" leadership style legacy: a new model of the impact of leadership inclusiveness on employee engagement. *Journal of Leadership and Organizational Studies*, 26(4), 510–525. https://doi.org/10.1177/1548051818810135.

Epstein, M., Oesterle, S., & Haggerty, K. P. (2019). Effectiveness of Facebook groups to boost participation in a parenting intervention. *Prevention Science*, 20(6), 894–903. https://doi.org/10.1007/s11121-019-01018-0.

Erford, B. T. (2018). *Group work: processes and applications* (2nd edition). Oxford: Routledge.

Freeman, T., Baum, F., Javanparast, S., Labonté, R., Lawless, A., & Barton, E. (2020). The contribution of group work to the goals of comprehensive primary health care. *Health Promotion Journal of Australia*, 32, 126–136. https://doi.org/10.1002/hpja.323.

Gavin, M. (2019). *Authentic leadership: what it is & why it's important*. online.hbs.edu/blog/post/authentic-leadership

Hampson, S. (2021). *The Johari window model: how to improve communication and productivity at work*. https://www.tsw.co.uk/blog/leadership-and-management/the-johari-window/

NHS England. (2022). Social media and comment moderation policy. https://www.england.nhs.uk/comment-policy/.

Nicholls, K. (2019). *Group therapy*. http://www.counselling-directory.org.uk/group-therapy.html

Prochaska, J. J., Coughlin, S. S., & Lyons, E. J. (2017). Social media and mobile technology for cancer prevention and treatment. *American Society of Clinical Oncology Educational Book*, 37, 128–137. https://doi.org/10.1200/EDBK_173841.

Reid, T. (2020). *Writing a ground rules agreement for group work*. https://blogs.bath.ac.uk/academic-and-employability-skills/2020/10/30/writing-a-ground-rules-agreement-for-group-work/

Tuckman, B. W. (1965). Developmental sequence in small groups. *Psychological Bulletin*, 65(6), 384–399. https://doi.org/10.1037/h0022100.

Tuckman, B. W., & Jensen, M. A. (1977). Stages of small-group development revisited. *Group and Organisation Studies*, 2(4), 419–427. https://doi.org/10.1177/105960117700200404.

Zupa, M. F., Krall, J., Collins, K., Marroquin, O., Ng, J. M., & Siminerio, L. (2022). A risk stratification approach to allocating diabetes education and support services. *Diabetes Technology and Therapeutics*, *24*(1), 75–78. https://doi.org/10.1089/dia.2021.0253.

YouTube

How to Create a Facebook Group – Facebook tutorial. https://www.youtube.com/watch?v=8KO3tK8YBJc

Websites

Facebook Help Centre. https://www.facebook.com/help/_220336891328465

Merton Council. (2022). *Social media protocol*. http://www.merton.gov.uk/council-and-local-democracy/plans-and-policies/social-media

Blog

Gavin. (2019). *Authentic leadership*. online.hbs.edu/blog/post/authentic-leadership

Enabling Healthier Living Through Behaviour Change

Angela Scriven

SUMMARY

This chapter considers some of the approaches that are used to support people in making changes to their health-related behaviour. In the first section, there is an exploration and application of two behaviour change models. This is followed by an overview of key factors that can underpin successful change, such as motivation, working towards self-empowerment, increasing self-awareness, clarifying values and changing attitudes. Public health strategies for decision making and changing behaviour are considered as are the principles for using behaviour change approaches effectively and overcoming barriers to change. Consistent with the format of other chapters, exercises, examples and a case study are interspersed throughout the chapter.

Lifestyle factors play a key role in the global burden of non-communicable disease, disability and death, with behaviours such as alcohol misuse, smoking, poor dietary habits and physical inactivity being particularly important (Li et al., 2020). Because of this, enabling healthier living through behaviour change approaches has been a consistent focus in promoting public health.

Individual health behaviour may have developed without conscious decision making and in response to various personal circumstances and external factors. Efforts to actively control or change behaviour involves committing time and effort to understand the factors that influence health choices and the associated behaviours. In exploring what influences behaviour, there is an opportunity to make and take considered decisions and actions that relate to health.

Some people may continue with behaviours that are unhealthy as, to them, the benefits may outweigh the risks. For example, a person who drinks alcohol to excess may put a lot of value on the short term benefits of alcohol and be less concerned with the long term impacts on their health. Furthermore, the socioeconomic circumstances in which a person lives might have resulted in them having limited choices and drinking may be their way of coping.

The Marmot review into health inequalities in England demonstrates that the social determinants of health – the conditions in which people are born, grow, live, work, and age – may lead to certain behaviours, such as dietary choices and substance use, and ultimately to health inequalities, making their ability to change more complex (Marmot et al., 2020). In contrast, if professional perceptions on what influences health focuses on the individual, their behaviours and their negative health choices, and ignores any socioeconomic inhibitors to change, then a behavioural change approach becomes more complex (Kane et al., 2022).

Respect for people's values, opinions and right to choose are fundamental to establishing relationships between practitioners and the individuals or groups they work with. There is a balance between considering a person's autonomy to individual freedom of choice against the effect of that choice on other people. For example, a parent with an unhealthy diet who rarely takes exercise could affect their children's health through role modelling, leading to overweight children (Coto et al., 2019).

Changes such as taking more exercise, eating healthier foods and stopping smoking can require self-discipline and overcoming barriers which make these changes difficult. It is important, therefore, to enable people to look at their motivations, beliefs, values and attitudes relating to health. In doing so, this creates opportunities to make and implement decisions that will lead to improved health and wellbeing.

MODELS OF BEHAVIOUR CHANGE

Health-related behaviour change is a very complex process involving a web of psychological, social and environmental factors. Positive health behaviour change refers to a replacement of health-compromising behaviours, such as sedentary behaviour, with health-enhancing behaviours, such as physical exercise. By contrast, a negative behaviour change implies the reverse, which in the above case would be a physically active person becoming sedentary.

To describe, predict, and explain the behaviour change process, a number of theories or models have been developed. For an example of the use of a behaviour change model in promoting dietary changes in people who have survived cancer, see Sremanakova et al. (2021).

Behaviour change theories and models are tools to help you to clarify your thinking and make your practice more effective. Models are simplified ways of describing reality and provide frameworks and routes to help you know where to start and what to do. The health action process approach (HAPA) and the stages of change model are examples of models that can be used by health promoters and public health practitioners.

The Health Action Process Approach

HAPA is a psychological theory and an open framework of various motivational and volitional constructs that explain and predict individual changes in health behaviours, such as quitting smoking or improving physical activity levels. HAPA suggests that the adoption, initiation and maintenance of health behaviours should be conceived of as a structured process, including a motivation phase and a volition phase. The former describes the intention formation, while the latter refers to planning and action (initiative, maintenance, recovery). The model emphasises the particular role of perceived self-efficacy at different stages of health behaviour change (see Fig. 14.1 and the user page for HAPA in the webpages in the references at the end of this chapter). The following explanation of the model is adapted from the HAPA user page:

The Motivation Phase

In the motivation phase, the individual forms an intention to change risk behaviours in favour of other behaviours. Self-efficacy and outcome expectancies are seen as the major predictors of intentions. Outcome expectancies can be seen as precursors of self-efficacy because people usually make assumptions about the possible consequences

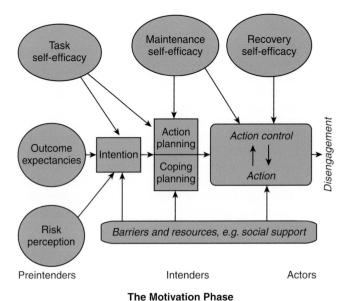

The Motivation Phase

Fig. 14.1 The health action process approach (HAPA). (Source: Schwarzer, 2016).

of behaviours before inquiring whether they can really take the action themselves. The influential role of risk perception (or threat) in the motivation and volition process may have been overestimated in past research and interventions. Fear appeals are of limited value; rather, the message must be framed in a way that allows individuals to draw on their coping resources and exercise skills to control health threats. In persuasive communications, a focus should be made on self-percepts of personal coping capabilities to manage effective precaution strategies. This suggests a causal order where a threat is specified as a distal antecedent that helps stimulate outcome expectancies which further stimulate self-efficacy. A minimum level of threat or concern must exist before people start contemplating the benefits of possible actions. The direct path from threat to intention may become negligible if expectancies are already well established.

In establishing a rank order among the three direct paths that lead to intention, it is assumed that self-efficacy and outcome expectancies dominate, whereas threat (or risk perceptions) may fail to contribute any additional direct influence. As indirect factors, however, a threat may be of considerable significance within the motivation phase (Zhang et al., 2019).

The Volition Phase

Correlations between intentions and behaviours vary tremendously. The right-hand part of Fig. 14.1 consists of three levels: cognitive, behavioural, and situational. The focus is on cognitions that instigate and control the action, a volitional process which is subdivided into action plans and action control. When a preference for health behaviour has been shaped, the intention has to be transformed into detailed instructions on how to perform the desired action. If, for example, someone intends to lose weight, it must be planned how to do it: what foods to buy, when and how often to eat which amounts, and when and where to exercise. Thus, a global intention can be specified by a set of subordinate intentions and action plans that contain proximal goals and action sequences. Self-efficacy beliefs influence the cognitive construction of specific action plans, for example, by visualising scenarios that may guide goal attainment. Once an action has been initiated, it must be controlled by cognitions to be maintained. The action has to be protected from being interrupted and abandoned prematurely due to incompatible competing intentions, which may become dominant while the behaviour is being performed. Daily physical exercise, for example, requires self-regulatory processes to secure effort and persistence and to keep other motivational tendencies at a distance (such as the desire to eat or socialise).

When an action is being performed, self-efficacy determines the amount of effort invested and perseverance. People with self-doubts are more inclined to anticipate failure scenarios, worry about possible performance deficiencies and abort their attempts prematurely. People with an optimistic sense of self-efficacy, however, visualise success scenarios that guide the action and let them persevere in the face of obstacles. When running into unforeseen difficulties, they quickly recover.

Performing intended health behaviour is an action. The suppression of health-detrimental actions requires effort and persistence as well and therefore is also guided by a volitional process that includes action plans and action control. If one intends to quit smoking, one has to plan how to do it. For example, it is important to avoid high-risk situations where there are pressures to relapse. If someone is craving a cigarette, action control helps him or her to survive the critical situation. For example, individuals can make favourable social comparisons, refer to their self-concept or simply pull themselves together. The more these meta-cognitive skills and internal coping dialogues are developed, and the better they are matched to specific risk situations, the easier the urges can be controlled. Finally, situational barriers and opportunities must be considered. If situational cues are overwhelming, the temptation cannot be resisted. Actions are not only a function of intentions and cognitive control, but they are also influenced by the perceived and the actual environment. A social network, for example, that ignores the coping process of a quitter by smoking in their presence creates a difficult stress situation which taxes the quitter's volitional strength. If, on the other hand, a friend or partner decides to quit too, then a social support situation is created that enables the quitter to remain abstinent despite lower levels of volitional strength.

In summary, the action phase can be described along three levels: cognitive, behavioural and situational. The cognitive level refers to a self-regulatory process that mediates between the intentions and the actions. This volitional process contains action planning and action control and is strongly influenced by self-efficacy and also by situational barriers and support (Zhang et al., 2019).

Transtheoretical Model and Stages of Change

One way of supporting people in making health-related decisions and changing their behaviour is to consider all the stages in the process and how people move from one stage to another. The transtheoretical model (TTM) developed by Prochaska and DiClemente (1982) is rooted in extensive research and integrates a range of psychological theories. The TTM has evolved over time and now contains five core stages: pre-contemplation, contemplation, preparation, action and maintenance, which provide a valuable conceptual framework for how people change their behaviour (Raiham and Cogburn, 2022). However, there is debate about whether the stages can be consistently translated into an intervention programme. For example, de Freitas et al. (2020) show success in using the model for changing behaviour amongst obese patients and a systematic review has demonstrated the value of TTM in changing the behaviour of people with chronic diseases (Hashemzadah et al., 2019). However, it is important before using the approach to be abreast of the model's efficacy for your particular intervention and the systematic reviews on its general effectiveness.

The stages of change component of the TTM identifies a number of stages that a person can go through during the process of behaviour change. It takes a holistic approach, integrating factors such as the role of personal responsibility and choices and the impact of social and environmental forces that set very real limits on the individual potential for change. It provides a framework for a wide range of potential interventions by health promoters, as well as describing the process individuals go through when acting as their own agents of change, for example, when someone stops smoking without any professional support. The main stages identified in the model are set out in Fig. 14.2.

The key to the model is to regard the cycle in the centre as a series of stages that people go through in the process of changing health behaviour, such as stopping smoking, taking more exercise regularly or adopting healthier eating. A crucial point is that the cycle can be thought of as a revolving door because people usually go around more than once before emerging to a permanently changed state. It is also important to recognise that some people may never get as far as entering the revolving door.

Pre-contemplation stage. The stage that precedes entry into the change cycle is referred to as pre-contemplation. At this stage, a person has no awareness of a need for change or does not accept it and has no motivation to change habits or lifestyle.

Contemplation stage. This stage is the way into the revolving door cycle of stages of change. People enter this stage when they have enough motivation to contemplate seriously changing their habits; the entry stage is therefore called contemplation.

Commitment stage. If people continue to progress around the cycle, they enter the commitment stage in which they make a serious decision to change the particular habit concerned, such as stopping smoking or doing more exercise.

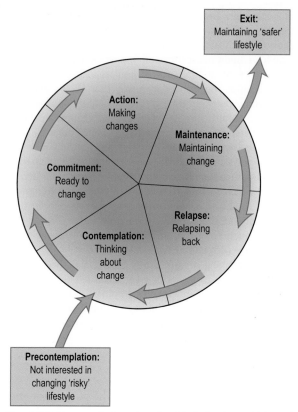

Fig. 14.2 Stages of changing health behaviour. (Adapted from Prochaska and DiClemente, 1984 and Neesham, 1983).

Action stage. They next enter the action stage as they actively begin to change the habit.

Maintenance stage. At this stage, people struggle to maintain the change and may experiment with a variety of coping strategies.

Relapse stage. Although individuals experience the satisfaction of a changed lifestyle for varying amounts of time, most of them cannot exit from the revolving door the first time around. Typically, they relapse; for example, they start smoking again. Of great importance, however, is that they do not stop there but move back into the contemplation stage, engaging in the cycle all over again. Prochaska et al. (1992) found that, on average, successful former smokers take three revolutions of change before they find a way to become fully free of the habit and exit from the revolving door.

Exit stage. This is the stage in which people are settled into a changed behaviour, such as stopping smoking permanently.

By identifying where clients are in the stages of change, health promoters can tailor their interventions to the stage. For example, behaviour change strategies are appropriate for someone in the action or maintenance stages; education and awareness raising are appropriate for someone in the pre-contemplation stage; working for client self-empowerment is appropriate for someone in the contemplation stage; strategies to help people to make decisions are useful for those in the commitment stage.

The model can be useful in primary healthcare settings because clients' needs can be assessed, and appropriate advice or information given within the constraints of a short consultation.

WORKING WITH A CLIENT'S MOTIVATION

Motivation is a state that changes frequently depending on many different factors. If people are struggling to maintain their new behaviour, what gets them through this difficult time without relapsing? It is thought that both the importance of the new behaviour (in terms of the expectation of costs and benefits) and the confidence of the person being able to maintain the new behaviour are essential to prevent relapse. To determine the client's attitude to change is an important first step. To give advice, you need to gauge your clients' understanding of how their behaviour is impacting on their health and their interest in changing. To explore the benefits of changing and to find ways of dealing with potential barriers, the following pointers may be useful:

1. Start where your client is and try to see the situation from their point of view.
2. If they want to change, encourage a realistic first step.
3. If a person is unsure, you could ask them to consider the pros and cons of making the change. People are more likely to change when they can see the benefit of changing.
4. If they are not ready for a change, you should respect their decision.
5. Build on their existing strengths and positive past experiences.
6. Use small measurements to assess and track their progress.

It is essential to listen actively to the client when exploring readiness to change. Confidence can be divided into self-efficacy and self-esteem. Self-efficacy is concerned with a person's confidence in being able to make a specific change in behaviour, whereas self-esteem is a more general sense of wellbeing that a person has about themselves. Self-efficacy can vary in different situations, and you can help your clients look at different approaches for improving self-efficacy in situations where they feel less confident.

Assumptions About Motivation

Health promoters and public health practitioners can become very focused on health issues and may forget that there are other motives for change and that health might not be one of them. The following list illustrates some of the other assumptions that are easy to make when counselling clients:

- This person ought to change.
- This person wants to change.
- It is the right time for this person to change.
- If this person decides not to change, this intervention has failed.
- A tough approach is always best.
- For this person, health is a prime motivator.
- I am the expert. This person must follow my advice.

Rollnick et al. (2022) (See also the Rollnick website under the website list at the end of the chapter.)

WORKING FOR CLIENT SELF-EMPOWERMENT

Making health choices, setting health goals, and carrying them out can bring benefits. These are not only the benefits that go with a healthier lifestyle, such as improved health and wellbeing, but also increased self-esteem from the feeling of taking active control over a part of life, such as being in control of the smoking habit rather than cigarettes being in control. In other words, making a positive choice about health can be a self-empowering process.

There are a number of different ways of working towards self-empowerment. Using the stages of change is empowering because people can follow their own progress. It may encourage them to try to get to the next stage of the cycle. Also, the recognition that relapse can be part of the process of changing behaviour is important (see Prochaska et al., 2013 for a discussion of the stages of changes and the position of relapse).

Methods of working with clients in an empowering way include group work and experiential learning, individual counselling, therapy, and advocacy, all of which are considered in the following sections, except therapy, which is beyond the scope of this book. Unless you are a mental health specialist, most people you work with probably do not need in-depth therapy.

The process of empowerment involves helping clients to become more self-aware and have greater insight into and understanding of themselves, their attitudes, values, motivations and feelings.

STRATEGIES FOR INCREASING SELF-AWARENESS, CLARIFYING VALUES AND CHANGING ATTITUDES

Many of the strategies that are useful for increasing self-awareness, clarifying values, developing belief systems and changing attitudes for the contemplation stage of change are designed for group work. However, some of them can be adapted for health promoters and public health practitioners to use in one-to-one situations (see Chapter 12, helping people learn, and Chapter 13, working with groups).

Deciding What to Change

Some clients could benefit from making several lifestyle changes to improve their health, and it can be tempting to try to address all of them at the same time. But people are often at different stages of readiness to change on different issues. For example, a person considering making improvements to their diet might be ready to make one change (such as eating more fruit and vegetables) but not ready to make others, such as changing to lower fat milk. As another example, an overweight person may be ready to do more exercise but not change their eating habits.

Ranking or Categorising

Ranking is a way of analysing an issue to distinguish the relative importance of different aspects. It is, therefore, useful for clarifying values. For example, in Exercise 1.1 in Chapter 1, readers are asked to rank aspects of being healthy. Health is a value, and that exercise is designed to help readers to clarify which aspects of health they value most (see Chapter 1, the section on what does being healthy mean to you).

Another approach to increasing self-awareness and value clarification is to generate a list of items and then code them into different categories. Exercise 14.1 illustrates this approach; it is designed to raise awareness of the link between enjoyment and health.

Using Polarised Views

This is a way of getting people to clarify their views about a particular issue. Views about the issue are polarised and phrased to reflect extremely different views. For example, if the issue was 'Is jogging good for you?' polarised views could be summed up as 'Jogging kills people and only very fit athletes should do it' or 'Jogging is very beneficial to health, and all people would be fitter if they took it up'. Examples of polarised views can be described by the health promoter or public health practitioner or taken from writings that express opposite views.

> ## EXERCISE 14.1   Enjoyment and Health
>
> Quickly list as many things as you can think of that you enjoy doing. Write them down on the left-hand side of a piece of paper. On the right-hand side, code each item according to the following categories:
>
> £ – any items that involve spending money.
> A – any items that you do alone.
> P – any items you do with other people.
> R – any items that involve some kind of risk.
> F – any items that help to keep you fit.
> C – any items that involve creativity.
> D – any items that involve the consumption of drugs (including alcohol and tobacco).
> H+ – any items that positively affect your health.
> H− – any items that negatively affect your health.
>
> Items may be coded in more than one category. For example, if one of the things you enjoy is going out to the pub for a drink, this may be coded £, P, and D, as well as H+ and/or H−.
>
> What have you learnt about enjoyment and health through doing this exercise?

If working with a group, the public health facilitator may ask people to work in pairs with one individual acting as if they fully adopted one of the points of view for the duration of the exercise, whatever their personal opinions. First, each person writes down all the arguments they can think of that support their position without discussing it with their partner at this stage. After a few minutes, the partners are asked to start arguing the case, usually for about 15 min. The leader then lists the points in favour of each view by asking each pair, in turn, to contribute one point until all the points have been collected. They then ask the group to comment on what they have learnt. In this way, members of the group can consider a whole range of arguments, which helps them to understand other people's points of view, tolerate differences of opinion, clarify their own views and perhaps see the issue in a new light.

Another example of a values clarification exercise using the polarised arguments approach is Exercise 4.1 in Chapter 4.

Using a Values Continuum

This is an extension of the polarised argument technique. It helps people to understand the spread of opinion on a particular issue and to clarify where they stand.

The leader describes two extremes of opinion and asks the group to imagine that these can be represented by two points, A and B, joined by a straight line. With a small group, this line can be across a room and with a large group, it could be drawn on the blackboard. The group members are then asked to mark or place themselves at a point along the line that best reflects their own view. For instance, in the jogging example discussed previously, pro-joggers place themselves at one end, with the most extreme at the farthest point, whereas people with moderate views stand around the middle, and the most ardent anti-joggers stand at the other end. The leader asks each person to state their views briefly as they take up their position. Other people are asked not to interrupt or comment until everyone has taken up a position or has passed if they choose not to participate.

This technique can encourage a more detailed discussion of the range of possible options than the polarised argument technique. On the other hand, if everyone seems moderate, a better discussion may be stimulated by the polarised argument technique. The values continuum technique is used in the last task of Exercise 4.1 in Chapter 4.

Using Role-Play

Role-play generally means taking on the role of another person in a specified situation and acting out what that other person might do and say in that situation. This helps people to understand what it feels like to be in another person's shoes. For example, health promoters or public health practitioners role-playing non-English-speaking patients visiting a clinic may be helped to understand how those patients feel, especially if the role-play is given added authenticity by using a foreign language that the health promoters do not speak.

It is also possible to role-play oneself in a new situation. This is a useful way of practising a new skill or rehearsing for a future event. For example, patients can role-play a consultation with a doctor to practise the skills of presenting their health problems to doctors.

Using Structured Activities

Structured activities, usually for a group of people but sometimes for one or two people only, can be used to meet a variety of aims. One is to help people to get to know each other – icebreakers. Other activities are devised to help people trust each other or communicate more openly or to increase self-awareness (see Chapter 13, the section on getting groups going, for icebreaker ideas).

For example, activities can be used to help people to identify irrational beliefs. Irrational beliefs are misconceptions that hinder people from achieving their goals. For an interesting discussion of irrational beliefs and COVID-19, see Magarini et al. (2021). These beliefs lead to self-defeating thinking, which in turn can affect health. It can lead to health-related behaviour with destructive consequences, such as emotional disorders, heavy drinking, and physical ailments, or in the case of COVID-19, not wearing a mask or refusing vaccinations. The quiz in Exercise 14.2 aims to help you identify your own irrational beliefs.

EXERCISE 14.2   Beliefs Quiz

Look at the following statements and put a tick in the appropriate column:

	Agree	Disagree
1. I believe in the saying, 'A leopard cannot change his spots'.	☐	☐
2. I believe that 'wait and see' is a good philosophy for life.	☐	☐
3. I want everyone to like me.	☐	☐
4. I usually put off important decisions.	☐	☐

Now identify your rational beliefs and your irrational beliefs (misconceptions):

Q1. If you agreed with this statement, you might believe that the past has much to do with determining the present and that people are largely unchangeable. 'I'm made that way.' The idea that you are no good at playing sports, for example, can be used to avoid trying out new behaviour and learning the skills necessary to participate in a sport. The truth is that people who take risks, experiment and work on things generally find that they can become reasonably competent at most of the things they attempt; not necessarily perfect, but good enough.

Q2. If you agreed with this statement, you might believe that human happiness can be achieved by hoping for the best and waiting to see what happens. This belief could result in you becoming merely a spectator in life, watching television every night and somnolent on a sun-lounger for the whole of your holidays. Getting more actively involved could be more satisfying and actually provide you with more energy. If you feel too exhausted, now may be the time to take

(Continued)

a close look at how you are managing your life and make some changes.

Q3. If you agree with this statement, you may believe you are only as good as other people think you are. Because of this, you may feel worthless if, despite your efforts, people do not seem to like you. Having the approval of others is pleasant, but to run our own lives, we shall almost certainly have to do some things some people do not like. Work on giving yourself the approval you deserve.

Q4. If you agreed with this statement, you might believe that life's problems will go away if you avoid them. Do not waste your time hoping that things will work out; make them.

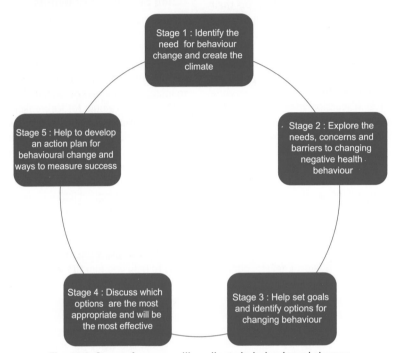

Fig. 14.3 Stages for counselling clients in behavioural change.

STRATEGIES FOR DECISION MAKING

As a health promoter or public health practitioner, you may be involved in counselling with the aim of enabling people to make a choice, such as which treatment to have, whether to have a blood test for a blood born virus or how to select healthy foods in particular circumstances (see Chapter 10 on fundamentals of communication).

Basic skills of counselling to help people make decisions at the commitment stage of change are those discussed in Chapter 10: Understanding nonverbal communication, listening, helping people to talk, asking questions and obtaining feedback. For those of you who require a level of counselling skill but are not trained counsellors or therapists, see Saunders et al. (2021) for an introduction to counselling techniques.

There are at least five stages involved in a counselling approach to working with clients in a health-promoting, behavioural change capacity. This includes a framework of planning and evaluating, which is similar to the stages of change discussed above. See Fig. 14.3 for an example of the stages involved.

Stage 1: Identify the Need and Create the Climate

Rogers (1983), an early pioneer of counselling, identified the qualities necessary for a counsellor to establish a climate in which a client can open up. These are warmth, openness, genuineness, empathy and unconditional positive regard. Unconditional positive regard is the quality of totally respecting the worth and dignity of a person, irrespective of whether you like the person or agree with their views or behaviour. The practical aspects of creating the climate include ensuring that you will not be interrupted and cannot be overheard, that you have sufficient time and that you are comfortably seated in chairs of the same height with the health promoter adopting an open posture and making direct eye contact when appropriate.

Stage 2: Explore the Needs and the Concerns

Through giving full attention and actively listening, encouraging the client to talk, and asking questions, the health professional begins to establish trust and enable the client to move from superficial issues to deeper needs and concerns.

Stage 3: Help the Client to Set Goals and Identify Options

Having gained a new perspective on the health issues and concerns, it becomes possible for the client to identify goals and ways these might be achieved. Ask the client to identify themes or to get a clearer vision of the future by asking key questions, such as:
'How would you feel if …?'
'If things were exactly how you wanted them to be, how would they be different from now …?'
'Have you ever felt like that on other occasions …?'
The health promoter may also provide the client with information to establish options:
'If you do X, what's likely to happen is …'
'If you do Y, the chances are that …'
'You might find it helpful to consider that …' and so on.

Stage 4: Help the Client to Decide Which Option to Choose

The important thing about this stage is that the choice must be the client's, not the health promoters. Making decisions – that is, choosing between alternative options – is a highly complex process. It involves:
- Weighing up the pros and cons of the alternative options.
- Considering the likely consequences of pursuing each alternative.
- Deciding which is the best alternative.
- Having the confidence to pursue the best alternative.

If the client is reluctant to commit to a decision, then both parties need to consider whether it is worth undertaking further work at stages 2 and 3.

If the client chooses an alternative that the health promoters feel may not work, they should nevertheless back the client's choice and help them to develop an action plan, knowing that if it does not work, there is still the possibility for exploring other options.

Stage 5: Help the Client to Develop an Action Plan

Having made a decision, the client now needs to think about turning that decision into action. They may need to identify coping strategies and sources of support. Once an action plan has been agreed upon, the final details are to set a review date and to clarify how progress will be monitored (see next section on strategies for changing behaviour).

STRATEGIES FOR CHANGING BEHAVIOUR

Having made a choice, people may need considerable help to carry their decision through into the action stage of change. Techniques developed from behavioural psychology are useful, and the philosophy behind them, that people are responsible for their own behaviour and are capable of exercising control over it, is as important as the techniques themselves.

A variety of material has been developed to help people to change different aspects of their behaviour. A good example of this is a behaviour change wheel (PHE, 2020) that has been used to address a very wide range of issues: for example reducing domestic water use, increasing physical activity in school children, reducing sitting time in desk-based office workers, promoting independent living in older adults, supporting parents to reduce the provision of unhealthy foods to children and reducing workplace energy use. For eight evidence-based strategies for changing behaviour, see Hooker et al. (2018).

Self-Monitoring

Self-monitoring involves keeping a detailed and precise account, often in the form of a diary, of behaviour that is to be changed. It aims to help people to analyse their pattern of behaviour and become fully aware of what they are doing, which is a starting point for gaining control. Secondly, the diary provides a baseline against which progress can be checked. Self-monitoring involves answering reflective questions, such as:
- How frequently does the problem or behaviour occur?
- When it does occur, what else is happening? This could consider both external factors, such as work-related stress, and internal factors, such as thoughts and feelings.
- What event leads up to the problem? How long beforehand did it occur?
- What happens afterwards in terms of the consequences?

Box 14.1 is an example of a smoker's diary.

BOX 14.1 A Smoker's Diary

Day........................ (Complete one of these charts every day.)
1. Each time you smoke a cigarette, note down in the columns: the time.
2. How urgent your craving for a cigarette is, on a scale of 1–10 (1, very little craving; 10, extremely high craving).
3. Where you smoke the cigarette.

4. Whether you are alone or who you are with.
5. Do you smoke it with drinks (coffee, tea, alcohol)?
6. Do you smoke it after a meal?
7. What else are you doing at the time (for example, chatting, reading the paper, working, talking on the phone)?
8. Why did you decide to smoke this cigarette?
9. What do you feel about it afterwards?

Time	Craving	Where	Who with	With drinks	After meal	Doing what	Why	Afterwards

---

Identifying Costs, Benefits and Rewards

The cost of changing behaviour can be considerable, involving deprivation of what might have become support mechanisms or pleasures, such as cigarettes, eating and drinking. There may also be a heavy price to pay in terms of time, effort and perhaps money. So it is helpful to identify the benefits clearly and set up a system of rewards to encourage perseverance.

Benefits may be long term, such as better health or increased life expectancy. They may be abstract: 'It will prove I've got willpower', or in other people's interests: 'For the family's sake'. These benefits may be important, but it is also necessary to find immediate, short term rewards that people genuinely enjoy, such as small treats or rewards.

Setting Targets and Evaluating Progress

Targets should be realistic rather than idealistic. Losing up to a kilo of weight a week is realistic for most people; losing 7 kg in a month usually is not. People may have unrealistic hopes and expectations about what can be achieved, which leads to disappointment and a sense of failure when they do not meet the target.

To evaluate progress, it is necessary to keep a record of behaviour so that achievements can be seen clearly. Progress should be assessed once the new behaviour has been given a fair trial, perhaps for two or three weeks, although short term reviews ('How have I done today?') can also be useful.

- If the target is not being achieved, possible reasons must be looked for and changes made. For example: is the target too difficult? Should it be lowered?
- Are the rewards too distant? Is there a more immediate reward that could be more encouraging?

- Is there an unforeseen crisis or illness? If so, encouragement to continue self-monitoring and to look at the setback as a learning experience may be needed.
- Are other people unhelpful? More strategies to cope with the negative influence of other people may be needed.
- Are there other problems which require support, such as learning to cope with anxiety or stress or a lack of the resources required to fund changes?

Devising Coping Strategies

Changing behaviour can mean coping with numerous difficulties for at least a short period of time until the new behaviour becomes a normal part of life. Someone who is stopping smoking has to cope with problems, such as the craving they feel, the need to put something in their mouth, not knowing what to do with their hands, doing without their accustomed tension reliever in moments of stress and resisting the offer of a cigarette.

People adopt a wide variety of coping strategies, and it is often useful to get a group to share their ideas about what helps them to cope. The list of strategies here is certainly not exhaustive:

- Finding a substitute, such as substituting chewing gum for cigarettes or eating low-calorie instead of high-calorie foods.
- Changing some routines and habits that are closely associated with unhealthy behaviour. Examples are drinking tea or fruit juice instead of coffee because coffee is closely associated with cigarettes.
- Making it difficult to carry on with the unhealthy behaviour by, for example, not keeping alcohol in the home or restricting eating to mealtimes, not between meals.

- What all these strategies have in common is that they require only a small step to achieve a large degree of help for self-control. Other strategies may be getting support from other people in the same situation, from a weight control group, a smoking cessation clinic or a self-help group. Another helpful way of getting support is by linking with another person on the understanding that each may telephone or meet the other if they need help.
- Practising ways of responding to unhelpful social pressures, for example, refusing the offer of a cigarette or a drink.
- Adopting a one-day-at-a-time approach. The prospect of the whole of the rest of life without a cigarette may be overwhelming, but the prospect of one day without one is far more tolerable. Even shorter time spans may be helpful, such as putting off eating, drinking or smoking for just 15 min at a time.
- Learning relaxation techniques and other ways, such as exercise, of relieving stress. Simple relaxation routines that can be practised at any time and place can be helpful in coping with stressful moments when the habit would have been to reach for a drink or a cigarette.

USING STRATEGIES EFFECTIVELY

A number of different strategies have been covered that you can use when you are trying to help clients increase their self-awareness, clarify their values and beliefs, change their attitudes and behaviour and maintain behaviour change, in other words, to move them through the stages of the change cycle. While it may be relatively easy to influence attitudes and behaviour in the short term, it can be difficult for people to sustain behaviour change over a longer period. To use these strategies with maximum effect, there are a number of principles to bear in mind.

Advocacy and Working in Partnership

Some people may need extra help to make health choices. Advocacy is generally taken to mean representing the interests of people who cannot speak up for themselves because of illness, disability or other disadvantages such as language issues. In the context of health promotion and public health, advocacy is better seen as a variety of ways of empowering those people who are disempowered in our society. It is concerned with using every possible means to assist people or disadvantaged groups in becoming independent and self-advocating. To reach and influence disadvantaged groups of people successfully, behavioural change interventions could involve professionals working in partnership with lay community groups and volunteers. See Mohajer and Singh (2018) for an examination of the factors enabling community health workers and volunteers to overcome sociocultural barriers to behaviour change to empower community members.

Making Healthier Choices Easy Choices

People make health choices in the context of their own environment, subject to all the pressures and influences that surround them. If this environment is conducive to a healthier lifestyle, clients have greater freedom to choose healthier alternatives and change their behaviour. For example, the provision of cycleways makes it easier to take regular exercise by cycling to work. National and local policies can create a climate where it is easier to adopt healthier behaviour. Nudging uses a combination of persuasion and environmental and legislative action to enable change, as shown in the examples in Fig. 14.4 (see Chapter 1, the section on what affects health and Chapter 16, the section on changing policy and practice).

Undertake Exercise 14.3 to apply some of these ideas to an example of a behaviour change scenario.

Relating to Clients

Clients are more likely to change if the health promoter or public health practitioner understands the client, sees things from their point of view and accepts them on their own terms. Achieving this relationship may be the most difficult part of helping people to change (see Chapter 10, the section on exploring relationships with clients).

Sometimes it is difficult to start a discussion about changing behaviour, and establishing a good rapport is essential for an honest discussion and openness to change. One way you can understand your client and also assess readiness to change is to ask the client to take you through a typical day with reference to a particular behaviour.

It is important to note that the attitude and behaviour of the health promoter may influence the outcome. For example, an obese health promoter may find it more difficult to encourage an obese client to adjust their dietary habits. The experiences of health promoters in trying to change their own behaviour, however, can be valuable in helping them understand the difficulties that their clients experience. It is important to remember that everyone is different and that, although for some people making a particular change may be easy, for others, a similar change may prove very difficult.

Dealing With Resistance

It is sometimes difficult for health promoters and public health practitioners to stop providing advice when they know that

Behavioural issue	Nudging	Shoving (regulating through legislative and fiscal action)
Smoking	Make nonsmoking more visible through mass media campaigns communicating that the majority do not smoke and the majority of smokers want to stop	Ban smoking in public places
	Reduce cues for smoking by keeping cigarettes and ashtrays out of sight	Increase price of cigarettes through taxation
Alcohol	Serve drinks in smaller glasses	Regulate pricing through duty or minimum pricing per unit
	Make lower alcohol consumption more visible through highlighting in mass media campaigns that the majority do not drink to excess	Raise the minimum age for purchase of alcohol
Diet	Designate sections of supermarket trolleys for fruit and vegetables	Restrict food advertising in media directed at children; introduce sugar tax.
	Make salad rather than chips the default side order in restaurants	Ban industrially produced trans fatty acids
Physical Activity	Make stairs, not lifts, more prominent and attractive in public buildings	Increase duty on petrol year on year (fuel price escalator)
	Make cycling more visible as a means of transport, e.g. through city bike hire schemes	Enforce car drop-off exclusion zones around schools

Fig. 14.4 Examples of nudging and legislative/regulating actions. (Source: Adjusted from Marteau, 2011).

EXERCISE 14.3 Changing Behaviour in Practice

Add to the table in Fig. 14.4 with further examples of nudging and shoving for COVID-19,
    Would nudging work for other health issues, such as sexual health or mental health? If so, how?
    What are the ethical issues linked to nudging? (see Schmidt and Engelen, 2020 for an overview of the ethics of nudging).

---

a particular behaviour, such as stopping smoking, can have huge benefits for the client. It is important to recognise when your clients are showing signs of resisting the suggestion to change. When you see this resistance, it is better to express empathy, emphasising that it is the client's personal choice and that they have control over their lifestyle choices. Useful strategies for these clients are to reassess their readiness to change, establish how important the behaviour change is to them and how confident they feel about making the change.

Using Methods Sensitively

People invest a great deal of emotion in their values and attitudes, which means that the exercises described here,

especially those that are designed to encourage people to explore feelings, need to be handled with care and sensitivity. Special training in the use of experiential methods is recommended, but at the very least, health promoters should not attempt to use them unless they have experienced them first themselves. Some points to remember are as follows:

- Explain the activities carefully and thoroughly and check to ensure that everybody understands what the exercise is for and what they are expected to do.
- Emphasise that participation is entirely voluntary.
- Allow plenty of time for discussion at the end. If people's opinions and cherished ideas have been challenged, they are likely to feel strongly about it. Increased self-awareness may be a very uncomfortable experience too. The group leader should ensure that people have time to express their feelings and get any support that they need before they leave the group.
- Ensure that there is an atmosphere of confidentiality and trust so that people feel free to explore their views and feelings safely.
- Save your own views to the end after the group members have had a chance to think things through for themselves. Be open and honest about yourself and

your beliefs, and be non-judgemental of values that might conflict with your own.

BRIEF INTERVENTIONS

A brief intervention is a technique used to initiate change for unhealthy or risky behaviour such as smoking, lack of exercise or alcohol misuse. As an alcohol intervention, it is typically targeted to nondependent drinkers whose drinking may still be harmful. Brief interventions involve opportunistic advice, discussion, negotiation or encouragement. They are commonly used in many areas of health promotion and public health and are delivered by a range of primary and community care professionals, including GPs (see Case study 14.1).

For smoking cessation, brief interventions typically take between 5 and 10 min and may include one or more of the following:

- Simple opportunistic advice to stop.
- An assessment of the patient's commitment to quit.
- An offer of pharmacotherapy and/or behavioural support.
- The provision of self-help material and referral to more intensive support such as the NHS stop smoking services.

The particular package that is provided will depend on a number of factors, including the individual's willingness to quit, how acceptable they find the intervention on offer and the previous ways they have tried to quit. UKGov (2021) provides support to healthcare professionals to deliver brief interventions for alcohol, smoking, and Making Every Contact Count programmes. It includes examples of the barriers and facilitators that affect whether healthcare professionals deliver brief interventions. The report also includes examples of behaviour change techniques that could be used to support and encourage health promoters to deliver brief interventions.

CASE STUDY 14.1 Brief Interventions in Primary Care

Case study produced by Dr Laura Jarvie, General Practitioner (GP), The Nelson Medical Practice, London (UK)

Alec is a 55-year-old window cleaner. He attended about some bothersome tendonitis in his shoulder, and my computer system prompted me to complete an AUDIT questionnaire in which he scored 14. Alec was surprised to hear that his current level of drinking could be damaging to his health; like most of his friends, he had a couple of beers in the evening, a bit more at the weekend and the occasional 'binge'. He had never seen his drinking as a problem and, at that stage, had no intentions of changing.

Alec is a 55-year-old window cleaner. He attended about some bothersome tendonitis in his shoulder, and my computer system prompted me to complete an AUDIT questionnaire in which he scored 14. Alec was surprised to hear that his current level of drinking could be damaging to his health; like most of his friends, he had a couple of beers in the evening, a bit more at the weekend and the occasional 'binge'. He had never seen his drinking as a problem and, at that stage, had no intentions of changing.

A few weeks later, he returned with indigestion which he thought was caused by the painkillers prescribed for his shoulder. We discussed how alcohol can also cause inflammation in the stomach and his current levels of drinking may also be contributing. I encouraged Alec to think about the benefits he might find by reducing his drinking including improved sleep and weight loss, as well as pointing out some of the longer term health benefits. We stopped the painkillers and arranged some routine blood tests and to meet again.

Alec's blood results showed evidence of excessive alcohol in both his blood count and liver function. I called him on the phone, explaining that this was nothing irreversible, and that small changes could result in big improvements in his health in both the long and short term. I explored his ideas about reducing his drinking and any strategies he had tried in the past. He seemed to recognise the problems.

I didn't see Alec for a while. When he did return many months later, his opening line was 'you've told me a few times I need to look at my drinking, now I realise I do'. It wasn't his health that had prompted this change of heart; Alec had been to the pub after work with his mates, had a few too many and got into an altercation. The police had been called, and Alec had spent a night in the cells. This had given him a fright; he had remembered the brief interventions I had employed and he now returned to me as he was ready to make the necessary changes.

As a GP, it sometimes feels like I am constantly talking to patients about their unhealthy behaviours, be it drinking, smoking, drugs or obesity. Not everyone is ready to change, and it is easy to become disheartened, prescriptive or rehearsed in your advice. However, because we see patients repeatedly, our brief interventions stand a better chance of catching them at the right point in the cycle of change, and even if they aren't there yet, our interventions, if executed effectively, may sow a seed which is remembered in the future.

BARRIERS TO BEHAVIOUR CHANGE

To successfully enable people to take up healthy behaviours, it is important to understand and take account of some of the obstacles that might be encountered. There is considerable research evidence which highlights some of these barriers. In a systematic review which looked at the barriers and facilitators to the uptake and maintenance of healthy behaviours by people at mid-life (aged 40 to 64), evidence was found relating to uptake and maintenance of physical activity, diet, and eating behaviours, smoking, alcohol, eye care and other health-promoting behaviours and grouped into six themes: health and quality of life, sociocultural factors, the physical environment, access, psychological factors and evidence relating to health inequalities. Barriers that recurred across the different health behaviours included lack of time (due to family, household and occupational responsibilities), access issues (to transport, facilities and resources), financial costs, entrenched attitudes and behaviours, restrictions in the physical environment, low socioeconomic status and lack of knowledge. Facilitators included a focus on enjoyment, and health benefits, including healthy ageing, social support, clear messages and integration of behaviours into lifestyle (see Kelly et al. (2016) for the full results). Kelly and Barker (2016) offer an excellent and important discussion of what they see as the six common errors that result in unsuccessful behaviour change interventions, including the notions that behaviour change is just common sense and that when people are given health information, they will make rational choices. The complexity of behaviour change as an approach should be noted, and efforts should be made to overcome some of the barriers and to challenge some of the assumptions on which behaviour change approaches are based.

Finally, for detailed guidance and evidence on behavioural change approaches, see the NICE website in the website section at the end of the chapter, and for details on social marketing as a behavioural change approach, see Chapter 2.

PRACTICE POINTS

- For individuals to be ready to change a particular behaviour, they need to feel confident in being able to adopt the new behaviour. The new behaviour also needs to be important to them and have clear benefits. You may need to help clients develop a number of competencies or life skills to do with social interaction, assertiveness and time management, and possibly specific skills (such as those needed to participate in a physical exercise programme).

- To devise the appropriate strategy for each individual, you need to start by exploring clients' health knowledge and beliefs related to the issue of concern, the stage of change they are at and what outcomes they desire. Asking the client to describe a typical day in relation to the behaviour is a useful approach.

- You need to be aware that clients may be resistant to change. In these situations, it is best to emphasise that it is the client's personal choice and that they are in control. At a later date, you could go back to explore again the individual's confidence about changing and how important the change is to them.

- You need to tailor an action plan to the specific needs of each client and provide positive consequences for the desired healthy behaviour (such as praise or rewards) to maintain behaviour change.

- You can improve success by combining a number of strategies. For example, a patient who is being rehabilitated after a heart attack could have an interview with a hospital doctor, a home visit from a nurse to encourage support from family members and small group self-help sessions to help patients to manage their problems.

- Records are important for follow-up. They are most effective if they are kept and owned by the individual concerned, for example, in the form of a diary.

- Equally important is the provision of environmental and socioeconomic circumstances that facilitate health choices rather than acting as barriers. At a broader level, national and local policy needs to address the broader socioeconomic determinants of health, such as poverty and deprivation.

References

Coto, J., Elizabeth, M. S., Pulgaron, R., & Delamater, A. (2019). Parents as role models: Associations between parent and young children's weight, dietary intake and physical intake in a minority sample. *Maternal Child Health Journal, 23*(7), 943–950. https://doi.org/10.1007/s10995-018-02722-z.

de Freitas, P. P., de Menezes, M. C., dos Santos, L. C., et al. (2020). The transtheoretical model is an effective weight management intervention: a randomised controlled trial. *BMC, 20,* 652. https://doi.org/10.1186/s12889-020-08796-1.

Hashemzadeh, M., Rahimi, A., Zare-Farashbandi, F., Alavi-Naeini, A. M., & Daei, A. (2019). Transtheoretical model of health behavioral change: a systematic review. *Iranian Journal of Nursing and Midwifery Research, 24*(2), 83–90. https://doi.org/10.4103/ijnmr.IJNMR_94_17.

Hooker S, Punjabi A, Justesen K, Boyle L, Sherman MD. Encouraging Health Behavior Change: Eight Evidence-Based Strategies. *Fam Pract Manag.* 2018 Mar/Apr;*25*(2):31–36. PMID:29537244.

Kane, M., Thornton, J., & Bibby, J. (2022). *Building public understanding of health and health inequalities.* The Health Foundation London.

Kelly, M. P., & Barker, M. (2016). Why is changing health-related behaviour so difficult? *Public Health*, *36*, 109–116. https://doi.org/10.1016/j.puhe.2016.03.030.

Kelly, S., Martin, S., Kuhn, I., Cowan, A., Brain, C., & Lafortune, L. (2016). Barriers and facilitators to the uptake and maintenance of healthy behaviours by people at mid-life: a rapid systematic review. *PLoS One*, *11*(1), e0145074. https://doi.org/10.1371/journal.pone.0145074.

Li, Y., Schoufour, J., Wang, D. D., Dhana, K., Pan, A., Liu, X., et al. (2020). Healthy lifestyle and life expectancy free of cancer, cardiovascular disease, and type 2 diabetes: prospective cohort study. *British Medical Journal*, *368*, l6669. https://doi.org/10.1136/bmj.l6669.

Magarini, F. M., Pinelli, M., Sinisi, A., Ferrari, S., De Fazio, G. L., & Galeazzi, G. M. (2021). Irrational beliefs about COVID-19: a scoping review. *International Journal of Environmental Research and Public Health*, *18*(19), 9839. https://doi.org/10.3390/ijerph18199839.

Marmot, M., Allen, J., Boyce, T., Goldblatt, P., & Morrison, J. (2020). *Health equity in England: the Marmot review 10 years on*. London: Institute of Health Equity.

Marteau, T. (2011). Judging nudging: can nudging improve population health? *British Medical Journal*, *342*, 263–264. https://doi.org/10.1136/bmj.d228.

Mohajer, N., Singh, D. Factors enabling community health workers and volunteers to overcome socio-cultural barriers to behaviour change: meta-synthesis using the concept of social capital. Hum Resour Health 16, 63 (2018). https://doi.org/10.1186/s12960-018-0331-7.

Prochaska, J. O., & DiClemente, C. C. (1982). Transtheoretical therapy: Toward a more integrative model of change. Psychotherapy: *Theory, Research & Practice*, *19*(3), 276–288. https://psycnet.apa.org/fulltext/1984-26566-001.pdf.

Prochaska, J. O., DiClemente, C. C., & Norcross, J. C. (1992). In search of how people change. *Application to addictive behaviors. American Psychology*, *47*(9), 1102–1114. https://doi.org/10.1037//0003-066x.47.9.1102.

Prochaska, J. O., Norcross, J. C., & DiClemente, C. C. (2013). Applying the stages of change. *Psychotherapy in Australia*, *19*(2), 10–15. https://search.informit.org/doi/10.3316/informit.254435778545597.

Public Health England. (2020). *Achieving behaviour change: a guide for national government*. https://assets.publishing.service.gov.uk/government/uploads/system/uploads/attachment_data/file/933328/UFG_National_Guide_v04.00__1___1_.pdf

Raiham, N., Cogburn, M. (2022). *Stages of change theory*. https://www.ncbi.nlm.nih.gov/books/NBK556005/

Rogers, C. R. (1983). *Freedom to learn for the eighties*. Columbus, Ohio: Charles E Merril.

Schmidt, A. T., & Engelen, B. (2020). The ethics of nudging: an overview. *Philosophy Compass*, *15*(4). https://doi.org/10.1111/phc3.12658.

Saunders, P., Williams, P. J., & Rogers, A. (2021). *First steps in counselling: an introductory companion, fifth edition*. Monmouth: PCCS Books.

Schwarzer, R. (2016). *The health action process approach (HAPA)*. *30*(121), 119–130. https://doi.org/10.15517/ap.v30i121.23458.

Rollnick, S., Miller, W., & Butler, C. C. (2022). *Motivational interviewing in health care, second edition*. Guildford: Guildford Press.

Sremanakova, J., Sowerbutts, A. M., Todd, C., Cooke, R., & Burden, S. (2021). Change theories: intervention in dietary interventions for people who have survived cancer. *MPDI Journal*, *13*(2). https://doi.org/10.3390/nu13020612.

UKGov. (2021). *Making every contact count alcohol and smoking brief interventions: review and strategic behavioural analysis*. https://www.gov.uk/government/publications/behaviour-change-helping-health-professionals-deliver-brief-interventions

Zhang, C. Q., Zhang, R., Schwarzer, R., & Hagger, M. S. (2019). A meta-analysis of the health action process approach. *Health Psychology*, *38*(7), 623–637. https://doi.org/10.1037/hea0000728.

YouTube

Kings Fund. (2019). *Changing behaviours: what's available and what works. Online panel discussion. I hour*. https://www.kingsfund.org.uk/events/changing-behaviours

Websites

HAPA. The health action process approach (HAPA). https://www.hapa-model.de

Marmot Review. Fair society healthy lives. http://www.instituteofhealthequity.org/projects/fair-society-healthy-lives-the-marmot-review

NICE. Behaviour change: individual approaches. https://www.nice.org.uk/guidance/ph49

REBT. Network irrational beliefs. http://www.rebtnetwork.org/library/ideas.html

Rollnick, S. For motivational interviewing. https://www.stephen-rollnick.com

Working With Communities

James Woodall

SUMMARY

This chapter begins with a discussion of community-based work in health promotion and public health and an overview of the range of activities it may include. Some key terms and principles are explained before an examination of three particular ways of working with communities: community participation, community development, and community health projects. Each of these includes an exercise, and there is also a case study of a community development project. The chapter finishes with a consideration of the competencies health promoters and public health practitioners need to work effectively with communities.

The challenge of promoting public health is considerable when working with people in the community who may be disadvantaged and discriminated against and who may feel powerless to do anything about their health. This chapter is about engaging with communities in ways that enable them to take more control over their health.

COMMUNITY ENGAGEMENT IN HEALTH PROMOTION AND PUBLIC HEALTH

Community-based work in health promotion and public health involves engaging with groups of the public in a sustained way which will enable them to increase control over their health and its determinants to improve their health.

Key Terms

Community

Traditionally, a community is seen as a group of interacting people living in a common location. The word is often used to refer to a group that is organised around common values and social cohesion within a shared geographical location, generally in social units larger than a household. Essentially, a community is a network of people. The link between them may be:

- Where they live (such as a housing estate or neighbourhood).
- The work they do (such as the farming community or school community).
- The way they live (such as new-age travellers or homeless people).
- Common interests, shared values or beliefs (such as a church community).
- Other factors they have in common (such as sexual preferences, so the gay community).

The people in the network come together based on a shared experience or concern and identify for themselves which communities they feel they belong to. Networks may be formal or informal, and since the advent of the internet, the concept of community no longer has geographical limitations as people can now virtually gather in an online community and share common interests regardless of physical location. 38 Degrees is an excellent example of a virtual community that demonstrates community empowerment and action by community-identified campaigns that put pressure on politicians and those in power. See the 38 Degrees website and Facebook pages referred to in the references at the end of the chapter, and watch the video of the work of 38 Degrees.

Community Work

This means working with community groups and organisations to overcome the community's problems. Community work aims to enhance the sense of solidarity and competence in the community. For example, a community development worker may promote health by working with particular communities to collectively bring about social change and improve quality of life. This involves working with individuals, families or whole communities to empower them to:

- Identify their needs, opportunities, rights, and responsibilities.
- Plan what they want to achieve and take appropriate action.
- Develop activities and services to improve their lives.

Community Health Work

This is community work with a focus on health concerns, but generally, health is defined broadly to include social

and economic aspects so that community health work may encompass almost as broad a range of activities as community development work.

Community Action

This means an activity carried out by members of the community under their own control to improve their collective conditions. It may involve campaigning, negotiating with, or challenging authorities and those with power.

Community Participation

This is about involving the community in health work that is led by someone outside the community, for example, a worker employed by a statutory agency. The degree of participation may vary (see Fig. 15.1).

Community Development

This means working to stimulate and encourage communities to express their needs and to support them in

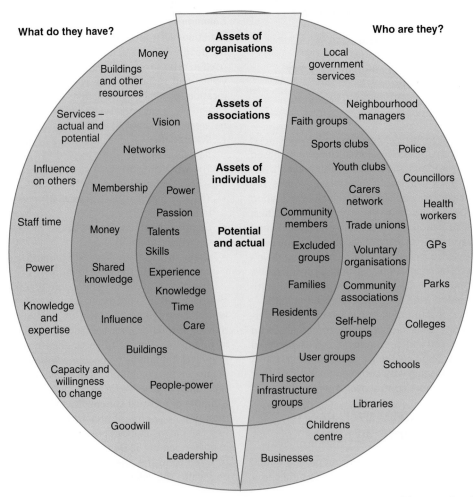

Fig. 15.1 What are health assets? Source: Asset mapping and more – an outline proposal for a pan-Scotland Learning Set; Slide share. http://www.slideshare.net/pashe/asset-mapping-and-more.

their collective action. It is not about dealing with people's problems on a one-to-one basis; it aims to develop the potential of a community as a whole. A community development approach to health involves working with groups of people to identify their own health concerns and to take appropriate action. Community development health workers are essentially facilitators, locally based, whose role is to help people in the community to acquire the skills, knowledge, and confidence to act on health issues. They are usually community workers by background rather than health professionals.

Community Health Projects

This is a loose term applied to programmes of work that are organised by agencies for the improvement of health in a community or applied to local organisations aiming to improve health by supporting some combination of community activity, self-help, community action, and/or community development.

Community Health Services

There are many community health services, with the word 'community' often used as an adjective to describe anything that is not based in a hospital. Most community health care takes place in people's homes. Teams of nurses and therapists coordinate care, working with professionals, including GPs and social care. Additionally, community health provides preventative and health improvement services, often with partners from the local government and the third sector. Although less visible than hospitals, they deliver an extensive and varied range of services (for more information on the extent of community networks and health services in England, see NHS Confederation, 2022).

PRINCIPLES OF COMMUNITY-BASED ENGAGEMENT

There are four key principles, as follows:

1. The Centrality of the Community

It is the community which defines its own needs. Community-based work is essentially a bottom-up process, rather than being top-down expert-led, where those with power and authority make the decisions. Health promoters and public health practitioners recognise and value the health experience and knowledge that exists in the community and seek to use it for everyone's benefit. In the United Kingdom (UK), both legislation and policy recognise the importance of community participation in their own affairs. The UK Government

have renewed their focus on community and community participation and involvement in its 'levelling up' agenda, which seeks to tackle health and social inequalities (HM Government, 2022).

2. The Facilitator Role of Community Health Promoters and Public Health Practitioners

Community health promoters and public health practitioners do not perceive themselves as experts in health but as facilitators whose role it is to validate, encourage, and empower people to define their own health needs and to meet them. They start where the community is, recognising and valuing people's own abilities and experiences. They involve people in community health work from the very beginning, encouraging, and supporting them in working together. Knowledge and skills are shared and demystified. Community health promoters aim to make people's access to statutory agencies easier and make the agencies more accountable to the people they serve.

3. The Importance of Addressing Inequalities

A central concern in community-based health promotion and public health work is the need to challenge and change the many forms of disadvantage, oppression, discrimination, and inequalities that people face and which adversely affect their health (see Chapter 1, the section on inequalities in health). Work, therefore, has focused particularly on the needs of disadvantaged groups. A central way of working is to bring people in such groups together for support and information sharing and to enable them to bring about change through collective action. The work can be political because it often involves working towards equality, social inclusion, and social justice with people who experience powerlessness and inequality as part of their everyday lives. Most recently, inequalities in health have been exposed through COVID-19, with sections of the population facing greater challenges as a result of social and environmental barriers (Woodall, 2020) – working within communities to address fundamental inequalities around access to green space and digital resources as well as education concerning vaccination uptake has been critical.

4. A Broad Perspective on Health

A social model of health is adopted, where health is perceived broadly and holistically as positive wellbeing, including social, emotional, mental, and societal aspects, as well as physical. It is not seen merely as the absence of disease and is not limited by medical or epidemiological views of what constitutes a health problem or issue. Health is seen to be affected by social, environmental, economic, and political factors.

COMMUNITY PARTICIPATION

Participation is a word that is used widely to mean a range of activities, from those that are merely tokenistic to those which are firmly rooted in the concept of empowerment. Partnership, public participation, and public decision-making are all key issues in health services and local authorities. However, in reality, some organisations may make decisions without having any wish to engage with the public (see Woodall and Cross, 2021, for a detailed overview of partnership working with communities).

Community Participation in Planning

The amount of community participation in planning health work organised by a statutory agency (such as an NHS or local authority) can vary along a spectrum of none to high, as shown in Table 15.1. In the health service, such participation can be called public involvement, engagement or service user involvement (see Haldane et al., 2019, for a systematic review of community participation and its

positive impact on health outcomes). See also Chapter 4, Fig. 4.1, Public Health Intervention Ladder, with examples.

Ways of Developing Community Participation

Community participation can be encouraged and supported in many ways at different levels. If you work for a public sector agency, such as a local authority or a health service, the following suggestions may be useful:

Be open about policies and plans. Publicise your policies, invite comments and recommendations on your plans, and involve representatives on planning and management groups. This is an intrinsic part of policy.

Plan for the community's expressed needs. When planning health promotion and public health services, help the community to express its own needs.

Decentralise planning. Set up planning and management of health-promoting and allied services on a neighbourhood basis, encouraging, and enabling the public's involvement.

Develop joint forums. Develop joint forums, such as patient participation groups in doctors' practices, where laypeople and professionals can work together in partnerships. Mental health services often have joint forums to involve service users in service development.

TABLE 15.1	Community Participation in Planning Public Health Promotion Work	
Level 1	No participation	The community is told nothing and is not involved in any way
Level 2	Very low participation	The community is informed. The agency makes a plan and announces it. The community is convened or notified in other ways to be informed; compliance is expected
Level 3	Low participation	The community is offered 'token' consultation. The agency tries to promote a plan and seeks support or at least sufficient sanction so that the plan can go ahead. It is unwilling to modify the plan unless absolutely necessary
Level 4	Moderate participation	The community advises through a consultation process. The agency presents a plan and invites questions, comments and recommendations. It is prepared to modify the plan
Level 5	High participation	The community plans jointly. Representatives of the agency and the community sit down together from the beginning to devise a plan
Level 6	Very high participation	The community has delegated decision-making authority. The agency identifies and presents an issue to the community, defines the limits, and asks the community to make a series of decisions that can be embodied in a plan which it will accept
Level 7	Highest participation	The community has control. The agency asks the community to identify the issue and make all the key decisions about goals and plans. It is willing to help the community at each step to accomplish its goals, even to the extent of delegating administrative control of the work
Level 8	Beyond participation	Community-owned health initiatives

Develop networks. Encourage individuals or groups to come together, thus increasing their collective knowledge and power to change things. Value interagency links and gain the support of workers from different organisations because competition and lack of understanding of each other's roles and cultures can hinder progress.

Use electronic/social media networking. Social media networks can provide community information and a means of communication within and between communities (email, Facebook, Twitter, Instagram, blogs, and websites), which go some way towards addressing the problem of social exclusion caused by lack of information. Not only can groups and individuals find and supply information on the internet, but they can also discuss issues and participate in democratic processes. See O'Neil (2019), who explains how to harness the potential of digital health promotion.

Provide support, advice, and training for community groups. Provide opportunities for laypeople to develop their knowledge, confidence, and skills.

Provide information. Provide information about health issues, details of useful local and national organisations, leaflets, posters, books, social media, and websites.

Provide help with funding and resources. Help local groups to obtain funding from statutory agencies and provide other sorts of practical help, such as a place to meet or facilities.

Provide help with evaluation. Being able to show real changes in community resources, services, and health outcomes increases respect and confidence from communities, funders, and agencies.

Support advocacy projects. Support projects that enable people who are otherwise excluded from having a voice, such as mental health advocacy schemes (see website under references).

Exercise 15.1 offers the opportunity for you to consider how you can encourage community participation in your work.

COMMUNITY DEVELOPMENT IN PRACTICE

However much you might seek people's participation, it may be that they feel so alienated, dissatisfied or overwhelmed with problems that they reject participation. In this situation, it is necessary to develop a climate and culture where participation can happen. You need to encourage, enable, and support people, and community development is a way of doing this. Asset-based approaches are a popular intervention strategy in health promotion and are seen as a legitimate way to address health inequalities by identifying strengths in communities

---

EXERCISE 15.1 Developing Community Participation in Your Health Promotion and Public Health Work

Consider the following list of ways in which you can encourage community participation in health improvement:

- Be open about policies and plans.
- Plan for the community's expressed needs.
- Decentralise planning.
- Develop joint forums and networks and social media activity.
- Offer support, advice, and training for community groups.
- Provide information.
- Facilitate coproduction and asset mapping.
- Provide help with funding and resources.
- Provide help with evaluation.
- Support advocacy projects.

(If you are not sure what is meant by these, look at the previous explanations and what follows).

To what extent do you think these things are desirable?

To what extent do you do these things already?

From this list, can you identify ways in which you would like to increase community participation in your work?

Can you identify any other ways in which you would like to increase community participation in your work?

What opportunities do virtual or online spaces bring to fostering greater community participation?

Given that there may be some obstacles to doing what you would ideally like to do, can you identify a practical way forward for acting on at least one of the things you would like to do?

Work individually, in pairs or in small groups.

---

and empowering people to increase control over their health and its determinants (Cassetti et al., 2020).

Asset-Based Community Development

Community development requires community participation but also involves working with people to identify their own health concerns and to support and facilitate them in their collective action. An asset-based approach to community health improvement makes value of, enhances, and develops community capacity, skills, knowledge, connections, and potential (Foot and Hopkins, 2010). Community assets were exemplified during the recent pandemic, where community and faith groups would find innovative ways to support people using digital and creative methods. It has been argued that an asset-based approach provides an opportunity for

---

EXERCISE 15.2   Thinking About Community Development and Asset-Based Approaches

Working individually, or in pairs or small groups, work through the following questionnaire. If you are working with other people, discuss the reasons for the answers you give. You do not have to reach a consensus. When you have listened to each other's views, you can agree to disagree.

Tick whether you think each of the following statements is true or false:

Community development is about:

	True	False
1. Fostering community cohesion and social capital.	☐	☐
2. Helping people to understand the root causes of their ill health.	☐	☐
3. Enabling a statutory authority to show it cares.	☐	☐
4. Getting involved in a political process to target inequalities in health.	☐	☐
5. Doing away with experts and professionals.	☐	☐
6. Confronting forms of discrimination such as racism and sexism.	☐	☐
7. Saving money on services by helping people to help themselves and to utilise available assets.	☐	☐
8. Promoting equal access to resources, such as health services.	☐	☐

Community development is about:

	True	False
9. Enabling a community worker to become a leader/spokesperson for the community.	☐	☐
10. Helping people to develop confidence and become more articulate about their needs.	☐	☐
11. Campaigning for a better environment, such as improved housing, transport and play facilities.	☐	☐
12. Controlling social unrest by providing, for example, activities for bored young people.	☐	☐
13. Helping people from lower socio-economic groups to change their attitudes and behaviour.	☐	☐
14. Recognising and valuing the assets of skills, knowledge, and expertise of individuals and groups in the community.	☐	☐
15. Beginning a process of redistributing wealth, power, and resources.	☐	☐

Now add any other points you think 1) community development and 2) asset-based approaches to community health improvement is, or is not, about.

(Adapted from a questionnaire by Adams and Hawkins (undated and unpublished) and reproduced by kind permission).

---

local authorities to respond to community inequalities (Nesta, 2020), and at the core of an asset-based approach is building community capacity to support health outcomes (see Cassetti et al., 2020, and Woodward et al., 2021, for evidence-reviews on this approach).

Exercise 15.2 is designed to help you to consider what community development work and asset-based approach means in practice.

Asset-based community health development approach means adhering firmly to the principles of community-based work. See Box 15.1 for some of the key principles of an asset-based approach. Health promoters or public health practitioners adopting an asset-based approach act as facilitators in a coproduction process, similar in many ways to traditional ways of working in community development (Hubley et al., 2020). The Scottish Coproduction Network has been active in the development of this approach and set up a range of tools to enable the

BOX 15.1   Asset-Based Approach to Community Health Development

- Working with people on their own terms.
- Helping people to identify and focus on the assets and strengths within themselves and their communities.
- Shifting control from the state to individuals and communities.
- Supporting individuals to develop their own potential.
- Seeing community residents as solutions.

Adapted from Woodward, J., South, J., Coan, S., Bagnall, A. M., and Rippon, S. (2021). Asset based community development: a review of current evidence. Leeds: Leeds Beckett University.

facilitation process (Scottish Coproduction Network, 2022). See Case study 15.1 as an example of coproduction in action and also the work of Woodward et al. (2021), who provide a range of illustrative examples.

CASE STUDY 15.1   Coproduction in Action

In Coventry, UK, 905 families were identified as having some challenges and required support. These challenges might include children not attending school, young people committing crime and involved in anti-social behaviour, and the parents or other significant others being out of work. Coventry City Council wanted to work in coproduction with these identified families and work *with* rather than *on* these groups to support and intervene early.

There is a strong empowerment element to the intervention with a coproduced action plan agreed upon with the family. This includes working with fathers to build resilience and sustainable behavioural change. The philosophy of coproduction is central to the whole approach. Coventry City Council now promotes strength-based approaches, which means that the whole early intervention approach seeks to work with and help to develop the capabilities of families and all their members.

Working in collaborative ways has achieved a number of positive outcomes:

- 632 families have children with improved attendance and behaviour at school.
- 334 families have committed at least 60% less anti-social behaviour.
- Youth offending has decreased by at least 33% in 76 families.
- 31 families have seen at least one adult move into continuous employment.

Governance International (2022).

Recent developments in enabling communities to understand their own needs and to identify the community resources that can be drawn on to meet those needs have included a number of innovations, such as asset mapping, and to enable asset mapping, WITTY, and Social Mirror:

1. Asset Mapping

Asset mapping is a key process in an asset-based approach to working with communities for health improvement. Community assets are seen as any factor or resource which enhances the ability of individuals, communities, and populations to maintain and sustain health and wellbeing and to reduce health inequalities. These assets can operate at the level of the individual, family or community as health-protective and promoting factors and are categorised into the social, financial, physical, environmental or human (employment opportunities, education, and social networks) within a community and which enhance health and wellbeing:

Asset Categorisation (adapted from Evans and Winson, 2014, and Foot and Hopkins, 2010):

Assets of Individuals (e.g. knowledge, networks, time, interests, passions, self-esteem, resilience).

Associational Assets (e.g. formal and voluntary organisations and informal networks).

Organisation Assets (e.g. local services within the community and staff assets).

Physical Assets (e.g. green spaces, land, buildings, streets, markets, transport links).

Economic Assets (e.g. skills and talents, such as employment generation).

Environmental Assets (e.g. a community that delivers security, social justice, sense of cohesion and harmony).

Cultural Assets (e.g. music, drama, creative expression opportunities).

See Fig. 15.1 for more details on community asset categorisation.

Mapping the assets within a community will require a number of processes, including data analysis, questionnaires, community mobilisation through social media and coproduction. A range of tools have been developed to assist with asset mapping and are available online (North Yorkshire Partnership, 2022). An excellent example of asset mapping is given in Case study 15.2.

2. WITTY (What's Important To You?)

WITTY is an app for iPad that can help community members understand the positive assets and factors which they have and can better use in their day-to-day life. WITTY was developed as an output of the empowerment and coproduction with families in Coventry.

'Social Assets in Action Project', a partnership project between the Institute for Research and Innovation in Social Services (IRISS), East Dunbartonshire Community Health Partnership and East Dunbartonshire Council, with support from the third sector (IRISS, 2013).

3. Social Mirror

Social networks reach into all areas of life, yet drawing insights from network information is often complex. The Social Mirror project looked at the transformative power of social networks and tested a social prescribing tool to see the potential for its use in the context of community health and wellbeing.

Starting in January 2012, the The Royal Society for the Encouragement of Arts, Manufactures and Commerce

CASE STUDY 15.2   Asset Mapping With Young People in Virginia: The Wellness Engagement (We) Project

Mosavel et al. (2018) report on the WE project in Virginia, United States. Local young people and university students mapped community assets relating to physical activity and healthy food options to inform obesity prevention interventions.

The asset mapping process was guided by the following underpinning questions:

- What types of health and health-related assets exist in the community?
- Which assets could be cultivated to increase physical activity and promote healthy food options?
- Which assets can people use to facilitate becoming more physically active?

Local young people were considered well-placed to uncover insights into the research questions. Young people were eligible to participate if they were a local resident, a student in grade 11 or above, living at home with their family and had availability to do asset mapping. Multiple recruitment methods were used and included: flyers, word of mouth, and enlisting the support of local schools who informed students of this opportunity.

Various strategies were used to identify assets, such as engaging community members around a map or conducting a focus group. A "community walk" also formed part of the strategy. While on these community mapping walks, the team members would interview willing community members about a particular asset. This approach also allowed teams to take pictures or videos of local assets.

Teams were tasked with locating tangible (i.e., structures, natural resources, land areas) and intangible (i.e., institutions, clubs, community leaders) community health assets. Existing and potential assets were grouped into 12 categories – these included: transportation; recreation; green space; education; retail, and tourism – significant for promoting physical activity and healthy food options. Young people identified 358 separate factors in their community, and of these, 18% were considered potential assets to support health outcomes.

This study demonstrated the importance of using asset mapping. It was shown to be a method with maximum potential for engagement, especially in highlighting available resources to assist with improving health outcomes. In addition, engaging young people in the process can lead to positive community changes, including fostering more positive perceptions about their community.

developed a tablet application prototype to measure and visualise social networks and ran a pilot study to test the impact of community prescriptions on the subjective well-being of individuals in the Knowle West area of Bristol (UK). By testing the app's effectiveness in different contexts, such as among GPs and other health practitioners, the RSA evaluated the impact of social prescriptions on people's mental wellbeing, their sense of attachment to and participation in the local community, and their use of public services (RSA, 2016).

Some Implications of the Community Engagement Approach

If you choose to adopt a community engagement approach, it is important to appreciate the implications and that areas of tension are likely to surface. These are identified in the following section as are suggestions for trying to prevent them.

1. Different Priorities and Agendas

Priorities chosen by communities may not be the same as those of local statutory agencies or funding organisations. For example, health priorities for health promoters may be influenced by government targets with lifestyle risk factors for major illnesses and low uptake of health services dominating the agenda. Community priorities, on the other hand, may be about social conditions, such as poor housing and lack of good public transport. Conflicting agendas must be clearly understood and dealt with at the outset of any community development work.

2. Threat to Local Health Workers

If local people gain confidence, become assertive and more articulate through the process of community development, they could voice concern and criticism about local health services. Furthermore, the prospect of members of the community taking an active role in policy-making and planning may be alien to many managers in statutory agencies. A thorough educational grounding in the rationale and principles of community-based work is required, although setting this up and getting people to listen may in itself be a difficult task.

3. No Instant Results

It takes time to get to know a community and to build up trust with local people, and it may be years before there is any tangible outcome. A common problem is that projects with fixed-term funding for a year or two are often expected to achieve substantial outcomes in these short timescales, which is unrealistic. Securing long-term funding with achievable objectives is fundamental to success.

4. A Token Gesture or an Easy Option

Well-meaning authorities who prioritise inequalities in health may consider a community health project as a way of addressing the issue. The inequalities issue is complex, involving deeply rooted causes of poor health; a community health project can make a valuable contribution, but it can also divert attention from political solutions to the problems.

5. Evaluation Conflicts

Outside agencies may expect to see results in terms of normative outcomes such as improved immunisation rates, a measurable change in community behaviour (less binge drinking, vandalism or crime, for example) or lower rates of hospital admission. However, the objectives of a community development project are rarely couched in such terms and are more likely to be concerned with far less easily measured results, such as increased public participation in health planning or better communication between the community and statutory agencies. Open debate about the process, principles, aims, and possible outcomes is essential if community involvement strategies are to be evidenced accurately (Rippon and South, 2017).

COMMUNITY HEALTH PROJECTS

A community health project aims to improve health usually by combining a number of approaches such as self-help, community action, and/or community engagement and development. They are generally expert-led rather than initiated by the community but should involve participatory approaches and can also employ asset mapping (see Chapter 5, planning and evaluating health promotion and public health).

It is important to adopt a systematic approach to planning a community health project. Fig. 15.2 summarises the planning and evaluation flowchart taken from Chapter 5, highlighting issues relevant to community health project work. This is not a comprehensive guide to setting up and running community health projects; it is intended to be complementary to the information in Chapter 5.

See Chapter 5 for more details on planning and evaluation methods.

Stage 1. Identifying Needs and Priorities

At this stage, two particular issues are: how do you get to know the community, and who do you consult?

Getting to know the community and its needs. An asset mapping process would be appropriate here. Get all the relevant information you can about the health of the community. Search out data from local health services and the local authority. Try contacting neighbourhood centres, community groups, voluntary organisations and tenants' associations. People who might be able to put you in touch with these include those working in health and social services, local churches and schools, the local Council for voluntary service, and the local Council for racial equality. Talk to members of the public, perhaps at local markets and festivals, or conduct a small survey. It might be necessary to hold public meetings to elicit full participation.

Talk to local professionals, but bear in mind that professional perceptions will often stem from a problem-centred view of a locality. For example, police may talk about crime, and social workers may talk about the number of children on the at-risk register.

Local newspapers are a useful source of information about the needs, interests, and activities of a locality. Social media and websites can also be exceptionally informative in understanding local concerns. Another approach is to walk, not drive, around the neighbourhood. Groups of young people on street corners, smells from fast-food shops, and the range and price of goods in shop windows can reveal a lot about local lifestyle and socioeconomic conditions.

Consulting before setting up. Consult with local health and social service workers at a very early stage and also elicit community participation so that they have ownership of the project. Only do this if you are confident the project is likely to secure funding, as you could raise community members' expectations falsely and diminish their trust.

Stages 2 and 3. Setting Aims and Objectives and Deciding the Best Way of Achieving Them

The key issues here are about being flexible and realistic. It is important to have full participation from the people you have already made contact with and the management group/steering group of the project (if there is one). These people are vital to setting realistic, achievable aims and objectives, and working out the best means of achieving them.

Flexibility is vital because community health improvement work is essentially a developmental process, so you need to review and, if necessary, modify your objectives regularly. Objectives may change, and indeed should change, if new opportunities arise and/or previous objectives no longer seem achievable or compatible with changing needs.

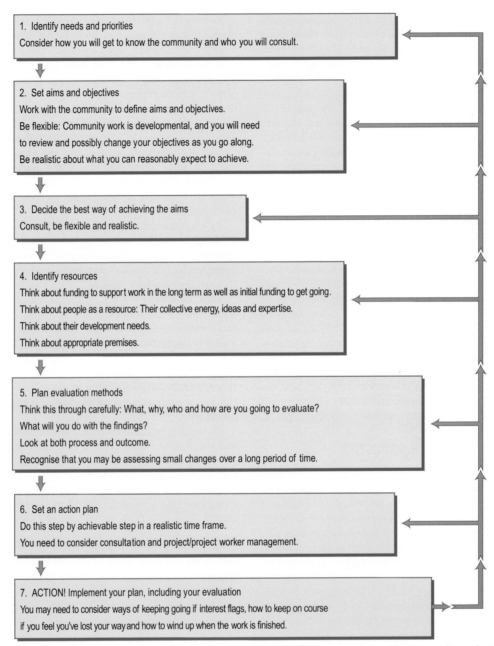

1. Identify needs and priorities
Consider how you will get to know the community and who you will consult.

2. Set aims and objectives
Work with the community to define aims and objectives.
Be flexible: Community work is developmental, and you will need
to review and possibly change your objectives as you go along.
Be realistic about what you can reasonably expect to achieve.

3. Decide the best way of achieving the aims
Consult, be flexible and realistic.

4. Identify resources
Think about funding to support work in the long term as well as initial funding to get going.
Think about people as a resource: Their collective energy, ideas and expertise.
Think about their development needs.
Think about appropriate premises.

5. Plan evaluation methods
Think this through carefully: What, why, who and how are you going to evaluate?
What will you do with the findings?
Look at both process and outcome.
Recognise that you may be assessing small changes over a long period of time.

6. Set an action plan
Do this step by achievable step in a realistic time frame.
You need to consider consultation and project/project worker management.

7. ACTION! Implement your plan, including your evaluation
You may need to consider ways of keeping going if interest flags, how to keep on course
if you feel you've lost your way and how to wind up when the work is finished.

Fig. 15.2 Flowchart for planning and evaluating a health promotion and public health community project.

Be realistic: this applies to identifying what you plan to achieve and when. For example, if you are planning a community development approach, ensure that you have a realistic time scale; three years is suggested as a reasonable minimum.

Stage 4. Identifying Resources

Funding. There are some global concerns about funding community health work and the scarcity of financial resources (Gichaga et al., 2021). That said, funding can come from a range of sources, such as statutory providers (local authorities or the health service). Projects may also be funded from the voluntary sector through funding from government grants and independent funds, such as The National Lottery Community Fund (https://www.tnlcommunityfund.org.uk/funding). When preparing a budget as part of an application for funding, it will be necessary to offer some justification for expenditures and explain why you need particular equipment, staffing, training, etc. (Hubley et al., 2020). Uncertain funding arrangements can increase difficulties in planning and evaluating work and can divert efforts from project work to fundraising. It is important to think about long-term funding; otherwise, there is a danger of work being dropped when funding runs out.

People. By bringing people with a common interest or experience together, you may find that the collective energy of the group generates ideas for future action. Your role may also begin to change from being an initiator/facilitator to being a supporter.

It is also important to think about what training and development is needed, who will do it and how it will be funded. Not only project workers but also the project management committee (if there is one), local laypeople, and health professionals may need help in understanding what this type of work is all about.

Premises. You need to consider what premises you need: Rooms for large and small meetings, a room for a crèche, a place to keep and use equipment such as video equipment and photocopiers, a library/place where people can look up information, and use computers with access to the internet and email. Is there access for wheelchairs, pushchairs and prams? Running water and toilets? Facilities for making refreshments or meals? Good access by public transport? Well-lit premises so that people feel safe going there after dark?

You also need to consider the nature of possible premises. If you are offered space in a clinic, for example, this may mean that people perceive the project to be part of the statutory health services.

Webpage/Facebook and other social media. Many community health projects now have webpages and other social media presence, so it is important to consider who will fund and develop this resource. See, as an example, the Pilton Community Health Project Facebook page in the references section at the end of this chapter.

Stage 5. Planning Evaluation Methods

It is vital that evaluation is planned at the outset, as this will avoid misunderstandings and false expectations. All parties (funders, managers, workers, and participants) need to agree on key issues. It is important to note that good health impact assessments move beyond the purely technical assessment of impacts on outcomes to include community views (Woodall and Rowlands, 2020). These views include:

- Why are you undertaking an evaluation? Who and what is it for?
- What will you be evaluating?
- How will you do it? What methods will you use?
- Who will do it? Will you evaluate yourselves, or will you use someone who is not involved in the work as an external evaluator?
- Who will be involved in the evaluation process? Will it involve the community, the workers, the funders, and the steering group?
- What will you do with your evaluation findings? Will you publish a report or disseminate it via social media? Who will the evaluation report be distributed to? Who will own it? Will findings be widely disseminated to the community?

Identify evaluation conflicts and ensure that your evaluation looks at process, impact, and outcome and identifies realistic ways of assessing what may be very small changes over long periods of time. It will probably not be possible to evaluate every element of a project, so it may be necessary to prioritise which elements will be assessed.

It may be helpful to think in terms of charting changes as they occur, using a framework to record these systematically.

Stage 6. Setting an Action Plan

There are many things to consider here, but the main one is to identify what you plan to do, step by step.

You may need to build the following activities into an action plan:

Reviewing aims and priorities. It is necessary to continuously review the aims and priorities originally set down for the project and compare them with those of the people who are now involved. You may need to modify the original aims and regularly check that the agenda is meeting community needs.

Consulting and being accountable to the community. The community participation established at the outset needs to continue throughout. Once the project is established, you have a continuing responsibility to involve the community. This could be through meetings, newsletters, electronic networks, and open days, for example.

Arranging a management committee or steering group. A management committee or steering group should provide a secure foundation for the project, taking responsibility for its continued development, its policies and management tasks such as fundraising and recruiting. It should also provide support for the project workers.

Usually, these are members of the group; they should not be expected to run the management committee themselves, but sometimes this is the case. This is not desirable because it leads to confusion about who is managing whom and puts an unreasonable burden on the workers.

A management group could consist of both local workers, such as health visitors and social workers, and local people, perhaps representing the community groups involved in the project.

It may be helpful to get the members of a management committee/steering committee together for a day to talk through the issues, clarify aims, and foster a sense of teamwork.

Writing job descriptions. Paid project workers need clear job descriptions specifying what is included. For example, does the job include fundraising, doing your own typing, servicing or even running the management committee meetings, keeping the accounts, evaluating, and writing progress reports?

Ensuring support for the project workers. Recognise the value of networking as a means of informal training and support. Networking requires making time and other resources available to meet people doing similar work and to link with other community health projects in different parts of the country. This enables information and ideas to be shared and problems discussed. Access to email, social media, and the internet is essential. The need to ensure that project workers are not isolated is crucial.

Networking also means that more people will know about the project, and you may get more support.

Formalising your project group. It may be helpful at some stage to look at the costs and benefits of formalising a project group that started off as a loose collection of interested people. The advantages of having a formal organisation are that it can apply for financial help and for recognition as a legitimate body; the disadvantages might be that control could be exercised from outside.

Dealing with opposition. The health issues the project is concerned with will probably have a local history and be likely to have both won and lost support in the past. You need to identify opposition and plan a strategy for dealing with individuals or groups who may oppose the project.

Stage 7. Implementing Your Plan

As the project is implemented, it may run into difficulties because of a) flagging interest, b) lack of direction and c) the project coming to an end.

Keeping going. Over time, the community may lose its enthusiasm. You need to be sensitive to the many ways in which a project can lose direction and, in such circumstances, you may be able to help by:

- Drawing the issue to the attention of relevant statutory agencies and conveying the response to the group.
- Helping the group to produce its own public health materials, such as posters, leaflets, websites or videos, and distributing them.
- Looking at other public health material on topics of interest.
- Encouraging members of the project to talk about their work to other people, such as groups of interested professionals and students.
- Sending emails to everyone to remind them of meetings.
- Providing practical support, such as access to a computer.
- Introducing new members.

Working out what to do next. If you feel that you have lost direction, it can help to write down what information you have found, what contacts you have made, what needs and aims you have identified and what you have done so far. Then seek the views of your management/steering group (if there is one) or the impartial views of someone who has not been involved. Exercise 15.3 may help to provide a focus for working out what to do next.

Leavings and endings. There comes the point when your involvement has to stop, maybe because you change your job or the priorities of your work or because the project work has been taken on by local people. Occasionally, you will need to recognise that you have done all you

---

EXERCISE 15.3 **Planning Community Health Improvement Work**

The following exercise may be useful when you are starting community health work or taking stock part-way through a community health project.

Complete the following statements as fully as you can:
The key issue is …
The people I need to consult/participate with are …
The documents I need to read are …
I can get to know more about the community by …
The information that is likely to be available is …
I intend to look for this information by …
Work done on this issue elsewhere is …
The people who are likely to be supportive are …
The people I should avoid offending are …
The period of time I can spend on this issue is …
The amount of time I can give it during this period is …
The person/people I will consult/participate with to work out what to do next are …

could do and that there is now no potential in the project. Ending your involvement provides the opportunity for a final evaluation of what has been achieved and what your own contribution has been and for making recommendations for future action.

DEVELOPING COMPETENCE IN COMMUNITY WORK

To be a successful community health worker, you need a range of competencies. You will also need to be committed to the principles and ideals of community-based work: the centrality of the community, your own role as a facilitator rather than an expert, the importance of addressing inequalities and a broad perspective on health (see Chapter 1, the section on inequalities in health and on models of health).

To adhere to these principles, you will need knowledge of key issues, such as the extent and cause of inequalities in health, the effects of racism, sexism, and other forms of oppression on health, and awareness of the structures, policies and powers which influence the lives and health of communities. You will also need to be clear about your own particular political ideologies.

See the previous section on getting to know the community and its needs, Chapter 3, the section on agents and agencies of health promotion and Exercise 4.1 in Chapter 4, on analysing your philosophical position on health promotion and public health.

Other areas of knowledge include familiarity with local health resources: who and where to go for information, advice, and materials on health issues. Knowledge of local health services and social services is vital, and so is understanding how local statutory and voluntary agencies work and how to use the system effectively. An understanding of the community itself is, of course, vital.

A range of competencies are required. It is important to have competencies in raising awareness of inequalities and discrimination and being able to counter these by taking positive action when appropriate and working in an antidiscriminatory way.

See Chapters 5, 7, and 8 for planning and managing, Chapter 10 for communication, Chapter 11 for using communication tools and Chapter 13 for working with groups.

Other skills link to working with people: being able to communicate well, facilitate groups and run effective meetings, good team working, and partnership skills. You also need skills in planning and management, using and producing social media and public health materials, and advocacy skills for working for political change.

PRACTICE POINTS

- Community-based health promotion, and public health involves engaging with communities (rather than individuals) over a period of time to enable them to increase control over, and improve, their health. It may involve community development work, specific community health projects and group work.
- A key principle is that community work is bottom-up, not top-down. This means that you respond to issues that the community identifies rather than working on issues identified by people outside the community, such as health workers from statutory agencies.
- Community health workers take on the role of facilitators rather than health experts to develop the community's abilities to both identify their assets and meet health needs.
- Work is often focused on addressing inequalities and working with people who are disadvantaged.
- Health is interpreted holistically to encompass social, emotional, and societal wellbeing.
- Community participation is fundamental to health planning and health promotion activity.
- You need particular skills and processes for successful community engagement work and community health projects. You need to be aware of the potential conflicts and difficulties inherent in this kind of work.

References

Cassetti, V., Powell, K., Barnes, A., & Sanders, T. (2020). A systematic scoping review of asset-based approaches to promote health in communities: development of a framework. *Global Health Promotion, 27*(3), 15–23. https://doi.org/10.1177/1757975919848925.

Evans, M., & Winson, A. (2014). *Asset-based approaches to public health: a conceptual framework for measuring community assets*. Birmingham, Birmingham City Council: University of Birmingham.

Foot, J., & Hopkins, T. (2010). *A glass half-full: how an asset approach can improve community health and well-being*. London: Improvement and Development Agency.

Gichaga, A., Masis, L., Chandra, A., Palazuelos, D., & Wakaba, N. (2021). Mind the global community health funding gap. *Global Health: Science and Practice, 9*(Supplement 1), S9–S17. https://doi.org/10.9745/GHSP-D-20-00517.

Governance International. (2022). *Intensive family support through prevention and family empowerment in Coventry*. https://www.govint.org/good-practice/case-studies/intensive-family-support-through-prevention-and-family-empowerment-in-coventry/change-management/.

Haldane, V., Chuah, F. L., Srivastava, A., Singh, S. R., Koh, G. C., Seng, C. K., & Legido-Quigley, H. (2019). Community participation in health services development, implementation, and evaluation: a systematic review of empowerment, health, community, and process outcomes. *PloS One, 14*(5), e0216112. https://doi.org/10.1371/journal.pone.0216112.

HM Government. (2022). *Levelling up the United Kingdom.* London, Crown.

Hubley, J., Copeman, J., & Woodall, J. (2020). *Practical health promotion, third edition.* Cambridge: Polity Press.

IRISS. (2013). *WITTY (what's important to you?).* http://www.iriss.org.uk/resources/witty-whats-important-you

Mosavel, M., Gough, M. Z., & Ferrell, D. (2018). Using asset mapping to engage youth in community-based participatory research: the WE project. *Progress in Community Health Partnerships: Research, Education, and Action, 12*(2), 223–236. https://doi:10.1353/cpr.2018.0042.

Nesta, (2020). *Asset-based community development for local authorities.* London: Nesta.

NHS Confederation. (2022). *Community network.* https://www.nhsconfed.org/networks-countries/community-network

North Yorkshire Partnership. (2022). *Tools for asset mapping.* https://nypartnerships.org.uk/assetmappingtools

O'Neil, I. (2019). *Digital health promotion.* Cambridge: Polity.

Rippon, S., & South, J. (2017). *Promoting asset based approaches for health and wellbeing: exploring a theory of change and challenges in evaluation.* Leeds: Leeds Beckett University.

RSA. (2016). *Social mirror.* https://www.thersa.org/action-and-research/rsa-projects/public-services-and-communities-folder/social-mirror

Scottish Coproduction Network. (2022). *Resources.* https://www.coproductionscotland.org.uk/resources/

Woodall, J. (2020). COVID-19 and the role of health promoters and educators. *Emerald Open Research,* 2. https://doi.org/10.35241/emeraldopenres.13608.2.

Woodall, J., & Cross, R. (2021). *Essentials of health promotion.* London: Sage.

Woodall, J., & Rowlands, S. (2020). Professional practice. In R. Cross, S. Foster, I. O'Neil, S. Rowlands, J. Woodall, & L. Warwick-Booth (Eds.), *Health promotion: global principles and practice, second edition.* London: CABI.

Woodward, J., South, J., Coan, S., Bagnall, A. M., & Rippon, S. (2021). *Asset based community development: a review of current evidence.* Leeds: Leeds Beckett University.

Websites

38 Degrees. *Website with a video on the work of the organisation.* https://home.38degrees.org.uk/

Community health *network page.* https://www.nhsconfed.org/networks-countries/community-network

Community Organisers. *Case studies and stories.* http://www.corganisers.org.uk/stories

For a list *of tools for asset mapping, see the North Yorkshire Partnership website.* http://www.nypartnerships.org.uk/index.aspx?articleid=29644.

For a range *of information on community action, see the National Association for Voluntary and Community Action (NAVCA).* https://www.navca.org.uk/.

Mental Health Advocacy Scheme. http://www.advocacyscheme.co.uk/

Scottish Coproduction Network. *Coproduction case studies.* https://www.coproductionscotland.org.uk/co-pro-resources

Video case *studies – IRISS what is coproduction.* http://www.coproductionscotland.org.uk/resources/video-case-studies/

YouTube

Nesta. (2020). *Asset-based community development for local authorities.* https://www.youtube.com/watch?v=kwbJieCRe9o&t=8s

UK Health Security Agency. (2018). *Health matters: community-centred approaches for health and wellbeing.* https://www.youtube.com/watch?v=KCQJTu2MrWk&t=17s

Twitter

Asset-based community *development in Leeds.* https://twitter.com/ABCD_in_Leeds

National Association for Voluntary and Community Action. https://twitter.com/navca

Facebook

38 Degrees. *People/power/change.* https://www.facebook.com/peoplepowerchange

Pilton Community Health Project. https://www.facebook.com/PiltonCommunityHealthProject/

Influencing and Implementing Public Health Policy

James Woodall

CHAPTER OUTLINE

SUMMARY

The focus of this chapter is on how public health policy at the local and national levels is made, how it can be influenced and how health promoters and public health practitioners can challenge health-damaging policies. The characteristics of power and the politics of influence are discussed and illustrated with a case study. There are sections on developing and implementing policies, a case study on the politics of influence and an exercise on policy implementation. The chapter ends with a section on planning a policy campaign (see Chapter 7, the section on linking your work to broader health promotion plans and strategies).

Health promoters and public health practitioners have an important role in influencing and implementing policies that affect health. A policy is a broad statement of the principles of how to proceed in relation to a specific issue and can be at a number of levels, from international to the national, regional, and organisational levels. At the international level, the World Health Organization (WHO) has produced a number of directives designed to influence national policy, such as the Working for Health 2022–2030 Action Plan (WHO, 2022).

GLOBAL HEALTH POLICY DIRECTIVES

The Working for Health Action Plan (2022–2030) suggests ways in which policy can support WHO Member States and stakeholders to maximise, increase capacity, and strengthen their health and care workforce. The document is geared to a range of countries, and therefore its guidance is used as a framework for informal national conversations with Ministers and decision-makers. The framework was developed to provide a clear pathway for progress that, therefore, can be made bespoke according to context and to catalysing new and sustainable investments in the health and care workforce. It suggests three core areas to focus on:

- Planning and financing.
- Education and employment.
- Protection and performance.

WHO notes the complexity of moving the action plan to political and practical reality, suggesting that it has a heightened likelihood of success when implemented through government-led multisectoral partnership and where there is effective cooperation between education, finance, health, labour and employment, and social affairs sectors, as well as collaboration with professional associations, workers' unions, and employers (public and private), along with other stakeholders (WHO, 2022). Given this example, it is very apparent that to influence policy, health promoters and public health practitioners need to understand international policy imperatives, how power is distributed and exercised between people at various levels and be able to use that knowledge to further shape policy decisions. In other words, a key skill of a health promoter is to be politically astute and savvy. Being a policy activist involves working with statutory, voluntary, and commercial organisations to influence the development of health-promoting public health policies. It also includes working for healthy public policies and economic and regulatory changes that might require campaigning, lobbying, and taking political action.

MAKING AND INFLUENCING LOCAL AND NATIONAL HEALTH POLICY

Working for policy change is an integral part of public health action, with health promoters and public health practitioners well placed to press for the introduction of policies at both national and local levels and influence how they are implemented. The development of local health policies cannot be divorced from the central government's policies that shape the organisation and funding of health services, local authority, and voluntary agency work at a local level. National policy is, in turn, influenced by consultation with and representations from a wide range of stakeholders, including health services, local authorities and voluntary agencies, and key public health member organisations. In the United Kingdom (UK), these will include the Faculty of Public Health (FPH) and the Royal Society of Public Health (RSPH), who advocate on key public health issues, influence policy change at the highest level, and work closely with policymakers. Public health research is also a key influence on policies and should form an essential step in the policy development process (Fig. 16.1). However, we know that there can be a whole series of challenges in translating research into policy responses – most notably the inconsistency between the immediacy of decision-making often necessary *versus* the time taken to undertake robust and rigorous research (Homer et al., 2022).

It is vital that those working to promote health have a good understanding of national public health policy and the various drivers that shape public health policy

statements and strategies. Given the scale of the challenge presented by the global growth in noncommunicable diseases and communicable diseases and the complexity of inequalities in health, all governments need to draw on the range of available policy tactics, from strong state action, including welfare and regulation, to behaviour and environmental approaches.

Local and National Public Health Policy Themes

Politics is a major influence on public health and the policies that affect population health, particularly policies linked to welfare and health service reforms. The UK government's "Levelling Up" (HM Government, 2022) agenda has come in for major criticism. Despite laudable intentions to improve life expectancy and reduce inequalities, the policy has been criticised heavily for being little more than a slogan and rhetoric (Forbes et al., 2022). Little progress has been made, and funding for the scheme consistently reduced (Forbes et al., 2022).

National health policies have a major impact on action at the local level. Currently, there are a number of strategies permeating UK health policy agendas which guide or determine health-promoting interventions. These are summed up in Fig. 16.2 and include directives that range from encouraging behavioural change to those that restrict choices through legislative and fiscal action.

Behavioural Change as a Policy Directive

Influencing people's behaviour is nothing new to governments, which often use tools such as legislation (such as a ban on smoking in public places), regulation (legislation is a directive proposed by a legislative body while a regulation is a specific requirement within the legislation, such as fines for adults smoking in cars that contain children

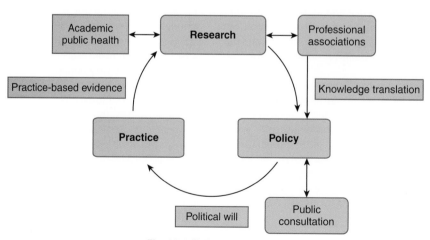

Fig. 16.1 Policy continuum.

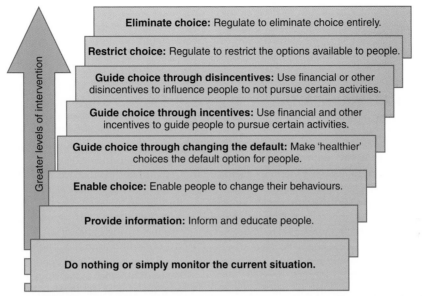

Greater levels of intervention →

Eliminate choice: Regulate to eliminate choice entirely.

Restrict choice: Regulate to restrict the options available to people.

Guide choice through disincentives: Use financial or other disincentives to influence people to not pursue certain activities.

Guide choice through incentives: Use financial and other incentives to guide people to pursue certain activities.

Guide choice through changing the default: Make 'healthier' choices the default option for people.

Enable choice: Enable people to change their behaviours.

Provide information: Inform and educate people.

Do nothing or simply monitor the current situation.

Fig. 16.2 Ladder of health-promoting strategies embedded in public health policy and practice. (Source: Local Government Association (2013) and Nuffield Council on Bioethics. (2007). *Full report public health: ethical issues.* http://nuffieldbioethics.org/wp-content/uploads/2014/07/Public-health-ethical-issues.pdf).

under 18) or taxation (a tax on cigarettes) to achieve desired behavioural change policy outcomes. Behaviour change ideology even permeates discussion of the broader determinants of health: 'A high-performing health system supports individuals to make positive decisions about their own health and acts to maximise its positive impact on the broader determinants of people's health' (Gregory et al., 2012). Government-sponsored campaigns, such as Change4Life (see websites and Facebook pages in the references at the end of the chapter), now called 'Better health. Healthier Families', and approaches, such as social marketing, contribute to the prevention agenda by driving lifestyle change across a wide range of health-related behaviours. Such approaches were seen as a key instrument of prevention at the heart of the National Health Service (NHS) five-year forward plan.

Nudging and choice architecture is another approach visible in some policy directives (DoH Ireland, 2015; Oe and Yamaoka, 2021). Choice architecture refers to the design of different ways in which choices can be presented to consumers and the impact of that presentation on consumer decision-making (see Ensaff's (2021) description of a choice architecture in relation to dietary choice). Fig. 14.3 in Chapter 14 has examples of nudging. It is important to note that behaviours do not exist at the individual level only. When replicated across a community or society, they are referred to as culture, such as the binge drinking

culture or the differences in smoking culture across socio-economic groups in the UK. Policy history suggests that wide scale cultural and behavioural change is driven by a mix of both broad social argument and small policy steps. Smoking is perhaps the best example. In the UK, the behavioural equilibrium has shifted from widespread smoking to a minority activity. A combination of nudging, choice architecture, and restricting choice, including health information; effective national media campaigns (and the prohibition of pro-smoking advertising); expanding bans on smoking in public places; and changing social norms have formed a mutually reinforcing thread of policy tactics to change smoking behaviour at a national level (Flor et al., 2021).

Place-Based Health

This is a dominant tactic in current health policy in England which involves planning by place for local populations in a way which is sustainable and transformative. Sustainability and transformation plans will cover (i) specialised services, (ii) primary medical care, and (iii) better integration between health and local authority services, including prevention and social care, reflecting local agreed health and wellbeing strategies (NHS England, 2015). Selby and Kippen (2016) argue that place-based health will result in energy, money, and power shifting from institutions to citizens and communities. They envisage that place-based health will become an enabler for a reform programme that starts to deliver on joining up health and social care for a population in a place with the ultimate aim to improve the public's health and wellbeing and reduce health inequalities.

IMPLEMENTING NATIONAL HEALTH POLICIES AT A LOCAL LEVEL

National strategies for health are outlined and referred to in Chapters 1 and 4. Public health and health promotion is a significant component of the UK government's health policy agenda. It is important to be up-to-date with your government's policy directives and the dominant themes and, from these, to interpret the sort of policies that would need to be implemented at a local level to improve the health of communities and local population groups.

The role that local government can play in improving population health is recognised internationally. The transfer of public health functions in England from the NHS to the local government in 2013 aimed to bring about improvements to population-level health and reduce health inequalities (Homer et al., 2022). While the delivery of public health can vary in local authorities, this reorganisation saw a change in culture from a narrow focus on healthcare pathways to one of a politically led environment with an opportunity to influence the wider determinants of health and wellbeing. As part of this, Health and Wellbeing strategies are a vehicle for local governments to act on the wider determinants of health and wellbeing and provide an opportunity to adopt an evidence-based approach to local decision-making and prioritisation of limited resources across local government. The rationale is that leadership and delivery of public services should be made as locally as possible, involving people who use them and the wider local community. The COVID-19 pandemic was an illustration of how national policy directives had to be transferred swiftly into local areas. This included behavioural messaging, decisions around resource use to support vulnerable groups, and the vaccine roll-out.

CHALLENGING POLICY

As a health promoter or public health practitioner, you may find you are expected to implement policies that you perceive as health-damaging or contrary to health promotion or public health principles. This can be difficult because such policies can emanate from the national government, your employing organisation or even your direct manager. To challenge may create a conflict of loyalty between wanting to press for what you see as right and what is decreed to be right by the government and/or your employing authority. To protest may be seen as too political. There is no easy answer to this issue, but there are some positive steps worth considering:

- Use your vote. At the next general or local election, look at the health implications in the policy manifestos. Raise questions about health policy with doorstep canvassers, at public meetings and by writing to candidates. All this can be done in your capacity as a private citizen rather than a health worker.
- Use your professional association or trade union. These groups can raise issues at a national and local level and be a powerful voice. You can play your part by joining and supporting their activities and raising the issues you feel strongly about.
- Use your representative. There are many people whose job is to represent your interests. At the national level, it is your Member of Parliament (MP). So if you want to raise an issue at this level, lobby your MP: send letters, telephone, attend politicians' surgeries. At the local level, do the same with your local elected councillor. You could also contact your professional association or union local branch representative.
- Use your collective power. If you are concerned about a health-related policy issue at your place of work, it may help to find out if colleagues feel the same. If they do, join together so that you raise the issue collectively: this can give it more impact. Or, at a national level, join with others who share your concern to improve health and challenge health-damaging policies. For example, the RSPH have more than 6000 members drawn from every area and profession across public health, including environmental health, nursing, food hygiene, health promotion, health protection, and dentistry, forming an international network of public health professionals committed to influencing policy and practice. 38 Degrees is a virtual collective people power organisation that enables individuals and groups to network and to establish campaigns or to vote on policy issues of importance to public health (for further information on 38 Degrees, see the 38 Degrees website reference at the end of the chapter).

However, many areas of policy development are not controversial and can be a positive and rewarding part of the day-to-day work of health promoters and public health practitioners. The main thrust is likely to be in developing, changing, and implementing local policies. To do this, you need to understand the characteristics of power and influence and be competent at exerting influence when necessary.

Characteristics of Power and Influence

Power is the ability to influence others. There are four generally recognised types of power that are relevant to health promotion and public health policy work:

1. **Position power** is the power vested in someone because of their position in an organisation. For example, a Director of Public Health has position power.
2. **Resource power** is the power to allocate or limit resources, including money and staff. It often goes hand-in-hand with position power. For example, a senior health service manager has both position power and the power to regulate the use of resources. You have a source of power if you have the authority to control the allocation of any resources. Every health promoter and public health practitioner will have some power because people want the skills or services on offer.
3. **Expert power** is power related to expertise. Directors of Public Health and health promotion specialists have the expert power associated with their specialty.
4. **Personal power** is the power that comes from the personal attributes of a person, including strong personality, charisma, and ability to inspire. It is closely related to leadership qualities and intelligence, initiative, self-confidence, and the ability to rise above a situation and see it in perspective. However, effective leaders are not always charismatic, and what makes a leader effective in one situation may cause them to be less effective in changed circumstances.

You may sometimes be in the position of wanting or needing to exert influence on people who have a stronger power base. For example, a health visitor may wish to influence a general practitioner to adopt a policy of supporting the running of antenatal clinics in the local ethnic minority group's community centre, or a community worker may want to lobby local councillors about the need for more recreational facilities for young people on a housing estate. To do this requires skills in influencing and negotiation (see Enix, 2016).

Before attempting to influence someone with position or resource power, consider the basic questions in the planning process, such as: what are your aims? What resources do you need? Is the investment of your time in influencing others going to be worth it? Could the aim be achieved more easily in another way? (see Chapter 5, the section on planning and evaluating health promotion).

The Politics of Influence

There are four key elements of a strategy aiming to change policy:

1. Planning.
2. Making allies.
3. Networking.
4. Making deals and negotiating.

Planning

Three particular aspects of planning are useful to consider: undertaking a force field analysis, identifying stakeholders and considering your timing:

Undertake a force field analysis. A force field analysis identifies the helping and hindering forces and helps pinpoint how you can influence the process to make progress towards policy change or implementation. You identify how you can increase the power of the helping forces and decrease the power of the hindering forces. Use the diagram in Fig. 16.3 to set out your own force field analysis.

Identify the stakeholders. The stakeholders are those people with a vested interest in the issue who wish to influence what is done and how it is done. They are obviously powerful forces in the situation. It could be difficult to identify all the stakeholders because some of them may not wish to be visible and try to work covertly through others.

Time your action. It is also important to consider when to introduce a proposal or when to delay it. If people are already preoccupied with other major issues, it might not be the right time to make a new proposal. On the other hand, if a proposal will help other people to attain their own objectives, it will be a good time.

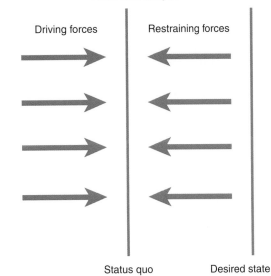

Fig. 16.3 Illustrating a force field analysis. (Source: The Bates Blog, 2013).

Making Allies

Identify which of the stakeholders could be allies and gain their trust and confidence to establish and maintain an alliance. It helps to pay attention to their concerns, values, beliefs, and behaviour patterns and to see what you need to do to form an effective working alliance.

For example, if you are concerned about the way in which people with disabilities are treated in an organisation, you might identify the person in charge of human resources as a key stakeholder. So find out if they are concerned about it and if they think it is important for the organisation. What kind of way do they work? Are they likely to respond best to a lively discussion on the subject or to a well-argued paper on the need for policy, backed up with facts and figures? Do they like time to make decisions? Will they be happy to leave you to take the lead, or will they want ownership of the initiative?

Networking

Many people working in organisations belong to one or more interest groups that meet to discuss, debate, and exchange information on issues that concern the members. By playing an active role in these networks, people can extend their influence. Networks provide access to information that can help with making a case, to people with experience of successfully influencing and to other resources. There are different types of networks: professional networks. Members are from the same profession.

  Professional networks may attempt to influence government, employers, and organisations to reconsider their policies or to develop new policies for the future. Professional networks institute criteria for professional practice and are active in the professional development of their members. The FPH is a professional network.

  Elitist networks. Membership is normally by invitation only. Members of such networks may have considerable power and influence, often through their position in organisations. An example of such a network might be the UK Public Health Network, which is a collaboration of umbrella organisations representing public health across the four nations that make up the United Kingdom. The four Chief Executives of the FPH, RSPH, Association of Directors of Public Health and UK Health Forum act as a coordinating group to oversee the network, which prioritises mapping the policy priorities and work priorities for the organisations in the network and developing a collective view of key UK-wide priorities for public health (see website references at the end of the chapter for details).

  Pressure groups. Members wish to pursue certain objectives, which may be environmental, social or political. There are a number of public health pressure groups, such as Action on Sugar, which have been influential in the introduction of a UK government childhood obesity strategy, which unfortunately, the pressure group feels does not go far enough in tackling some of the major issues (Wollaston, 2016). See the website and Twitter pages for the Action on Sugar pressure group in the references at the end of this page.

Influencing Policy by Making Deals and Negotiating

Making deals is common practice in most organisations. Individuals or groups agree to support a policy proposal in return for agreement on something that benefits them. To make deals successfully, it pays to know the person with whom you are dealing, paying careful attention to their values and intentions and what you could realistically expect from them.

Negotiation is the art of creating an agreement on a specific issue between two or more parties with different views. Successful negotiation takes place when there is a desire to solve problems, and the parties genuinely commit to going through a number of steps. There are many guides on how to improve your negotiation skills. While these are mainly written for the business community, the skills are also relevant to health promotion and public health. See, for example, Enix (2016).

On Being Political

A final point is about political behaviour, which refers to finding out about who holds power and working on using this information to change a situation. When is it acceptable, and when is it unethical?

Being political can be considered devious and manipulative. Some people may view it with suspicion and will, therefore, not be easily influenced by such behaviour. To manipulate covertly or coerce, lie or deliberately withhold information that affects others is unethical and unprofessional. But to ignore the politics within organisations is unwise because it results in failure to make a realistic appraisal of situations and failure to make the best of the opportunities for promoting health. Furthermore, it is possible to be political without losing professional integrity, for example, by ensuring deals are made as the outcome of open negotiations, and those relationships should be based on genuineness, trust, goodwill, and mutual respect. Case study 16.1 offers an example of the politics of influence in practice.

By joining a local network of people interested in health promotion, he is able to find out what is going on elsewhere, and this gives him some useful ideas, including sources of help in stress management training which he incorporates into the training plan.

CASE STUDY 16.1   The Politics of Influence – Health and Safety at Work

Bob is an environmental health officer working for Midshire City Council. His aim is to improve the implementation of the health and safety at work policy of the council. He makes a list of the *helping* forces and the *hindering* forces:

Helping
- The existing safety officers.
- Existing codes of practice, for example, sight checks for visual display unit operators.
- A councillor who is a health lecturer at the university.
- A human resources officer interested in improving the working environment for staff.
- An existing commitment to appoint an occupational health nurse.

Hindering
- The cost of any improvements (the council has severe financial constraints).
- Staff time to attend health and safety training.
- Problems with recruiting an occupational health nurse.
- Deficiencies in the structure of council buildings (poor ventilation, open-plan offices, lack of showers for those staff wishing to take physical exercise during the day).

- Lack of councillors' commitment to improve health and safety conditions for staff.
- Lack of access to council buildings for disabled people.

He identifies the stakeholders as
- The staff themselves.
- The trade unions.
- Departmental managers, senior and chief officers.
- The councillors.
- The public health specialist and the health promotion specialist from the local authority (LA).

He further identifies key stakeholders as
- Officers in the department of engineering because they enforce building regulations.
- Council members on the health committee.
- The director of personnel.

He then identifies ways of increasing the helping forces and decreasing the hindering forces. By making an ally of the interested human resources officer, he is able to increase the commitment of the director of human resources, who is also a chief officer. One short-term outcome is that an occupational health nurse is recruited. Another outcome is a plan agreed upon by the human resources department and the trade unions for training staff in health and safety.

He makes a deal with the engineering department by agreeing to assist with monitoring the construction sites of new buildings to prevent accidents on the site. In return, they agree to assist with a plan for improving soundproofing and modifications to open-plan offices. Their commitment grows after a report showed that accidents on construction sites are reduced. He discusses with them the issue of raising with council members the plan for modifying council buildings.

Finally, he makes an ally of the councillor at the university by offering to provide input to some of the courses. This councillor is on the health committee and provides him with useful advice on how to approach the committee and how to prepare documents for its consideration.

Developing and Implementing Policies

Many public health policies are about health issues that relate to workplaces or other settings such as schools, communities, and hospitals. Other policies focus on more specific issues, such as the government's approach to women's health and how women's voices can be better heard to influence a life-course approach to treatment

and prevention from adolescents and young adults to later life (Department of Health and Social Care, 2022).

Policies on Promoting Health in Workplaces

The benefits of promoting health at work are well established, and reviews of the literature identify major benefits that are also highly cost-effective (Vargas-Martínez et al., 2021). The European Network for Workplace Health Promotion (ENWH, 2018) has a range of publications that will support policy development that encourages employers and trade unions to take on a wider concept of health at work, including giving priority to issues such as smoking, alcohol, and stress. The WHO also has a number of guidelines on supporting workplace policy development (for example, WHO, 2010).

In the UK, there are a number of agencies that support the promotion of health and wellbeing in the workplace. The Health and Safety Executive is also a source of information on all statutory policies governing health and safety in the workplace (see the Health and Safety Executive free guides under the web references). Many other organisations have an interest in workplace health;

this includes voluntary sector and private sector providers (see websites and resources at the end of the chapter).

Policies on Promoting Health in Hospitals

Health Promoting Hospitals (HPH) is a WHO initiative designed to improve health and environmental conditions for both staff and patients by reviewing and implementing a range of health-promoting policies. HPH consists of 20 National/Regional Networks and individual hospitals and health services members. The International HPH Network totals more than 600 hospital and health service members all over the world (see website reference at the end of the chapter). It can be difficult in practice to inform and involve everyone in an institution as large and complex as a hospital, and with this in mind The New Haven Recommendations on partnering with patients, families, and citizens to enhance performance and quality in health-promoting hospitals and health services (INHPH, 2020) are designed to inform policy development linked to health-promoting hospitals.

Promoting Health in Urban Settings: Healthy Cities

The WHO's Healthy Cities initiative promotes comprehensive and systematic policy and planning with a special emphasis on health inequalities and urban poverty, the needs of vulnerable groups, participatory governance, and the social, economic, and environmental determinants of health. It also strives to include health considerations in economic, regeneration, and urban development efforts. It aims to work from the bottom up, not from the top down, and to involve collaborative work between local government, health authorities, local businesses, community organisations and, of course, individual citizens. The UK Healthy Cities Network is part of the global movement for urban health that is led and supported by the WHO. Its vision is to develop a creative, supportive, and motivating network for UK cities and towns that are tackling health inequalities and striving to put health improvement and health equity at the core of all local policies (see the website in the reference section; see also Chapter 15 for the principles of working with communities).

Policies on Promoting Health in Schools and Universities

The European Network of Health-Promoting Schools, now known as Schools for Health in Europe, sets out to show that schools can be powerful agents for change through the adoption of whole-school approaches. This means that the school promotes health not only by curriculum policies which include sufficient time for social, personal, economic, and health education for the pupils but also by wider school policies that ensure that the school promotes a sense of positive self-esteem and the health and wellbeing of teachers and other staff, parents, and the wider community who have contact with the school. Recent analysis has reviewed the policies and effectiveness of promoting health in schools, offering contemporary challenges, including COVID-19 and schools, but also providing an optimistic picture for future developments (Gugglberger, 2021).

The UK National Healthy Universities Network was established in 2006 and aims to offer a facilitative environment for the development of a whole university approach to health and wellbeing. The Okanagan Charter for Health Promoting Universities and Colleges was launched in 2015 at the International Conference on Health Promoting Universities and Colleges. The Charter sets out a radical and far-reaching vision designed to influence organisational policies within the university sector (see full details on the Schools for Health and Health Universities websites in the references at the end of the chapter).

Policies on Promoting Health in Prisons

In October 1995, an international meeting with senior prison health representatives from eight selected European countries agreed that the public health importance of prisoner health had been neglected. The settings approach to health promotion was recognised as a way of addressing the health of the prison population after observing the effectiveness of the settings approach in schools, workplaces, hospitals, and cities. However, despite the global endorsement for healthy cities and health-promoting schools, health-promoting prisons have to date, failed to penetrate beyond a few countries (Woodall and Cross, 2021). One of the key challenges for health promoters in this area has been how to translate policy directives in a setting where control and security dominate. This can cause considerable friction when trying to align health promotion in secure environments.

Guidelines on Developing and Implementing a Policy

Many health promoters and public health practitioners have a role in developing and implementing policies in specific settings such as those previously discussed. An example of such a policy is the workplace healthy eating draft policy outlined in Exercise 16.1.

Having read the sample policy, consider these questions:
- What steps are involved in the development of the policy?
- What else might have been done?
- What are the significant points to note about the development of a public health policy from this example?

EXERCISE 16.1 A Draft of a Workplace Healthy Eating Policy

Healthy eating at work policy for: **Workplace A**

Effective from: 00/00/00

Next review date: 00/00/00

Notes

This section of the policy could include information on some of the following topics:

- How and why a good diet affects productivity and performance at work.
- How the organisation can create an environment that supports and encourages healthy eating.
- How the support of health at work initiatives can demonstrate that the workforce is valued and the work-life balance is respected.

The need for a healthy eating at work policy

Healthy eating is essential for good health and contributes to positive wellbeing. Many of the leading causes of disease and disability in our society, such as obesity, coronary heart disease, diabetes, and certain forms of cancer, mental ill health, and osteoporosis, are associated with poor nutritional choices. A healthy, balanced diet contains a variety of different types of food, including lots of fruit and vegetables; plenty of starchy foods such as wholemeal bread and wholegrain cereals; some protein-rich foods such as meat, fish, eggs, and lentils; and some dairy foods. We should also be drinking about six to eight glasses (1.2 L) of water or other fluids every day to stop us from getting dehydrated. The workplace is an important setting in which people can increase their intake of healthy foods to benefit their health and protect against illness. A healthy, balanced diet also helps people to recover more quickly from illnesses they may get. What we eat and drink not only has a physical impact on our body but can also contribute to our mental health, resulting in improved levels of concentration, mental alertness, and ability to cope with everyday stresses and strains and therefore perform better in work.

Example aims are given on the right. These can also link to policies on mental wellbeing, smoking, and physical activity, as well as national public health policies and initiatives.

Aim of the policy:

- To support and encourage employees to make healthy eating choices.
- To increase the opportunities for employees to learn more about nutrition.
- To create a workplace culture that encourages employees to incorporate healthy eating into their daily routine, thus creating a lifestyle behaviour.
- To set out a coordinated approach to increase the availability of healthier eating options.
- To achieve recognition for a healthy workplace through the Workplace Wellbeing Charter, Healthier Catering Award or Public Health Responsibility Deal.

The objectives should be SMART (Specific, Measurable, Achievable, Realistic, and Time-specific). See the examples opposite. Each objective should be followed by what the organisation will do – 'policy actions' – to meet the objectives

Objectives

To implement a healthy eating policy that raises awareness of the benefits of healthy eating.

Policy actions:

- Develop healthy eating pages on an intranet and provide educational leaflets and resources on healthy eating.
- Appoint a healthy eating champion to be responsible for workplace healthy eating programmes.
- Ensure healthy eating is included in any health and wellbeing groups with senior management attendance.
- Provide courses and seminars on the benefits of healthy eating and the risks of poor nutrition.
- Hold healthy eating promotional events such as Fruity Friday.

(Continued)

EXERCISE 16.1   A Draft of a Workplace Healthy Eating Policy—Cont'd

Notes

	To implement a healthy eating policy that supports employees to make healthier eating choices in a variety of ways.

Policy actions:

- Encourage employees to make healthy eating choices through the use of promotional and motivational resources, e.g. encouraging employees to make healthy choices from the canteen menu.
- Provide food storage and preparation areas in all departments.
- Provide information on local or onsite weight management groups.
- Organise fruit and vegetable box delivery schemes.
- Investigate the demand for and feasibility of extending canteen opening times to include breakfast.
- Designate one week each year as a healthy eating week, with a range of organised activities.
- Provide access to water in all meeting and training rooms.

To remove barriers and enable employees to make healthy eating choices.

Policy actions:

- Review the current provision of services in vending and catering facilities.
- Engage senior management in the development of the policy.
- Provide cool storage areas for lunchboxes and snacks.
- Work with onsite caterers to trial more healthy choices, reducing salt and trans fats. Develop a traffic light system in canteens as an easy reference for employees to see the foods which are healthier.
- Increase access to healthy foods for shift workers by introducing healthy options in vending machines.
- Develop links with local food providers who will deliver healthy food options to the workplace.
- Endorse the eating of meals away from desks.
- Provide fruit bowls in each department.
- Offer fruit instead of biscuits during meetings.
- Provide access to cool drinking water for all employees.

Explain how this policy will be communicated throughout the organisation.

Communication

All employees will be made aware of the healthy eating policy and the facilities available. The healthy eating policy will be included in the employee handbook and employee information or induction packs.
A specific focus group will be established to take forward the actions from this policy to complement other health at work policies. Regular updates will be provided to all employees via their line management.

Regular review and monitoring are vital to assess the effectiveness of a healthy eating policy. How will you track progress?

Review and monitoring

Employees participating in any of the healthy eating activities will be regularly asked for feedback. Healthy eating will be integrated into a 'health at work audit', which will be undertaken annually. The policy, status updates, and evaluation reports will be circulated to management and be available on request through the workplace health champion. The policy will be reviewed six months from implementation and then annually after that to ensure that it remains relevant.

Date:
Signature:

Source: Rochdale Borough Council (2016).

1. Preparation of The Policy

The formulation of a policy by any organisation is a corporate matter, so the usual starting point is to convene a working group.

- This group clarifies its terms of reference and elects a Chair.
- Identifies the need for a policy.
- Identifies the committee, department or senior person who has overall responsibility for taking the policy forward.
- Identifies key personnel to consult with and convince of the need for a policy.
- Establishes a timescale for policy development.
- Prepares a draft policy and consults widely.
- Prepares the final draft policy for approval.

In the case of a workplace policy, it is important to involve trade unions. This can be achieved either by including trade union representatives on the working group or by setting up an effective framework for consultation and negotiation. This may be crucial in persuading the workforce to look positively on the new policy.

It is also important that an identified senior member of staff or manager with political influence acts as a champion for the policy. This person will be crucial in getting the commitment of other managers to the policy.

2. Implementation of The Policy

This starts with planning, which will include:

- Setting aims and objectives.
- Setting up a system for monitoring and evaluation.
- Identifying resources and defining key implementation tasks.
- Defining the role of key personnel.
- Developing an action plan.

Key personnel should be encouraged to participate actively in identifying their roles and in discussing boundaries and overlap in roles so that the potential for conflict and confusion is reduced. For example, managers have the primary responsibility of ensuring that their staff are fully conversant with workplace policies and understand what is expected of them. Nevertheless, the trade unions also have a role in informing the workforce of the policy. These sources of information hopefully will be complementary and spell out the same, not contradictory, messages. The open discussion of these issues will help to increase commitment to making the policy work.

Any policy that is not the subject of regular review risks becoming obsolete. So the working group must reconvene at intervals to consider issues such as the following:

- Does the workforce know about and understand the policy?
- Have attitudes changed to the health issue covered by the policy? If so, how? How do staff feel about the policy?

- Has the behaviour of individual staff changed? Does this include changes in working practices and/or individual lifestyles?
- Are staff getting the help they need?
- Are managers and trade unions supporting the policy?
- Are indicators showing that the policy is making progress towards the attainment of its aims and objectives? For example, in the case of a workplace policy, has sickness reduced? Has work performance improved? Is morale better?
- How can we improve the effectiveness of the policy?

3. Education and Training

This is a continuous process, not a one-off event. Wherever possible, it should be integrated into existing provisions for professional and managerial staff development. The purposes of education and training include the following:

- Securing the commitment of management (such as elected members, chief officers, and senior management in the case of a LA).
- Obtaining the commitment of the whole workforce or group at which the policy is aimed (such as the prison population or the staff of a business).
- Providing those responsible for implementing the policy with the necessary skills.
- Overcoming prejudices, discrimination, and stereotyping where relevant (for example, in policies on alcohol and HIV/AIDS).
- Encouraging and assisting the workforce, or the particular groups of people the policy is concerned with, to make choices and individual lifestyle changes.

4. Evaluation

This should include an evaluation of both process and outcomes. It will require the collection of information, both baseline and ongoing.

See Chapter 5, the section on planning evaluation methods, for further suggestions.

CAMPAIGNING

You, or clients with whom you work, may feel strongly about changing policy or practice about a public health issue and decide that the way forward is to mount a campaign.

Policy campaigns can range from short-lived local campaigns with the objective of making a single change to long-term national campaigns. An example of a national pressure group campaigning for policy change is Action on Smoking and Health (ASH), which is a campaigning public health charity that works to eliminate the harm caused by tobacco and e-cigarettes. ASH has a list of policy issues on its website (http://www.ash.org.uk), which includes inequalities in health.

Some pressure groups (such as Shelter) may provide direct services as well as acting as a pressure group.

Principles of Campaigning for Policy Change

Some important principles to keep in mind if you are setting up a policy campaign are the following:

- **Be persistent:** Success requires persistent effort, so you must be committed and prepared to put in a lot of time and energy over a long period.
- **Be professional:** Give care and attention to details (such as well-written campaign materials with the name of the campaign clearly evident), and ensure that activities such as keeping records are undertaken properly.
- **Keep a sense of perspective:** Your campaign may be vitally important to you, but being perceived as fanatical will do your cause no good.
- **Reflect your ideals:** It is no good, for example, campaigning for changes to equal opportunities policy if your own organisation does not have good access for people with disabilities.
- **Be positive:** Use positive rather than negative language and arguments.
- **Join with others:** Rival pressure groups campaigning on similar (or even identical) issues waste a lot of time, effort, and other resources. If someone is already campaigning on your issue, join them rather than setting up a rival organisation. Or, if there is more than one organisation working on similar issues, form a coalition.
- **Involve as many people as possible:** This not only harnesses support but also informs people about what is wrong and what needs to change.

Planning a Policy Campaign

When you plan a public health policy campaign, it helps to go through the same planning process as you would with any other kind of health promotion activity.

- See also Chapter 5 for help with planning that applies to planning a campaign: identify your aims clearly.
- Decide the best way of achieving them (public meetings? press coverage? lobbying MPs and local councillors? a petition? use of social media?).
- Identify your resources (do you need to fundraise?).
- Clarify how you will know if your aim is achieved (set milestones and specific outcomes?).
- Set an action plan of who is going to do what and when.

As a concluding point to this chapter on policy and to the book as a whole, I would like to share the views of Popejoy (2016). He argues that population health outcomes result from a complex interplay of variables, not all of which have

been studied adequately to help us arrive at a set of policy solutions. Health promoters and public health practitioners have much to do in developing and/or influencing the evidence base to underpin public health policy.

PRACTICE POINTS

- Recognise that you and all health promoters and public health practitioners have a role in influencing policy at the national, local, and organisational levels.
- Influencing policy requires careful planning and timing. You need to know how national and local health promotion and public health policy are created, developed, and changed and how you can have a voice by commenting on proposals and plans.
- Know the rights and standards you can expect from NHS and LA services, and comment on those which you and your clients receive.
- Challenge health-damaging policy by working with others, using your vote and by collective action.
- Identify how you could be more effective in influencing policy by reviewing your skills in planning, networking, negotiating, and joint working.
- Start policy change by identifying key stakeholders and looking at issues from each of their viewpoints; use techniques such as force field analysis to establish how to move forward.
- When campaigning on health issues, pay attention to careful planning and be persistent, professional and positive; involve as many other people as possible.
- Keep the ethical aspects of activities in mind when campaigning, lobbying, and working towards changing health policy and practice; work with other people to build up trust and mutual respect.

References

Department of Health and Social Care, (2022). *Women's health strategy for England*. United Kingdom: Crown.

Department of Health Ireland. (2015). *Nudging in public health – an ethical framework. A report by the National Advisory Committee on Bioethics*. http://health.gov.ie/wp-content/uploads/2016/04/Nudging-in-Public-Health-Ethical-Framework-Dec-2015.pdf

Enix, A. (2016). *Negotiation: 8 essential negotiation skills to increase your influence and persuasion*. CreateSpace Independent Publishing Platform.

Ensaff, H. (2021). A nudge in the right direction: The role of food choice architecture in changing populations' diets. *Proceedings of the Nutrition Society, 80*(2), 195–206. https://doi.org/10.1017/S0029665120007983.

ENWHP. (2018). *European network for workplace health promotion*. https://www.enwhp.org/

Flor, L. S., Reitsma, M. B., Gupta, V., Ng, M., & Gakidou, E. (2021). The effects of tobacco control policies on global smoking prevalence. *Nature Medicine*, 27(2), 239–243. https://doi.org/10.1038/s41591-020-01210-8.

Forbes, C., Liddle, J., & Shutt, J. (2022). *Levelling up in the North East region*. Newcastle: Northumbria University.

Gregory, S., Dixon, A., & Ham, C. (2012). *Health policy under the coalition: a midterm assessment*. London: Kings Fund.

Gugglberger, L. (2021). A brief overview of a wide framework— health promoting schools: a curated collection. *Health Promotion International*, 36(2), 297–302. https://doi.org/10.1093/heapro/daab037.

HM Government, (2022). *Levelling up the United Kingdom*. London: Crown.

Homer, C., Woodall, J., Freeman, C., South, J., Cooke, J., Holliday, J., Hartley, A., & Mullen, S. (2022). Changing the culture: a qualitative study exploring research capacity in local government. *BMC Public Health*, 22, 1341. https://doi.org/10.1186/s12889-022-13758-w.

INHPH. (2020). *The New Haven recommendations on partnering with patients, families and citizens to enhance performance and quality in health promoting hospitals and health services*. https://www.hphnet.org/wp-content/uploads/2021/07/New-Haven-Recommendations-TF.pdf

LGA, (2013). *Changing behaviours in public health: to nudge or to shove?*. London: Local Government Association.

NHS England, (2015). *Delivering the forward view: NHS planning guidance 2016/17–2020/21*. London: NHS England. https://www.england.nhs.uk/wp-content/uploads/2015/12/planning-guid-16-17-20-21.pdf.

Nuffield Council on Bioethics. (2007). *Public health: ethical issues*. http://nuffieldbioethics.org/project/public-health/

Oe, H., & Yamaoka, Y. (2021). Discussion of citizen behavioural change using the nudge effect: a perspective based on social policy interventions. *International Journal of Sociology and Social Policy*. https://doi.org/10.1108/IJSSP-08-2021-0210.

Popejoy, W. M. (2016). Book review of health inequalities: critical perspectives. *Perspectives in Public Health*, 136(5), 307.

Rochdale Borough Council. (2016). *Health eating at work policy: sample policy*. http://www.rochdale.gov.uk/pdf/2732_WelfareAtWork_EatingAtWork_HR.pdf

Selby, D., & Kippen, H. (2016). *The journey to place based health*. PHE Blog. https://publichealthmatters.blog.gov.uk/2016/03/17/the-journey-to-place-based-health/.

The Bates Blog. (2013). *Leading transformational change: using the force field analysis*. http://www.bates-communications.com/bates-blog/bid/94065/Leading-Transformational-Change-Using-the-Force-Field-Analysis.

Vargas-Martínez, A. M., Romero-Saldaña, M., & De Diego-Cordero, R. (2021). Economic evaluation of workplace health promotion interventions focused on lifestyle: systematic review and meta-analysis. *Journal of Advanced Nursing*, 77(9), 3657–3691. https://doi.org/10.1111/jan.14857.

Wollaston, S. (2016). *Public health is in crisis – and Theresa May is failing to act*. Health Policy, The Guardian Newspaper.

Woodall, J., & Cross, R. (2021). *Essentials of health promotion*. London: Sage.

World Health Organisation, (2010). *Healthy workplaces: a model for action: for employers, workers, policy-makers and practitioners*. Geneva: WHO.

WHO, (2022). *Working for health 2022–2030 action plan*. Geneva: WHO.

Websites

38 Degrees. *New campaign page*. https://you.38degrees.org.uk/petition/new?source=google-start-a-petition38&gclid=Cj0KEQjwr7S-BRD96_uw9JK8uNA-BEiQAujbffMIYBHvBZT7aoaSbpSqh2Pfsrsd3Kk0yz-gg73Rm-BR4aAtuE8P8HAQ

Action on Sugar. *Pressure group*. http://www.actiononsugar.org/

Collaborate. *A policy and practice hub supporting cross sector collaboration in services to the public*. http://collaboratei.com/2016/03/new-report-place-based-collaboration-that-can-transform-health-and-care/

Details of the Public Health Network. https://ukpublichealthnetwork.org.uk/about-us/.

HSE. Free guides on health and safety at work and other employment policy issues. https://www.citation.co.uk/free-guides

NHS. *Change4 Life*. https://www.nhs.uk/healthier-families/

The European Network for Workplace Health Promotion. https://www.enwhp.org /

The NHS Confederation Network Pages. *Meeting the specific needs of different specialist groups through its networks*. https://www.nhsconfed.org/networks-countries

WHO. (2020). Welcome to the UK Healthy Universities Network. http://www.euro.who.int/en/health-topics/health-policy/health-2020-the-european-policy-for-health-and-well-being/about-health-2020

Health Promoting Universities Network. http://www.healthyuniversities.ac.uk/

Public Health England Blog. *Public health matters. Duncan Selbie and Henry Kippin, 17 March 2016. The journey to place based health*. https://publichealthmatters.blog.gov.uk/2016/03/17/the-journey-to-place-based-health/

The European Schools for Health Network. http://www.schools-for-health.eu/she-network

The International Network of Health Promoting Hospitals and Health Services. http://www.hphnet.org/

Webinars

The Health Foundation. *Webinars on a range of health policy issues*. http://www.health.org.uk/about-the-health-foundation/get-involved/events

Twitter

Action on Sugar. *Pressure group*. https://twitter.com/actiononsugar?ref_src=twsrc%5Etfw

Office for Health Improvement and Disparities. https://twitter.com/OHID

Facebook

Change4Life Wales. https://www.facebook.com/C4LWales

INDEX

Note: Page numbers followed by "*f*" indicate figures, "*t*" indicate tables, and "*b*" indicate boxes.